Handbook of Pathogens and Diseases in Cephalopods

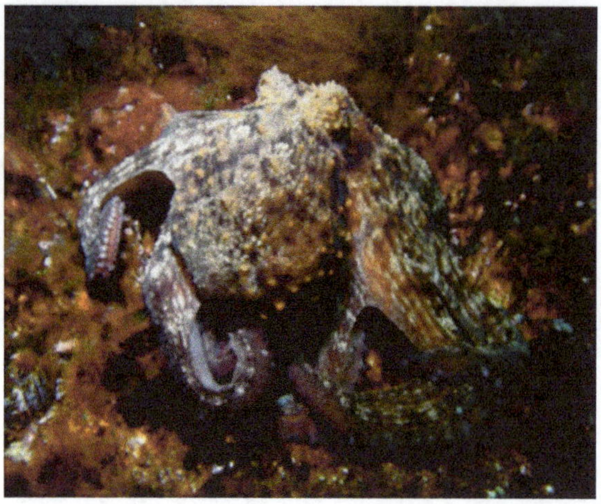

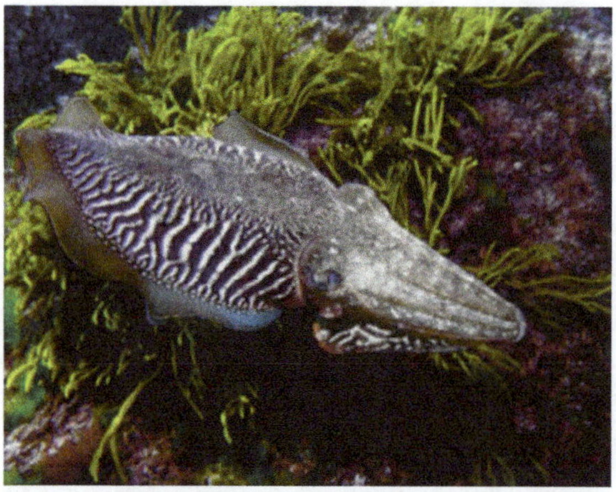

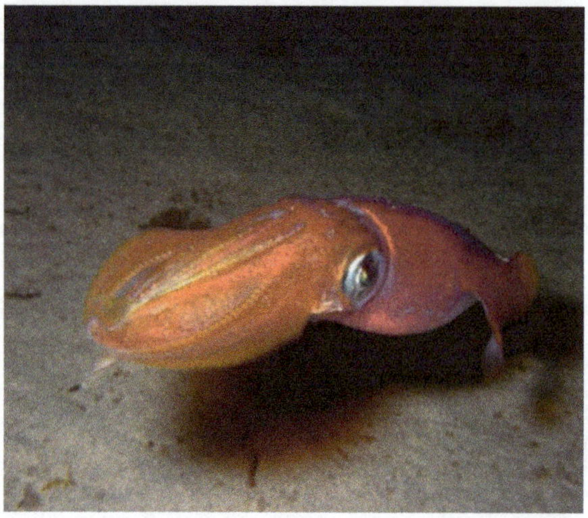

Octopus vulgaris and *Sepia officinalis* (by Jorge H. Urcera); *Loligo vulgaris* (by Felipe Escolano)

Camino Gestal • Santiago Pascual •
Ángel Guerra • Graziano Fiorito •
Juan M. Vieites
Editors

Handbook of Pathogens and Diseases in Cephalopods

Editors
Camino Gestal
Institute of Marine Research
Spanish National Research Council (CSIC)
Vigo, Pontevedra, Spain

Ángel Guerra
Institute of Marine Research
Spanish National Research Council (CSIC)
Vigo, Pontevedra, Spain

Juan M. Vieites
ANFACO-CECOPESCA
Vigo, Pontevedra, Spain

Santiago Pascual
Institute of Marine Research
Spanish National Research Council (CSIC)
Vigo, Pontevedra, Spain

Graziano Fiorito
Association for Cephalopod Research (CephRes)
Naples, Italy

https://doi.org/10.1007/978-3-030-11330-8

Dedicated to
Frederich G. Hochberg,
Roger T. Hanlon and
John W. Forsythe

Preface

Octopuses, cuttlefish, squids, and nautiluses compose a diverse and ancient class of Mollusca, the Cephalopoda. They play an important role in the trophic structure of marine ecosystems and are a valuable fishery resource sought in lucrative European and Asian markets.

Cephalopods have evolved highly advanced sensory systems with large, very sophisticated eyes and the most complex brain of the invertebrates. They have a demonstrated capacity for both short- and long-term memory and are able to perform impressive high-order cognitive tasks on a par with some of the lower vertebrates.

They also are distinguished by special anatomical and biological features. Octopuses, for example, have muscular arms capable of performing a range of delicate tasks. Their suckers are equipped with sensitive chemoreceptors that 'taste' minute changes in their immediate environment. Squid and cuttlefish, for their part, have a unique dual mode of locomotion: Pulsed jetting drives bursts of speed, and fin flapping allows high-precision maneuvering.

Cephalopods' delicate skin has peculiarities that contribute to their evolutionary success and add to their general air of intrigue. The epidermis is formed by a single-celled epithelium over a dermal layer of connective tissue. The latter has light-reflecting cells (iridophores and leucophores) and a remarkable array of pigmented cells, chromatophores, which are under direct control of the brain. With the exception of *Nautilus,* this allows the dramatic changes in skin color, pattern, and even texture that impress specialists and non-specialists alike and that make cephalopods the masters of marine camouflage.

Owing to these and other distinctive features, cephalopods have a long tradition as valuable experimental models in neurobiology and related disciplines. As might be expected, they also have great appeal as ornamental aquarium species. More recently, their short life cycles, high ratio of production to biomass, high protein content, and high market value have drawn attention to their aquaculture potential, and this has become an area of active research.

Because of their advanced sensory discrimination, extraordinary ability to learn and perform complex tasks, and their overall behavioral complexity, cephalopods are the only invertebrates recognized in European Union Directive 2010/63/EU that sets out welfare standards for animals used in scientific research. This directive applies to cephalopods used in laboratory studies, maintained in aquaria, and raised for aquaculture.

The increasing importance of cephalopods in scientific and commercial activities motivates the need to learn more about potential threats to their health, namely pathogens and disease vectors. Accurate disease identification and effective treatment are, in fact, essential for any program that may have an impact on cephalopod health and welfare. We presently are on the early part of that learning curve and would benefit from a user-friendly guide to cephalopod diseases. Such a guide would summarize important anatomical and histological structures required for necropsy, describe assertive histopathological analyses, and discuss the diagnosis of infectious and non-infectious diseases along with their pathologies.

That is, in fact, the aim of the timely *Handbook of Pathogens and Diseases in Cephalopods.* The *Handbook* provides the reader with current knowledge of cephalopod disease etiologies, diagnoses, and pathologies. It brings into the light many important facts that contribute to our understanding of cephalopod pathology that readers will find of great practical use, including accurate assessment of parasites and pathogens, and the effects of the cultural environment on the health and welfare of these truly captivating invertebrates. The *Handbook of Pathogens and Diseases in Cephalopods* is an essential reference for everyone in the field.

As one example, those who work in the field know very well that cephalopod skin is very fragile and prone to damage. Thus, physical contact during capture or any subsequent handling, and especially abrasions inflicted when scraping against a tank wall, can lead to the invasion of pathogens that result in serious infections. The highly active swimming habits of squid and cuttlefish thus impose strict design considerations to minimize skin and fin abrasions. To complicate matters further, the synergic effects of stressors while in captivity—such as high density or sub-optimal water quality—may adversely affect the immune system and so make disease outbreaks all the more likely. This common problem alone is a strong argument for studying the diagnosis and treatment of cephalopod pathologies covered so thoroughly in the *Handbook*.

Jointly written by 40 authors from research groups distributed over 3 continents, 18 chapters of the *Handbook of Pathogens and Diseases in Cephalopods* are a detailed and up-to-date reference that will prove to be useful in many disciplines. It comprises two parts. The first lays the foundation of accurate necropsy and histopathological analyses. It also describes the tissues of early life stages and adults of the more important European species: *Octopus vulgaris*, *Loligo vulgaris*, and *Sepia officinalis*.

The second part is a broad and thorough assessment of parasites, pathogens, and diseases found mainly in European cephalopods. Among other topics, it covers conditions caused by fungi and Labyrinthulomycetes, viruses and bacteria, Protists (coccidians and ciliates), Dicyemids, and Metazoans. For completeness, there also is a chapter on the pathogens and diseases in non-European cephalopods.

Other topics include valuable information on aquarium maintenance and a section on the cephalopods' remarkable ability to regenerate lost or damaged tissue. An additional chapter discusses senescence, the process by which cephalopods cease eating and live solely on their stored reserves during a period of self-imposed starvation.

Improving the health, maintenance, and survival of cephalopods in captivity is essential for advancing the field, and this is inextricably linked to the quick and accurate diagnosis and treatment of cephalopod diseases. In this very important respect, the cephalopod research community will welcome the *Handbook* as an authoritative reference that will play a critical part in furthering our knowledge of these enigmatic and ecologically important animals.

Dr. Erica A. G. Vidal
President, Cephalopod International Advisory Council

Acknowledgements

The authors would like to thank ANFACO-CECOPESCA and Regional Ministry for Maritime Affairs, Xunta de Galicia, for their collaboration in supporting the edition of this publication. We also thank the Spanish National Research Council (CSIC) and Institute of Marine Research (IIM-CSIC) for their support and facilities. We thank Graham Pierce for their comments and advice on specific sections of this book. In addition, we appreciate the help of Manuel E. Garci (IIM-CSIC) for photographic assistance of fresh specimens during necropsies, José Manuel Antonio Durán (IIM-CSIC) for his technical assistance in tissue processing for histological analysis of part of the material, and Lucía Sánchez (IIM-CSIC) for her technical assistance in image analysis and edition.

This work benefited from networking activities carried out under the COST Action FA1301 and is considered a contribution to the COST (European Cooperation on Science and Technology) Action FA1301 "A network for improvement of cephalopod welfare and husbandry in research, aquaculture and fisheries" (http://www.cephsinaction.org/).

Contents

Contributors

Elvira Abollo Centro Tecnológico del Mar, Fundación CETMAR, Vigo, Pontevedra, Spain

Ma. Leopoldina Aguirre-Macedo Laboratorio de Patología Acuática y Parasitología, CINVESTAV Unidad Mérida, Mérida, Yucatán, Mexico

Eduardo Almansa Centro Oceanográfico de Canarias, Instituto Español de Oceanografía, Santa Cruz de Tenerife, Canary Islands, Spain

Roberto C. Alonso ANFACO-CECOPESCA, Ctra. Colexio Universitario, Vigo, Pontevedra, Spain

Ramón Anadón Department of Functional Biology, University of Santiago de Compostela, Campus Vida, Santiago de Compostela, Spain

Carlos Azevedo Laboratory of Cell Biology, Institute of Biomedical Sciences (ICBAS/uP), University of Porto, Porto, Portugal

Sheila Castellanos-Martínez Instituto de Investigaciones Oceanológicas, UABC, Ensenada, Mexico

Yanis Cruz-Quintana Grupo de Investigación en Sanidad Acuícola, Inocuidad y Salud Ambiental, Escuela de Acuicultura y Pesquería, Facultad de Ciencias Veterinarias, Universidad Técnica de Manabí, Bahía de Caráquez, Ecuador

Sarah Culloty School of Biological, Earth and Environmental Sciences, Aquaculture and Fisheries Development Center, University College Cork, Cork, Ireland

Rosa Farto Marine Research Centre (CIM-UVIGO), University of Vigo, Vigo, Spain

Felicidad Fernández ANFACO-CECOPESCA, Ctra. Colexio Universitario, Vigo, Pontevedra, Spain

Raquel Fernández-Gago Department of Ecology and Animal Biology, University of Vigo, Lagoas-Marcosende, Vigo, Spain

Gianluca Fichi Istituto Zooprofilattico Sperimentale delle Regioni Lazio e Toscana, Pisa, Italy

Graziano Fiorito Association for Cephalopod Research (CephRes), Naples, Italy

Hidetaka Furuya Department of Biology, Graduate School of Science, Osaka University, Toyonaka, Osaka, Japan

Pablo García-Fernández Aquatic Molecular Pathobiology Group, Institute of Marine Research, Spanish National Research Council (CSIC), Vigo, Pontevedra, Spain

Camino Gestal Aquatic Molecular Pathobiology Group, Institute of Marine Research, Spanish National Research Council (CSIC), Vigo, Pontevedra, Spain

Panos Grigoriou HCMR, Gournes Pediados, Irakleion, Crete, Greece

Ángel Guerra Ecology and Biodiversity Department, Institute of Marine Research, Spanish National Research Council (CSIC), Vigo, Pontevedra, Spain

Pamela Imperadore Association for Cephalopod Research (CephRes), Naples, Italy
Stazione Zoologica Anton Dohrn, Biology and Evolution of Marine Organisms, Naples, Italy

Jonathan Fabricio Lucas Demera Grupo de Investigación en Sanidad Acuícola, Inocuidad y Salud Ambiental, Escuela de Acuicultura y Pesquería, Facultad de Ciencias Veterinarias, Universidad Técnica de Manabí, Bahía de Caráquez, Ecuador

Ivona Mladineo Institute of Oceanography and Fisheries, Split, Croatia

Pilar Molist Department of Functional Biology and Health Sciences, University of Vigo, Lagoas-Marcosende, Vigo, Spain

Leonela Griselda Muñoz-Chumo Grupo de Investigación en Sanidad Acuícola, Inocuidad y Salud Ambiental, Escuela de Acuicultura y Pesquería, Facultad de Ciencias Veterinarias, Universidad Técnica de Manabí, Bahía de Caráquez, Ecuador

Teresa Pérez Nieto Marine Research Centre (CIM-UVIGO), University of Vigo, Vigo, Pontevedra, Spain

Santiago Pascual Ecology and Biodiversity Department, Institute of Marine Research, Spanish National Research Council (CSIC), Vigo, Pontevedra, Spain

Kerry Perkins Sea Life Brighton—Merlin Entertainments, Brighton, UK

Jane L. Polglase Institute of Life and Earth Sciences, School of Energy, Geoscience, Infrastructure and Society, Heriot Watt University, Edinburgh, Scotland, UK

María Prado-Álvarez Aquatic Molecular Pathobiology Group, Institute of Marine Research, Spanish National Research Council (CSIC), Vigo, Pontevedra, Spain

Yaosen Qian Ganyu Institute of Fishery Science, Lianyungang, China

Jing Ren Key Laboratory of Mariculture, Ministry of Education, Institute of Evolution and Marine Biodiversity, Ocean University of China, Qingdao, China

Katina Roumbedakis Association for Cephalopod Research (CephRes), Naples, Italy

Carlos S. Ruiz ANFACO-CECOPESCA, Ctra. Colexio Universitario, Vigo, Pontevedra, Spain

Ana María Santana-Piñeros Grupo de Investigación en Sanidad Acuícola, Inocuidad y Salud Ambiental, Escuela de Acuicultura y Pesquería, Facultad de Ciencias Veterinarias, Universidad Técnica de Manabí, Bahía de Caráquez, Ecuador

Dhikra Souidenne National Museum of Natural History of Paris, Biologie des Organismes et Ecosystèmes Aquatiques (BOREA), Research Team: Reproduction and Development, Evolution Adaptation, Regulation CNRS 7208, Sorbonne Université, UCN, IRD 207, Paris, France

Antonio V. Sykes Centro de Ciências Do Mar, Universidade Do Algarve|CCMAR, Faro, Portugal

Juan M. Vieites ANFACO-CECOPESCA, Ctra. Colexio Universitario, Vigo, Pontevedra, Spain

Qingqi Zhang Ganyu Jiaxin Fishery Technical Development Co., Ltd., Lianyungang, China

Xiaodong Zheng Key Laboratory of Mariculture, Ministry of Education, Institute of Evolution and Marine Biodiversity, Ocean University of China, Qingdao, China

Letizia Zullo Centre for Synaptic Neuroscience and Technology, Fondazione Istituto Italiano Di Tecnologia, Genoa, Italy

1 Introduction

Camino Gestal, Santiago Pascual, Ángel Guerra, Graziano Fiorito, and Juan M. Vieites

Abstract

Cephalopods are valuable seafood for human consumption, and some of them are good candidates for aquaculture. In addition, they have evolved many characteristic features that make them interesting models for research. The recent inclusion of cephalopods in the Directive 2010/EU regulates the use of animals for scientific purposes and obliges cephalopod researchers to promote the best health and welfare practices during aquarium maintenance or aquaculture procedures. The identification of diseases of cephalopods, and the pathogens that cause them, is consequently of major interest to improve cephalopod welfare and husbandry. This work has been designed as a short, easy to follow 'handbook,' with the aim of presenting fundamental aspects of the anatomical and histological structures as well as the identification of different pathogens, the resulting histopathology, and the diagnosis of diseases in cephalopods. We hope it will provide a useful contribution that will also encourage marine pathologists, parasitologists, veterinarians and those involved in fishery sanitary assessment, aquarium maintenance, and aquaculture practice to increase our knowledge about the pathology of cephalopods further.

Keywords

Cephalopods • Pathology • Parasites • Infectious diseases • Fisheries • Aquaculture • Seafood

Knowledge of pathologies of cephalopod mollusks in the wild is very limited. The information available is mainly based on *postmortem* examination of animals after capture, which limits the identification of the etiological agent responsible for the disease. Most recently, pathologies of cephalopods have also been identified in laboratory and small-scale culture conditions; it is predicted that the increasing interest in industrial cephalopod aquaculture will increase the risks of their occurrence (Sykes and Gestal 2014).

Identifying pathogens and the resulting diseases, and the potential risks to animals' health due to mechanical damage or injuries from capture or in the laboratory are considered some of the main requisites for improving welfare and husbandry for these animals, as required in 'assessment of health and welfare' of the Directive 2010/63/EU.

Cephalopods (i.e., nautilus, cuttlefish, squid, and octopus) are members of the phylum mollusca. The taxon currently numbers about 800 species, representing a large diversity of

C. Gestal (✉)
Aquatic Molecular Pathobiology Group, Institute of Marine Research, Spanish National Research Council (CSIC), 36208 Vigo, Pontevedra, Spain
e-mail: cgestal@iim.csic.es

S. Pascual · Á. Guerra
Ecology and Biodiversity Department, Institute of Marine Research, Spanish National Research Council (CSIC), 36208 Vigo, Pontevedra, Spain
e-mail: spascual@iim.csic.es

Á. Guerra
e-mail: angelguerra@iim.csic.es

G. Fiorito
Association for Cephalopod Research (CephRes), Naples, Italy
e-mail: graziano.fiorito@gmail.com

J. M. Vieites
ANFACO-CECOPESCA. Ctra. Colexio Universitario, 16, 36310 Vigo, Pontevedra, Spain
e-mail: jvieites@anfaco.es

C. Gestal et al. (eds.), *Handbook of Pathogens and Diseases in Cephalopods*,
https://doi.org/10.1007/978-3-030-11330-8_1

forms and adaptations. These are exclusively marine invertebrates distributed in all areas of the world, from the intertidal areas to deep sea.

The interest in cephalopods has increased considerably over the last few decades, mainly because they (i) represent a very important target for fisheries with high market value; (ii) constitute an important resource of seafood for human consumption, with a high protein and polyunsaturated fatty acid content; (iii) are characterized by features of their biology and physiology which are novel in design and evolutionary adaptation (Albertin et al. 2015; Shigeno et al. 2018); (iv) are the sole invertebrates included in the list of regulated species by the Directive 2010/63/EU (Fiorito et al. 2015; Di Cristina et al. 2015).

Coleoid cephalopods have been used for millennia as seafood by humans across the world and across different food cultures (Mouritsen and Styrbæk 2018). Cephalopod landings reached about 4 million tons in 2016 (FAO 2017), although a fall of approximately one-quarter from that total was reported for 2017 (G. Pierce, pers. communication). The continuously increasing demand from the market, the decline in fishing overall, and the search for a more sustainable food resource have all contributed to promote a great interest in cephalopod aquaculture over the last decade, with an important, associated research effort in the field (Iglesias et al. 2014).

Considered classically as 'marine guinea pigs' (Grimpe 1928), cephalopods have been studied for more than one century for the uniqueness of their biology (Grimpe 1928; Packard 1972; Marini et al. 2017). They have evolved many characteristic features that make them 'organisms of interest' for the study of the evolution of neural and behavioral complexity. Despite their typical molluscan design and body plan, cephalopods possess a highly differentiated multi-lobular brain, a camera eye resembling that of vertebrates, a 'closed' circulatory system, a sophisticated set of sensory organs and fast jet-propelled locomotion. Cephalopods, and squid in particular, are also the animals that donated to neuroscience the giant axon, the classic preparation that allowed the discovery of how neuronal action potentials and nerve propagation worked, together with the ionic mechanism of action potentials.

The identification and management of diseases are some of the major hurdles in the development of the aquaculture industry. The accurate identification of the different organs at histological level and the knowledge and management of infectious and non-infectious diseases that may affect cultured species are a priority for both the aquarium maintenance and aquaculture of cephalopods.

A range of diseases has been described in cephalopods, caused by a wide variety of pathogens, belonging to many phyla, including fungi, viruses, bacteria, and protozoan and metazoan parasites. Bacterial infections have been identified in wild cephalopods, while the collection, transfer, aquarium maintenance and weakening of animals under stress may facilitate and increase the development of the diseases (Hanlon and Forsythe 1990; Hochberg 1990). Wild cephalopods are also intermediate, paratenic, or definitive hosts of a range of parasites with different life cycle strategies. They occupy an ecological niche that makes them vulnerable to infection by specific groups of parasites, which are transmitted to the definitive host, namely fish, marine mammals, or birds. An association between relative species diversity of parasites and cephalopod life cycle characteristics has been observed in Atlantic waters, suggesting that the ecological niche of a cephalopod species is more important in determining its risk of parasitic infection than its phylogeny (González et al. 2003).

Despite the increased interest in cephalopods as seafood and the recommendations of Food Safety Authorities on parasite risk in fishery products, currently only fragmentary information on pathogens and diseases in cephalopods exists. This information has been mainly gathered from opportunistic sampling plans within commercial fisheries or market surveys, and it is small in comparison with information available for other commercially important taxa (Pascual and Guerra 2003; González and Pascual 2018). At the present, there is no available information on the risk that cephalopod parasites pose to human consumers. In order to carry out good Regulatory Science, (which is described as the scientific and technical foundations upon which regulations are based) knowing what risks cephalopod disease pose to consumers will be a key point. Future research should be addressed to this, together with building the knowledge base overall, which is also a critical point in this research area. Although human consumption of cephalopods worldwide is much lower than that of fish, potential risk should be managed appropriately. As an example, González and Pascual (2018) pointed out that 'risk management should configure and consistently implement policies to ensure that scientific evidence is translated into action, while also considering aspects such as the key general principles established in EU food law (necessity, proportionality, minimum effect on competence, and guarantee of level playing field) that guarantee and protect the functioning of markets.' The use of certified biobanking in fish (González et al. 2018) can aid the establishment of a similar network for sampling and collection of traceable cephalopod parasites.

Knowledge of the most important pathogenic agents identified in cephalopods has been reviewed in volume III (1990) of the seminal serial work 'Diseases of Marine Animals,' edited by Otto Kinne. A general overview of each group of pathogens, together with a compilation of information on microorganisms and parasite species identified per cephalopod host species, is included in the original work (Hochberg 1990; Hanlon and Forsythe 1990). In more recent years, a review by Castellanos-Martínez and Gestal (2013), and some additional papers on specific pathogens or parasites added additional data on the knowledge of cephalopod parasitology and diseases.

However, to the best of our knowledge, no guide to histological identification has yet been published; this book aims to contribute to fill this gap. It originates as one of the outcomes of the activities of the COST Action FA1301, Cephs *In* Action, which established an interdisciplinary network for improvement of cephalopod welfare and husbandry in research, aquaculture, and fisheries.

The first part of the book offers tools that advise one on how to make an accurate pathological analysis. Several chapters provide a review of sampling methodology (including necropsy and postmortem examination), organ anatomy, as well as a detailed description of the histology of larval stages and adults for three species of cephalopods (*Sepia officinalis, Loligo vulgaris,* and *Octopus vulgaris*). We consider these species as valuable 'morphotype' models of the taxonomic groups Sepioidea, Myopsida, and Octopoda, which include most of the species with highest culture potential (Iglesias et al. 2014).

Additionally, knowledge of organ architecture and tissue structure at histological level is a key factor to identify and analyze pathological conditions. The histological identification of organs of the selected species of cephalopods is discussed for both larval stages and adults.

In the second part of this book, methods for assessment of parasites and pathogens in cephalopods are thoroughly described. Diseases conditions are diverse in the wild- and aquarium-maintained cephalopods, depending on the combination of physiological and immunological host factors, as well as the virulence of the pathogens. Current techniques involving molecular tools are being used to support the diagnosis of different pathologies. However, conventional diagnostic tools, including gross pathology, histopathology, and identification of signs of diseases, remain not only useful but also very valuable techniques. The combination of both approaches, i.e., diagnosis taxonomy and molecular biology, is needed for the accurate identification of pathogens. Aquarium maintenance and conditions (e.g., seawater quality, tank materials, density of individuals per tank) provoke stress that increases the susceptibility of cephalopods to suffer diseases. Consequently, knowledge of these disorders is a bottleneck for the assessment and improvement of the health status and welfare in cephalopods, as required by the European Directive 2010/EU (EU 2010; see also Fiorito et al. 2015).

The material selected for this compendium represents a comprehensive overview of the pathologies observed in wild- and aquarium-maintained cephalopods, in the form of a short, easy to follow handbook. We aim to present fundamental aspects of the anatomical and histological structures, as well as the identification of different pathogens, the resulting histopathologies and diagnosis of diseases in cephalopods.

We hope this will provide a useful contribution that will also encourage marine pathologists, parasitologists, veterinarians and those involved in fishery sanitary assessment, aquarium maintenance, and aquaculture practice, to increase our knowledge regarding the pathology of cephalopods further.

References

Albertin CB, Simakov O, Mitros T, Wang ZY, Pungor JR, Edsinger-Gonzales E, Brenner S, Ragsdale CW, Rokhsar DS (2015) The octopus genome and the evolution of cephalopod neural and morphological novelties. Nature 524:220–224

Castellanos-Martínez S, Gestal C (2013) Pathogens and immune response of cephalopods. J Exp Mar Bio Ecol 447:14–22

Di Cristina G, Andrews P, Ponte G, Galligioni V, Fiorito G (2015) The impact of Directive 2010/63/EU on cephalopod research. Invert Neurosci 15:8

EU (2010) Directive 2010/63/EU of the European Parliament and of the Council of 22 September 2010 on the Protection of Animals used for Scientific Purposes. Official J Euro Union 33–79

FAO (2017) Yearbook of fisheries and aquaculture statistics. FAO annuaire, November, 2017, Rome

Fiorito G, Affuso A, Basil J et al (2015) Guidelines for the care and welfare of cephalopods in research—a consensus based on an initiative by CephRes, FELASA and the Boyd Group. Lab Animal 49:90

González AF, Pascual S (eds) (2018) Parasite risk assessment in European fish stocks. Fish Res 202, p 160

González AF, Pascual S, Gestal C, Abollo E, Guerra A (2003) What makes a cephalopod a suitable host for parasites? The case of Galician waters. Fish Res 60:177–183

González AF, Rodríguez H, Outeriño L, Vello C, Larsson Ch, Pascual S (2018) A biobanking platform for fish-borne zoonotic parasites: a traceable system to preserve samples, data and money. Fish Res 202:29–37

Grimpe G (1928) Pflege, Behandlung und Zucht der Cephalopoden für zoologische und physiologische Zwecke. Handb Biol Arbeit 331–402

Hanlon RT, Forsythe JW (1990) Diseases Caused by Microorganisms. In: Kinne O (ed) Diseases of Mollusca: Cephalopoda. Diseases of Marine Animals, vol. III. Cephalopoda to Urochordata. Biologische Anstalt Helgoland, Hamburg, pp 23–46

Hochberg FG (1990) Diseases caused by protistans and metazoans. In: Kinne O (ed) Diseases of Mollusca: Cephalopoda. Diseases of Marine Animals, vol III. Cephalopoda to Urochordata. Biologische Anstalt Helgoland, Hamburg, pp 47–227

Iglesias J, Fuentes L (2014) *Octopus vulgaris*. Paralarval Culture. In: Iglesias J, Fuentes, L, Villanueva R (eds) Cephalopod culture. Springer, Netherlands, pp 427–450, 494

Iglesias J, Fuentes L, Villanueva R (eds) (2014) Cephalopod Culture. Springer, Netherlands, p 494

Marini G, De Sio F, Ponte G, Fiorito G (2017) Behavioral analysis of learning and memory in cephalopods. In: Byrne JH (ed) Learning and memory: a comprehensive reference, 2nd edn. Academic Press, Elsevier, Amsterdam, pp 441–462

Mouritsen O, Styrbæk K (2018) Cephalopod gastronomy. A promise for the future. Front Comm, New Jersey. https://doi.org/10.3389/fcomm.2018.00038

Packard A (1972) Cephalopods and fish: the limits of convergence. Biol Rev 47:241–307

Pascual S, Guerra A (2003) Vexing question on fisheries research: the study of cephalopods and their parasites. Iberus 19:87–95

Shigeno S, Andrews PL, Ponte G, Fiorito G (2018) Cephalopod brains: An overview of current knowledge to facilitate comparison with vertebrates. Front Physiol 9:952

Sykes A, Gestal C (2014) Welfare and diseases under culture conditions. In: Iglesias J, Fuentes L, Villanueva R (eds) Cephalopod Culture. Springer, Netherlands, pp 97–112

2 Importance of Cephalopod Health and Welfare for the Commercial Sector

Juan M. Vieites, Carlos S. Ruiz, Felicidad Fernández, and Roberto C. Alonso

Abstract

We witness the expansion of cephalopod fisheries and their growing importance in the world's fisheries production. Despite this, only 4 of the 28 taxonomic families are commercially exploited. The rational exploitation of resources could provide large quantities of high-quality cephalopods and would only require further development in harvesting techniques. The intrinsic nutritional value of the cephalopods and the progress of extraction and processing technologies would allow for an expansion of the range of products attractive to consumers, including current non-commercial species. This atlas presents a review of general pathology in octopus, cuttlefish, and squid from different regions of the world. This topic is closely linked to food safety concerns, and it can also be considered a tool for assessing the state of populations. This review provides a resource for teaching and guidance in universities, research centers, public and private laboratories, processing and transformation companies, as well as for administrations in their legislative processes.

Keywords

Cephalopods • Pathology guidance • Seafood • Commercial sector

The 2010 FAO review of cephalopods of the world (Jereb and Roper 2010), considers the existence of 28 families, although the most commercially available species are focused on the families Sepiidae, Loliginidae, Ommastrephidae, and Octopoteuthidae. The number of cephalopod species covered by commercial fishing has continued to grow significantly since 1984, as a result of the increasing market demand and the expansion of fishing activities in new fishing grounds and deeper waters. Species of the Ommastrephidae family are the most important commercial fishery among cephalopods. According to FAO (2016), during the decade from 1997 to 2007, the annual world catch of Ommastrephidae varied between 1 and more than 2 million tons, which represents 50% of the total catch of cephalopods worldwide. The impressive increase in squid production over the past 30 years is mainly due to the discovery and subsequent exploitation of resources in the southwestern Atlantic, mainly *Illex argentinus*, as well as an increase in the production of other target species, mainly *Dosidicus gigas* in the East Pacific and *Todarodes pacificus* in the Northwest Pacific.

Regarding the evolution of the catches of all cephalopods, Doubleday et al's (2016) data show a general upward trend in the period 1955–2012. Within this general trend, we highlight that, after reaching the maximum level of 4.3 million tons in 2007, the increase in total cephalopod catch slowed for some years. However, in 2012, catches surpassed again and, in 2014, they surpassed 4.5 million tons, according to the 2016 FAO report. In successive reports (FAO 2018), a dramatic drop in the cephalopod catch was recorded in 2016, although there seem to be signs of recovery in 2017. Catches of octopuses (family Octopoteuthidae) have been shown, in global figures to be more stable than those of squids. Since 2008, both catches of cuttlefish and octopuses have remained relatively

J. M. Vieites (✉) · C. S. Ruiz · F. Fernández · R. C. Alonso
ANFACO-CECOPESCA, Ctra. Colexio Universitario, 16, 36310 Vigo, Pontevedra, Spain
e-mail: jvieites@anfaco.es

C. S. Ruiz
e-mail: ffernandez@anfaco.es

F. Fernández
e-mail: cruiz@anfaco.es

R. C. Alonso
e-mail: robertocarlos@anfaco.es

C. Gestal et al. (eds.), *Handbook of Pathogens and Diseases in Cephalopods*,
https://doi.org/10.1007/978-3-030-11330-8_2

stable between 300 and 350,000 tons, respectively, although this represents a decrease in the case of cuttlefish and an increase in octopuses, as compared to previous years.

From the 2018 FAO report on the state of fisheries and aquaculture, we can mention that, after five years of continuous growth, which began in 2010, catches of cephalopods stabilized in 2015, but fell in 2016, when the three main species of squids recorded a combined loss of 1.2 million tons.

The potential for the fishery of all species of the exploitable Ommastrephidae family is estimated between 6 and 9 million tons. A large number of squids of this family, which lacks ammonium, are considered little exploited. These include *Sthenoteuthis pteropus, Ommastrephes bartramii, Martialia hyadesi, Todarodes sagittatus, Sthenoteuthis oualaniensis, Nototodarus philippinensis, Dosidicus gigas,* and the cir cumpolar and subantarctic species *Todarodes filippovae.*

The assessment of the availability of commercial and other less exploited species faces the difficulties derived from the short life of the cephalopods and their adaptive strategies to ensure survival against stressful environmental conditions, including those caused by intensive fishing. Therefore, both stock assessments and predicting important fluctuations in catches and landings are difficult (Pierce and Guerra 1994; Robert et al. 2010). Barring uncertainties in the assessment of fishing potential, the exploitation of these species could provide large quantities of high-quality cephalopods and would require only further development in harvesting techniques.

On the consumption forecast of products derived from cephalopods, the aforementioned FAO 2018 and 2016 reports show that Spain, Italy, and Japan are the main consumers and importers of these species. Thailand, Spain, China, Argentina, and Peru were the largest exporters of squid and cuttlefish, while Morocco, Mauritania, and China were the main exporters of octopus. Vietnam is expanding its cephalopod markets, including squid, in Southeast Asia. Other Asian countries such as the Republic of Korea and India are also important suppliers. In South America, there is an increasing interest in the Humboldt Squid (*Dosidicus gigas*), which is being exported from Peru to more than 50 countries, and efforts are being made to develop new products. In 2013, the main markets, especially Japan and the European Union, remained strong, despite the difficult economic situations and the high prices of these species. In the 2014–2015 period, the largest increases in the markets were of octopus, rather than of squid and cuttlefish. However, the reduction in catches resulted in a shortage of supply in 2016 and 2017.

On consumer preferences according to the FAO 2016 report, the use of squid for human consumption is extensive and diverse. There is an increasingly wide range of raw, refrigerated, frozen, dry, canned, and prepared products. Despite the aversion of cultural origin of the inhabitants of northern countries to the consumption of cephalopods, technological development allows to add value to cephalopod products, making them attractive to broader layers of consumers. In one of the last discussion forums (MAFE 2012) it became clear that, currently, consumers consider food as the guarantor of their future health. The high-protein content, the abundance of essential amino acids, and the low-fat content of cephalopods make them an ideal food to be part of healthy and balanced diets. The data collected in nutritional tables such as those prepared by ANFACO-CECOPESCA (2018) and the USDA (2018) show that the squid form a homogeneous group with high-protein content, in which essential amino acids abound (with slight differences in level with respect to octopuses) plus a low-fat content, giving a healthy profile. The significant numbers of authorized declarations of health properties, to which the products derived from cephalopods can be accepted under the provisions of the EU (2012), support the nutritional quality of cephalopods.

From the reports on the state of world fisheries, it should be noted that in the last 40 years the percentage of cephalopods production to world production increased from 2 to around 5%. The manufacturing industry requires constancy in purchases. The important fluctuations experienced by the main species of cephalopods of commercial interest raise practical issues in the control of conformity of the specifications of commercial quality of the raw materials since they condition the specifications of the final products. This entails the execution of a series of controls based on self-control, on the maximum content of certain contaminants and microbiological criteria, and on the organoleptic or sensorial characteristics that determine the acceptability of the raw material.

With this panoramic view it presents, our Atlas covers aspects directly linked to food safety and quality. The Atlas presents an overall review of the general pathology in octopus, cuttlefish, and squid from other regions of the world. Regarding morphological aspects, it describes macro and microscopic lesions and their consequences for organisms, both in the wild and from mariculture. In addition, there is a chapter on tissue and organ regeneration and others on viruses and parasites.

Given the expected future projection of cephalopods in the world diet, the Atlas is considered a reference publication for teaching and guidance in universities, research centers, public and private laboratories, processing and transformation companies, as well as for use by administrations in their legislative processes.

2.1 Concluding Remarks

The chapter justifies the importance of cephalopod health and welfare for the commercial sector and the usefulness of the handbook under the panoramic view presented.

References

ANFACO-CECOPESCA (2018) IV Forum of Innovation and Technology of Anfaco-Cecopesca: "Innovation and Biotechnology for a more competitive Marine and Food sector" 10.9.2018 (Available in http://www.anfaco.es/es/index.php)

Doubleday ZA, Prowse TA, Arkhipkin A, Pierce GJ, Semmens J, Steer M, Leporati SC, Lourenço S, Quetglas A, Sauer W, Gillanders BM (2016) Global proliferation of cephalopods. Curr Biol 26 (10):406–407. https://doi.org/10.1016/j.cub.2016.04.002

EU (2012) Commission Regulation No 432/2012 of 16 May 2012 establishing a list of permitted health claims made on foods, other than those referring to the reduction of disease risk and to children's development and health (Official Journal of the European Union L 136/1, https://eur-lex.europa.eu/LexUriServ/LexUriServ.do?uri=OJ:L:2012:136:0001:0040:en:PDF

FAO (2016) The state of world fisheries and aquaculture 2016. Contribution to food security and nutrition for all, Rome, p 224

FAO (2018) The state of world fisheries and aquaculture. Fulfilling the objectives of sustainable development, Rome, http://www.fao.org/3/i9540en/I9540EN.pdf

Jereb P, Roper CFE (2010) Cephalopods of the world: an annotated and illustrated catalogue of cephalopod species known to date. FAO Species Catalogue for Fishery Purposes 4:1– 4. FIR/Cat. 4/2 ISBN 92-5-105383-9

MAFE (2012) Guide of the nutritional qualities of products from Extractive Fisheries and Aquaculture: risk-Benefit Binomial. Ministry of Agriculture, Food and Environment (Spain), Spain

Pierce GJ, Guerra A (1994) Stock assessment methods used for cephalopod fisheries. Fis Res 21:255–285

Robert M, Faraj A, Mcallister MK, Rivot E (2010) Bayesian state-space modelling of the De Lury depletion model: strengths and limitations of the method, and application to the Moroccan octopus fishery. ICES J Mar Sci 67:1272–1290

USDA (2018) United States Department of Agriculture Agricultural Research Service National Nutrient Database for Standard Reference. Tables available in three web pages: https://ndb.nal.usda.gov/ndb/foods/show/4641?fgcd=Finfish+and+Shellfish+Products&manu=&lfacet=&format=&count=&max=35&offset=140&sort=&qlookup; https://ndb.nal.usda.gov/ndb/foods/show/4644?fgcd=Finfish+and+Shellfish+Products&manu=&lfacet=&format=&count=&max=35&offset=140&sort=&qlookup; https://ndb.nal.usda.gov/ndb/foods/show/4653?fgcd=Finfish+and+Shellfish+Products&manu=&lfacet=&format=&count=&max=35&offset=140&sort=&qlookup

Part I

Functional Anatomy and Histology

3 Functional Anatomy: Macroscopic Anatomy and Post-mortem Examination

Ángel Guerra

Abstract

Understanding the relationship between form and function of living beings is an intimidating challenge. The recognition and interpretation of physiological and pathological processes require a previous knowledge of regular morphology and anatomy of the external and internal structures and organs of any living creature. Cephalopods span an awesome range of shapes and scales, and the variations between species are crucial for correct interpretations. This chapter covers the gross morphological and anatomical main characteristics of different cephalopod species, as well as necropsy protocols and methods of euthanasia. This knowledge is decisive to a suitable understanding of the modifications caused by injury, infection, or disease, especially for those people who are not familiar with these remarkable marine molluscs.

Keywords

Cephalopods • Gross morphology • Functional anatomy • Euthanasia • Necropsy

3.1 Classification

The Cephalopoda is an ancient class of the Phylum Mollusca dating from the Upper Cambrian Period (around 500 million years ago; mya). Cephalopods constitute one of the most complex groups of invertebrates and the most evolved of molluscs. This group has been among the dominant large predators in the ocean at various times in geological history. Its evolution is related directly to the development of low-pressure buoyancy mechanisms. They have acquired the ability to regulate buoyancy, followed by reduction and internalization of the shell and the development of the mantle musculature. Some 17,000 fossil species are known, most of them provided with an outer calcareous shell, whose abundance and distribution have experience important fluctuations throughout the different geologic eras. Clearly, the lineages of extinct taxa were prolific and diverse. Palaeontologists have identified three distinct fossil clades that are entirely extinct. All members of these clades were squid-like, but had straight external shells. They flourished in Palaeozoic oceans between the Ordovician (488 mya) and Triassic periods (200 mya). The shells of some of these species reached nearly 10 m in length. The most well known of these fossil records are the nautiloids, ammonoids, and belemnites. Some of the shelled ammonites that were the dominant elements of the marine fauna during the Mesozoic were of 3 m in diameter. Increase in brain size and complexity, development of effective sense organs, and changes in the skin concurred to the development of sophisticated behaviours. These traits make cephalopods the most active and intriguing of the molluscs (Nixon and Young 2003).

There are two major divisions within present-day cephalopods: the Nautiloidea with six species of the pearly nautilus (Fig. 3.1), which are the only living cephalopods with outer shells, and the Coleoidea, which is represented by about 800 species, containing the cuttlefishes and bobtail squids (Fig. 3.2), long-fin and short-fin squids (Fig. 3.3), vampire squids, Dumbo octopuses and octopods. This last group includes *Argonauta* species whose females produce an

Á. Guerra (✉)
Ecology and Biodiversity Department, Institute of Marine Research, Spanish National Research Council (CSIC), 36208 Vigo, Pontevedra, Spain
e-mail: angelguerra@iim.csic.es

C. Gestal et al. (eds.), *Handbook of Pathogens and Diseases in Cephalopods*,
https://doi.org/10.1007/978-3-030-11330-8_3

Class: Cephalopoda Cuvier, 1797
Subclass: Nautiloidea Agassiz, 1847
Family: Nautilidae Blainville, 1825 (Pearly or chambered nautilus)
Subclass: Coleoidea Bather, 1888
- Superorder: Decapodiformes Leach, 1817
  - Order: Spirulida Haeckel, 1896
    - Fam: Spirulidae Owen, 1836
  - Order: Sepioidea Naef, 1916
    - Suborder: Sepiida Keferstein, 1866
      - Fam: Sepiidae Keferstein, 1866 (Cuttlefishes)
    - Suborder: Sepiolida Naef, 1916
      - Fam: Sepiadariidae Fischer, 1882
      - Fam: Sepiolidae Leach, 1817 (Bobtail squids)
  - Order: Myopsida Naef, 1916
    - Fam: Australiteuthidae Lu, 2005
    - Fam: Loliginidae Lesueur, 1821 (Long-fin squids)
  - Order: Oegopsida Orbigny, 1845
    - Fam: Architeuthidae Pfeffer, 1900 (Giant squid)
    - Fam: Brachioteuthidae Pfeffer, 1908
    - Fam: Batoteuthidae Young and Roper, 1968
    - Fam: Chiroteuthidae Gray, 1849
    - Fam: Joubiniteuthidae Naef, 1922
    - Fam: Magnapinnidae Vecchione and Young, 1998
    - Fam: Mastigoteuthidae Verrill, 1881
    - Fam: Promachoteuthidae Naef, 1912
    - Fam: Cranchiidae Prosch, 1847
    - Fam: Cycloteuthidae Naef, 1923
    - Fam: Ancistrocheiridae Pfeffer, 1912
    - Fam: Enoploteuthidae Pfeffer, 1900
    - Fam: Lycoteuthidae Pfeffer, 1908
    - Fam: Pyroteuthidae Pfeffer, 1912
    - Fam: Gonatidae Hoyle 1886
    - Fam: Histioteuthidae Verrill, 1881
    - Fam: Psychroteuthidae Thiele, 1920
    - Fam: Lepidoteuthidae Naef, 1912
    - Fam: Octopoteuthidae Berry, 1912
    - Fam: Pholidoteuthidae Voss, 1956
    - Fam: Neoteuthidae Naef, 1921
    - Fam: Ommastrephidae Steenstrup, 1857 (Short-fin squids)
    - Fam: Onychoteuthidae Gray, 1847
    - Fam: Thysanoteuthidae Keferstein, 1866
- Superorder: Octopodiformes Berthold and Engeser, 1987
  - Order: Vampyromorpha Robson, 1929
    - Fam: Vampyroteuthidae Thiele, in Chun, 1915 (Vampire squids)
  - Order: Octopoda Leach, 1818
    - Suborder: Cirrata Grimpe, 1916 (Dumbo octopuses or Cirroctopods)
      - Fam: Cirroteuthidae Keferstein, 1866
      - Fam: Stauroteuthidae Grimpe, 1916
      - Fam: Opisthoteuthidae Verrill, 1896
    - Suborder: Incirrata Grimpe, 1916
      - Fam: Alloposidae Verrill, 1881
      - Fam: Argonautidae Cantraine, 1841
      - Fam: Ocythoidae Gray, 1849
      - Fam: Tremoctopodidae Tryon, 1879
      - Fam: Eledonidae Grimpe, 1921
      - Fam: Octopodidae Orbigny, 1839 (Octopuses)
      - Fam: Enteroctopodidae Strugnell et al., 2013
      - Fam: Amphitretidae Hoyle, 1886
      - Fam: Bathypolypodidae Robson, 1932

Fam: Megaleledonidae Taki, 1961
Order uncertain
Superfamily: Bathyteuthoidea nov.
Fam: Bathyteuthidae Pfeffer, 1900
Fam: Chtenopterygidae Grimpe, 1922
Fam: Idiosepiidae Fischer, 1882

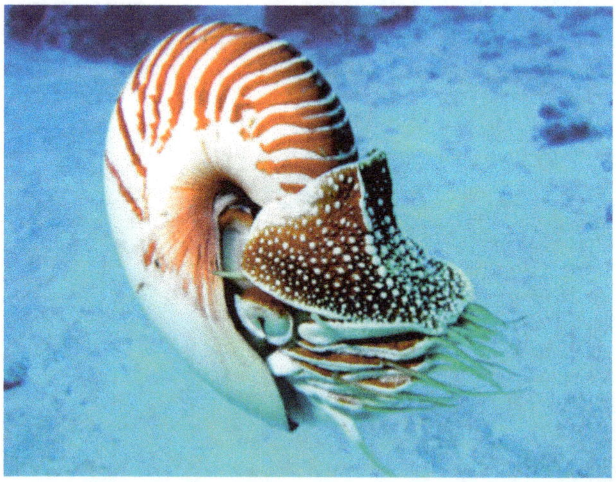

Fig. 3.1 Nautiluses or chambered nautiluses are the sole living cephalopods with an external shell

external calcareous structure (Fig. 3.4), which is not a true shell but a brood chamber.

Currently, the most widely accepted classification is the proposed by Young et al. (2018):

3.2 Ecology: General Aspects

As indicated by Boyle and Rodhouse (2005): «Any ecological approach always tries to take account of the interacting factors of evolution, genetics, physiology, and behaviour of the organisms as well as their relationships with the stochastics parameters of the environment. Consequently, these studies involve multidisciplinary approaches, which are not always easy to obtain for marine animals». This difficulty also affects cephalopods which occupy a great variety of habitats in all of the world's oceans (Fig. 3.5) and have a large variety of life history strategies. Another difficulty with these studies is the disparity of knowledge currently held about cephalopod species, which, on the other hand, increases day by day. For these reasons, we are going to provide here some generalities concerning the great ecological categories in which it is possible to classify living cephalopods.

The broad category of "coastal and shelf species" (neritic species) covers the relatively well-known cephalopod groups. The aphorism "live fast, die young" describes quite well the life history strategy of these coleoid cephalopods, which have epipelagic and benthic habitats. Nevertheless, as indicated by O'Dor (In Darmaillacq et al. 2014), «that phrase "live fast, die young" perhaps should be expanded to "live fast and smart, to leave offspring fewer enemies». Specifically, the available evidence of species of neritic cephalopods is that they complete their life cycle in one or two years and in some small species even in a shorter time. Beside this short lifespan, other characteristics shared by all members of this category are a similar type of predation, which places them at the upper trophic levels of the ecosystem. Like most cephalopods, neritic species have a single ovarian cycle. However, many of them have long spawning periods, in which the larger peak of new hatchlings is synchronized with environmental conditions providing them with suitable oceanographic factors and appropriate prey, which ensures high survival rates, but, conversely, noteworthy mass mortality. Consequently, cephalopod populations are highly unsteadied responsive to change in physical, chemical, and biological environment. Fecundity of the species within this category is very variable, from a few hundred eggs in cuttlefish, to several hundreds of thousands in octopus. Cephalopods do not have a true larva, because they lack of a distinct metamorphosis. Hatchlings of a number of species are planktonic and have a distinctively mode of life from older conspecifics (paralarvae). The neritic species share some degree of dependency on the seabed: some of them lay and eat at the bottom (demersal species, e.g. Loliginidae), but others, such as cuttlefish and octopuses, are truly benthic species.

The "oceanic and deep-sea category" of species encompasses the taxonomically diverse families of epi-, meso-, and bathypelagic, as well as bathybenthic cephalopods. The ecological knowledge about this group is still scarce. Although they share many basic characteristics, their lifestyles are more different between these taxa than with the neritic forms.

Like all division into categories, the one we present here is artificial and there are some species of difficult location, even within the same family. Thus, for example, in the Ommastrephidae, there are several species of different genera (*Ommastrephes, Sthenoteuthis, Martialia, Dosidicus*) that are truly ocean dwellers. Conversely, species of the genus *Illex, Todadores, Todaropsis,* and *Nototodarus*, although they typically have an offshore distribution, are frequently present on the continental shelves. There are many other examples of this or similar scenarios, and Jereb and Roper (2005, 2010) and Jereb et al. (2016) catalogues provide account for all families.

In any case, cephalopods are important to the ecosystem as both predator and prey as well as reservoirs of parasites.

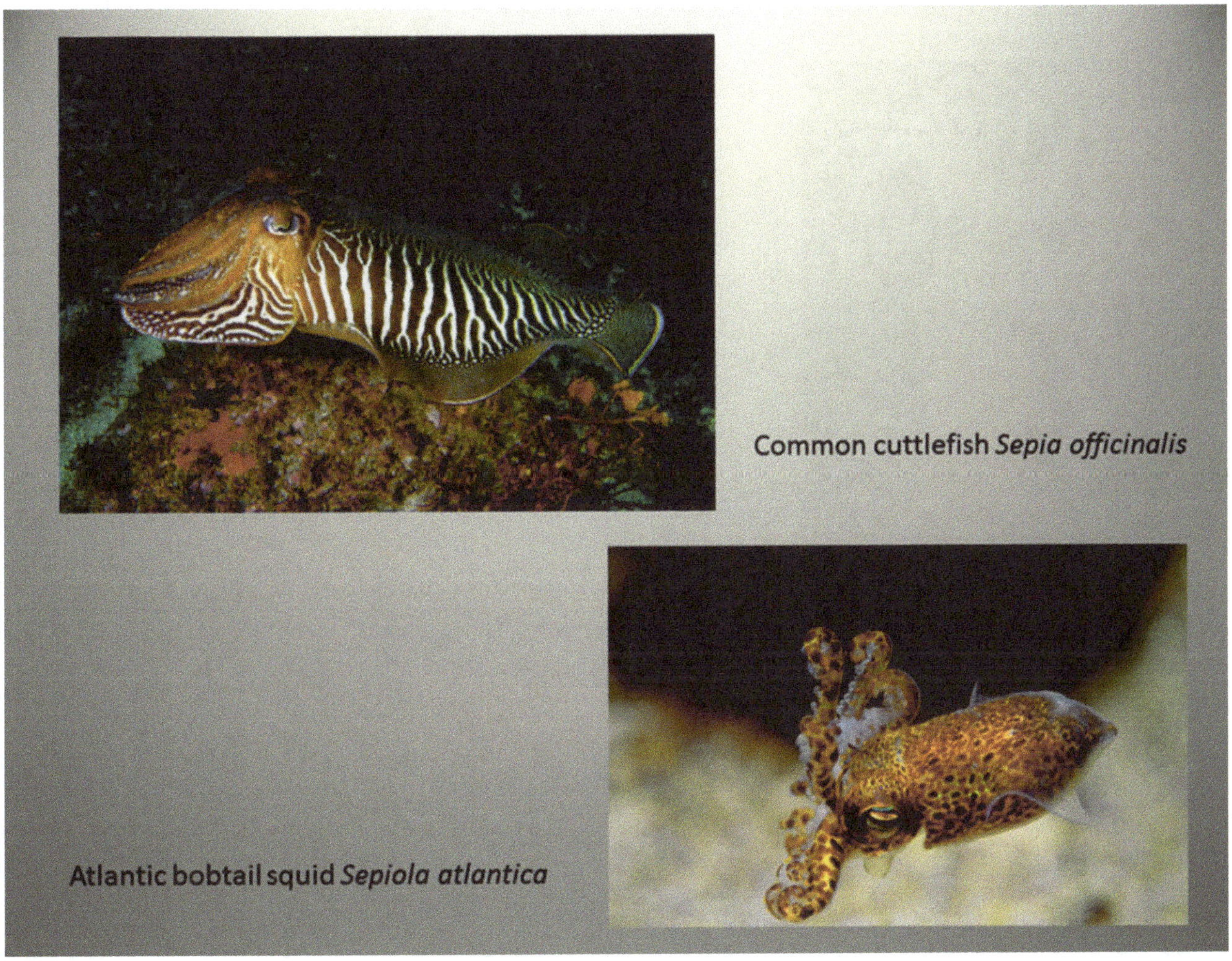

Fig. 3.2 Two species representatives of the order Sepioidea. Photographs by J. Hernández-Urcera and J. L. González

3.3 Fisheries and Aquaculture

Cephalopod catches worldwide account for around 4 million tons per year in 2016 (about 4% of total marine products). Although in recent times the total world catch from marine and freshwater fish stocks appears to have peaked and may be declining, the catch of cephalopods has continued to increase as fishers concentrate efforts away from more traditional finfish resources. Cephalopods fisheries can be divided between small-scale fisheries (SSFs) and industrial fisheries (IF). The SSFs are of great importance in terms of job opportunities, and they contribute significantly to the economy of many coastal communities. Methods of capture in SSFs are very diverse (pots, traps, lures, etc.), and the catches are mainly consumed in fresh. IF methods of capture are mainly jigging and trawling, and the catches are mainly commercialized frozen. Numerous species are caught in SSFs; however, IF are supported by a few species, mainly belonging to the families Loliginidae, Ommastrephidae, and Octopodidae (see Arkhipkin et al. 2015 for review).

Historically, the consumption of cephalopod products has been highest in the countries of Asia (Japan, Thailand, Taiwan, and China). Among European countries, Spain, Portugal, Italy, and Greece are the traditionally high consumers of cephalopods. In the rest of the globe, per capita cephalopod consumption is low.

The life cycle characteristics of cephalopods mean that their fisheries are intrinsically difficult to assess and manage. The level of exploitation of some stocks exploited in IF is quite high, and some of them are actually overexploited. Increasing of scientific knowledge for assessment and management purposes is needed.

The increasing demand of cephalopods and some of biological traits (high growth rates and short life spans) make cephalopods ideal candidates for commercial

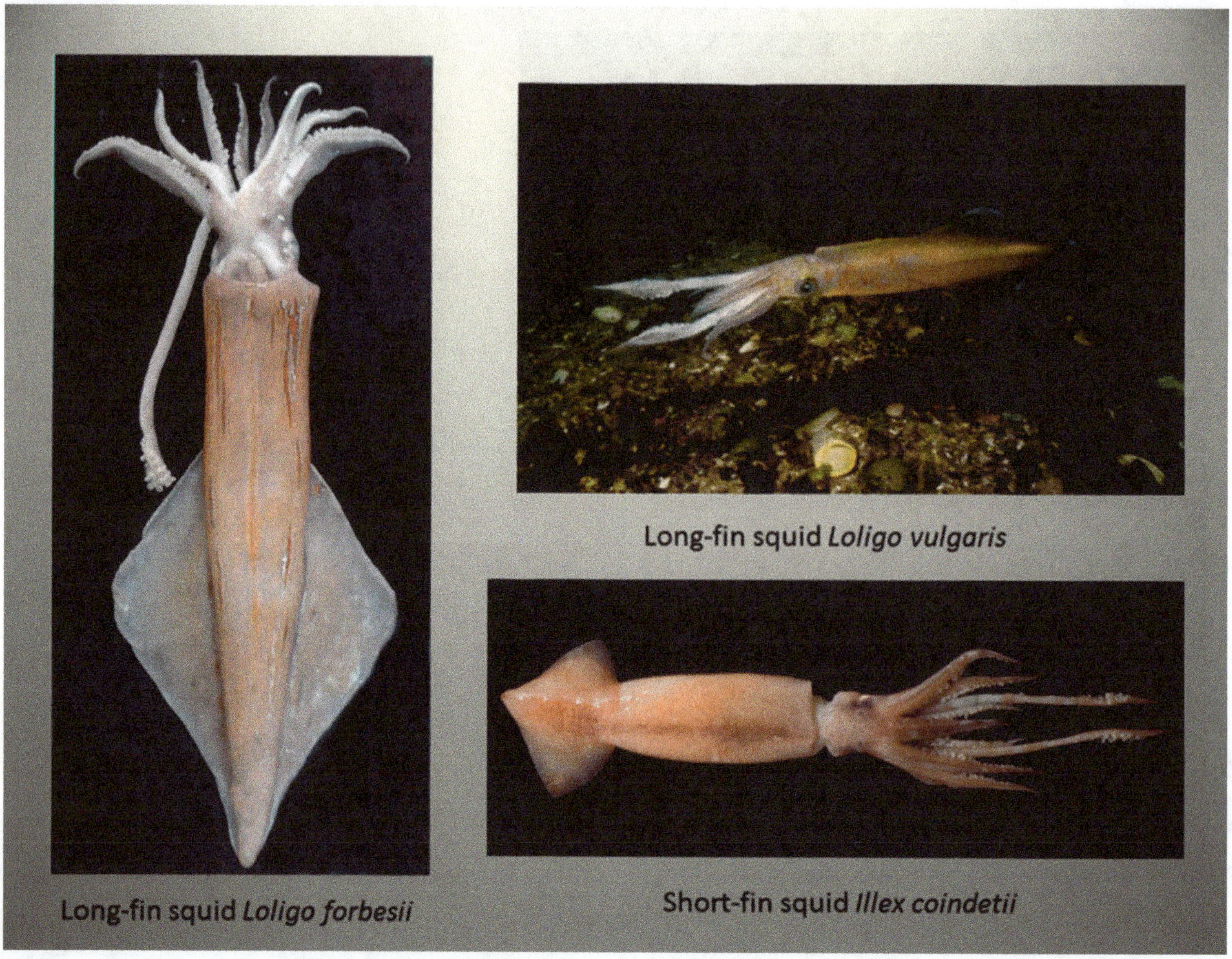

Fig. 3.3 Two species representatives of the order Myopsida (genus *Loligo*, family Loliginidae) and one of the order Oegopsida (genus *Illex*, family Ommastrephidae). Courtesy of A. Escánez and J.L. González

aquaculture since they have the potential to rapidly reach market size. As pointed out by Louise Allcock, former President of the Cephalopod International Council (CIAC), in the preface of the book "Cephalopod Culture" by Iglesias et al. (2014), «this is a pioneering text, which draws together a vast array of knowledge on cephalopod culture and provides the foundations for further advances in this significant field». Moreover, some species are used as model organisms in neurobiology, robotics, restocking, pharmaceutical exploitation of antibacterial anticancer activities reported from the ink sac, the use of modified cuttlebone in tissue engineering, the many and varied used of cuttlefish oil, and to study the cephalopod immune system. In consequence, small-scale culture of some species has become scientifically important in the latter half of the twentieth century. Nevertheless, the industrial culture of cephalopods is still in an incipient state. There are, however, some advances; one of them is successfully culture octopuses with large hatchlings using a completely artificial diet. As a result of the numerous studies carried out since 1990 to present days, many culture protocols had been optimized. At present, only 19 species of cephalopods are being cultivated worldwide: three *Nautilus and Allonautilus* species, four cuttlefish, two sepiolids, three loliginid squids, and seven octopods. The main bottlenecks in cephalopod culture were identified to be nutrition and physiology.

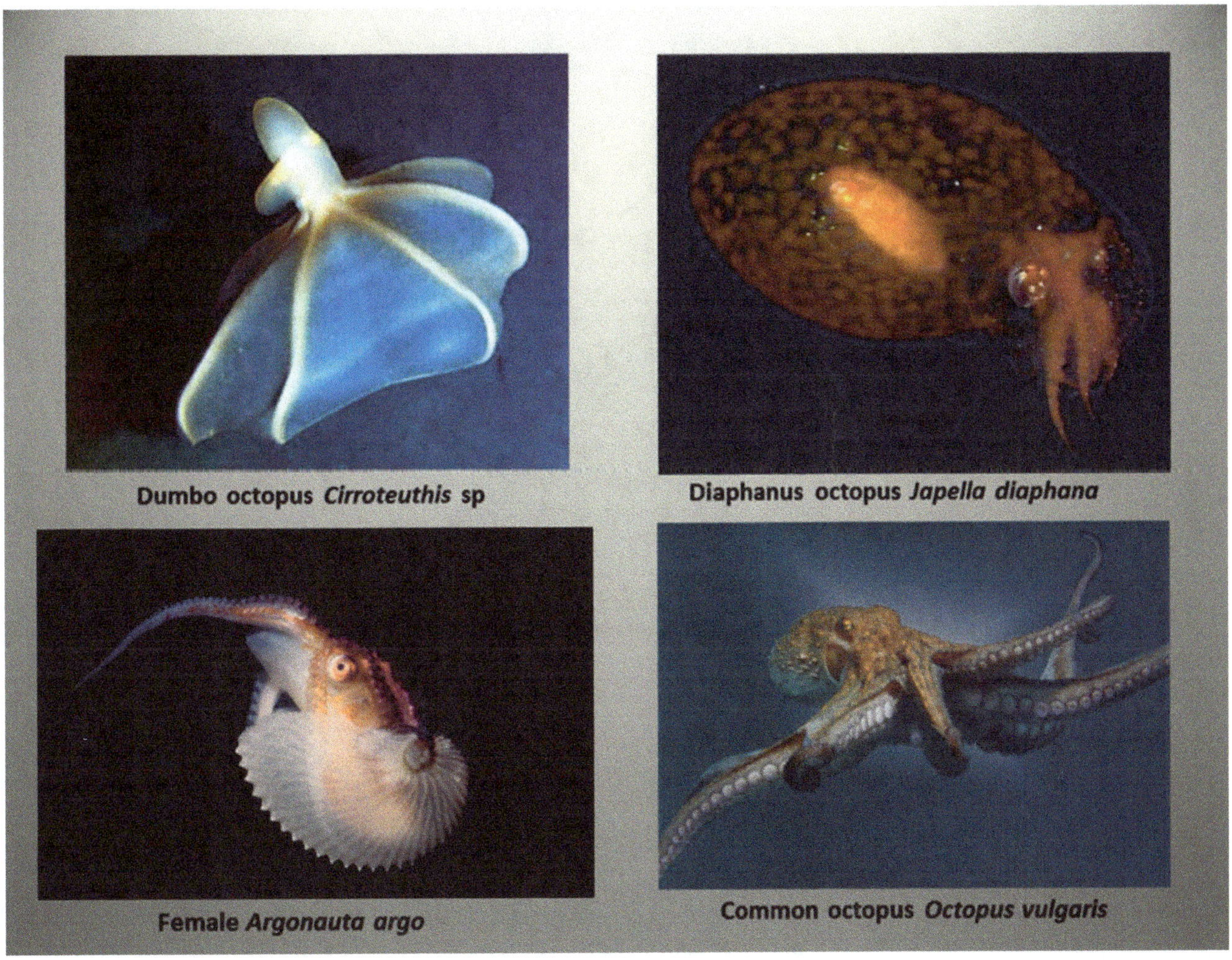

Fig. 3.4 Dumbo octopus (*Cirroteuthis* sp) is representative of the order Octopoda, suborder Cirrata; *Japetella diaphana* is a pelagic Octopoda; *Argonatuta argo* and *Octopus vulgaris* are representatives of the order Octopoda, suborder Incirrata. Courtesy of J.L. González

3.4 Morphology and Anatomy of the Adult

Modern cephalopods (subclass Coleoidea) have bilateral symmetry, and the body is divided into two defined parts: the cephalopodium or anterior part and the visceropalium or posterior part. The cephalopodium includes the head, the appendages that surround the mouth and the funnel; the visceropalium comprises the mantle, the cavity of the mantle and its organs, as well as the shell and the fins, the latter if present (Mangold 1989).

3.4.1 External Morphology

3.4.1.1 Size

The basic measure of cephalopods is the dorsal length of the mantle (ML), but also ventral mantle length (VML) can be used. In Sepioidea, Myopsida, and Oegopsida, ML is the distance between the antero-dorsal margin of the mantle and the posterior apex of the mantle (Fig. 3.6). In the Octopodiformes, ML is measured from the back of the body to an imaginary line that would connect the centre of both eyes (Fig. 3.7). Sometimes, other measures such as the total length (TL), which is the distance between the longest arm, or the extended tentacle, and the back of the animal's mantle, are used. Mantle length of adult cephalopods varies between 6 mm in the genus *Idiosepius* to around 2 m in the giant squid *Architeuthis dux*.

3.4.1.2 External Form

The head is usually separated from the mantle by the nuchal constriction. It carries the oral appendices and the eyes, which are usually spherical and of similar size, although in *Histioteuthis* the left eye is much larger than the right. In the occipital region, the head may be completely fused with the mantle or attached to it by a nuchal cartilage. A cartilaginous capsule contributes to the shape and volume of the head.

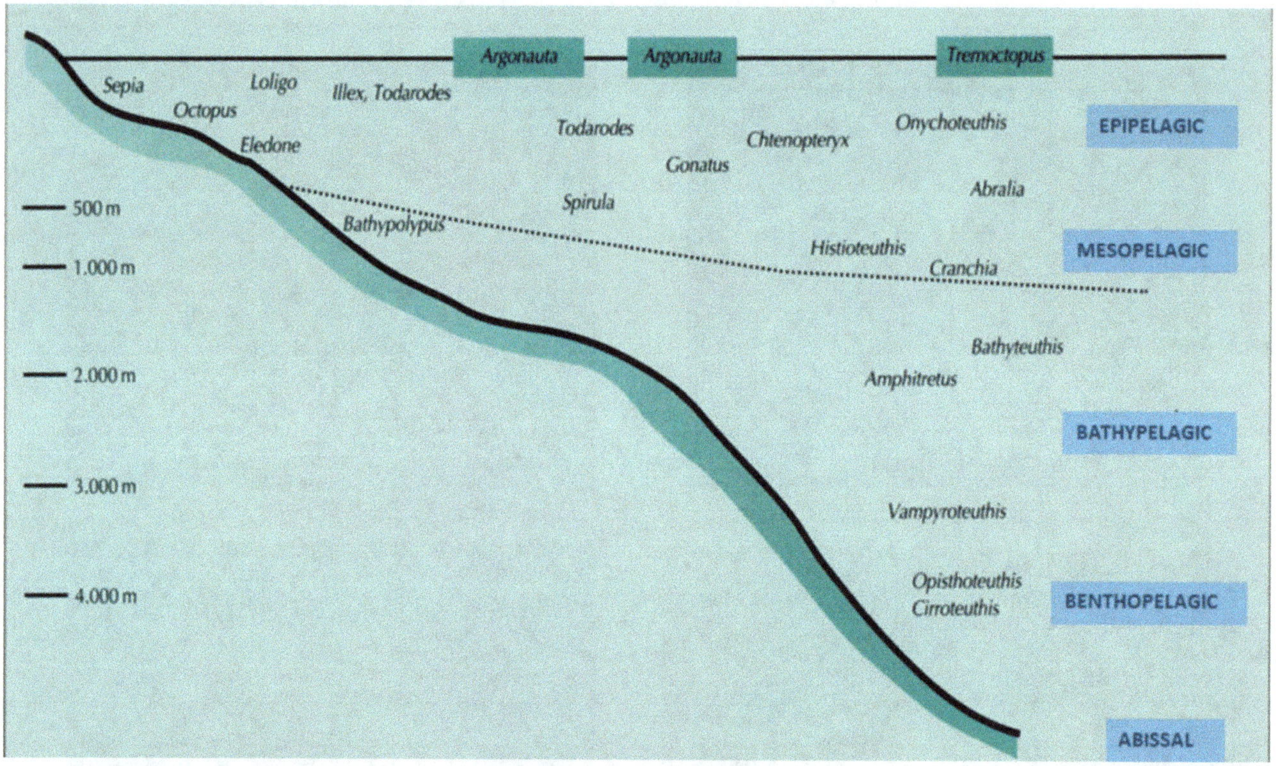

Fig. 3.5 Distribution with habitat and depth of selected genera characteristics of different marine zones

This capsule is like a skull that surrounds and protects the brain. On both sides of the head, near the neck, the olfactory organs are located.

Decapodiformes cephalopods have ten muscular appendages of two types, differing according to their length: eight arms (shorter) and two tentacles (longer). In contrast, Octopodiformes have only eight arms, lacking tentacles, although the arms are usually longer in proportion to body size than Decapodiformes. Each pair of arms is generally different in size from the other pairs. In *Vampyroteuthis,* two of its ten arms have been transformed into long and thin filaments that are retracted in a pair of bags placed between the dorsal and dorso-lateral arms. The species of *Nautilus* have 63–94 arms or short tentacles. The arms are often numbered from the dorsal pair to the ventral (which is well defined because it is the side of the animal where the funnel opens). This gives rise to the "brachial formula" (Figs. 3.6 and 3.7). A brachial formula such as 4.13.2 indicates that the fourth pair of arms (or ventral) to the right of the animal's body is longer than the second (or dorso-lateral), and this one longer than the first (or dorsal), which is longer than the third. The numbers of the brachial formula can be Arabic or Roman (Figs. 3.6 and 3.7). This formula has taxonomic value, especially the Octopodiformes (Jereb and Roper 2005, 2010 and Jereb et al. 2016 catalogues provide illustrated glossaries of technical terms and measurements).

The arms of Sepioidea, Myopsida, and Oegopsida are attached to the outer lip by a buccal membrane that has six, seven, or eight folds. These folds are attached to the dorsal and ventral margins of the arms through the buccal connectives. The arrangement of such bonds has taxonomic value and is also expressed by a formula. Thus, a DDVV formula indicates that the buccal connectives are attached to the dorsal margin of the first two pairs of arms and to the ventral of the following two pairs. *Vampyroteuthis* and all Octopodiformes lack buccal connectives.

The cross section of the arms of Sepioidea, Myopsida, and Oegopsida is generally triangular. The inner surface (oral) is flattened, while the outer (aboral) surface is angular. The suckers are arranged on the oral surface, usually in two rows, although there may be more. Suckers are provided with denticulate or smooth chitinous rings. Arm suckers have been converted into hooks in some oceanic species of Oegopsida (e.g. *Taningia danae*). Along the lateral angle of the oral surface of the arms, there are web-like integument protective membranes, generally supported by muscular rods called trabeculae. These protective membranes are well developed in some species. Thus, for example, in *Histioteuthis* species join two pairs or more arms, while in some Ommastrephidae (e.g. *Ommastrephes bartramii*), the ventral protective membranes of arm III are very wide and in adult females expand into a large, triangular, membranous lobe.

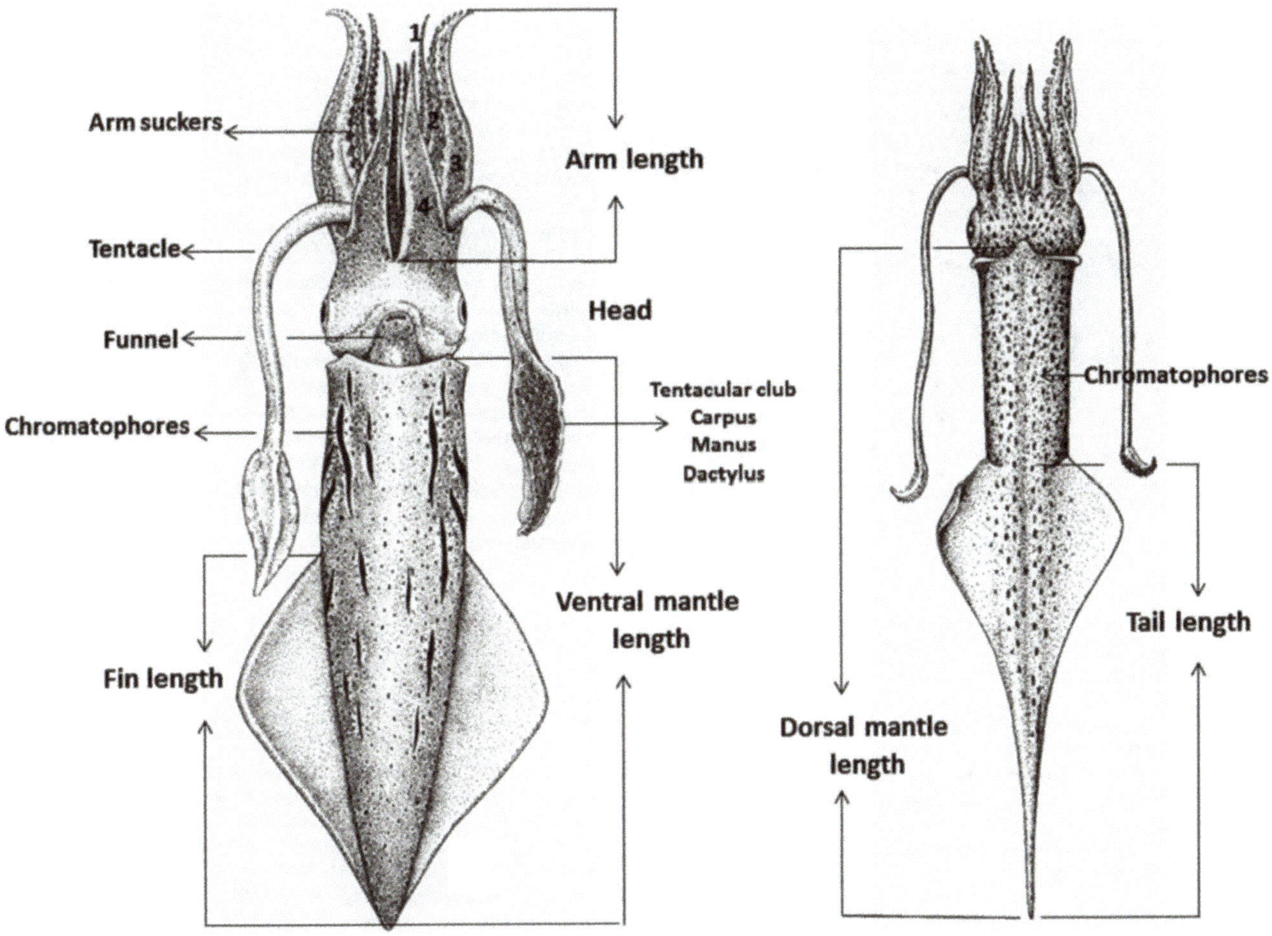

Fig. 3.6 Nomenclature of diverse parts of the body of Loliginidae and points between which the body measurements should be taken (Drawings from Guerra 1992)

The so-called swimming keels are flattened and muscular expansions located on the aboral side of some arms to render them more hydrodynamic.

Vampyroteuthis and Octopodiformes cross section of the arms is, generally, circular. All arm suckers of Octopodiformes lack of chitinous rings. In certain cases, as in the males of some species of Octopoda Incirrata, there are several modified suckers, generally larger than the others, which play a role in courtship. Both Vampyromorpha and Octopoda Cirrata have elongate, fleshy, finger-like papillae (cirri) along the lateral edges of the oral surface of the arms, which length is variable. Cirri are mechanoreceptors. A membranous sheet of greater or lesser extent can be present between the arms of many Octopodiformes (Fig. 3.7a); this web gives an umbrella-like appearance when the arms are spread out.

One (or more) arm in male cephalopods is modified to be used transferring spermatophores to the female. This arm (s) is called hectocotilized arm and the modified portion hectocotylus. Modifications may involve suckers, sucker stalks, protective membranes, trabeculae, and a section of the arm. The last occurs in the distal tip of the Cirrata and Incirrata Octopodiformes. In these cases, along the hectocotilized arm, there is a spermatophore groove, which end open into a structure formed by the ligula and the calamus (Fig. 3.7b). The ligula is a spatulate or spoon-shaped, terminal structure of the hectocotylus, which usually contains a series of transverse ridges and grooves on the oral surface. The calamus is a conical papilla or projection of the base of the ligula at the distal terminus of the sperm groove, distal to the last sucker.

The tentacles are two long appendages in Decapodiformes, used for prey capture and capable of considerable extension and contraction. The tentacles can be retracted into open depression or pockets located in the antero-ventral surface of the head between the bases of the ventro-lateral (3) and ventral pair of arms (4) in all Sepioidea species, but not in Myopsid and Oegopsid squids. A tentacle is composed by a peduncle, the carpus or fixing apparatus, and the tentacular club, which is an expansion of the distal part

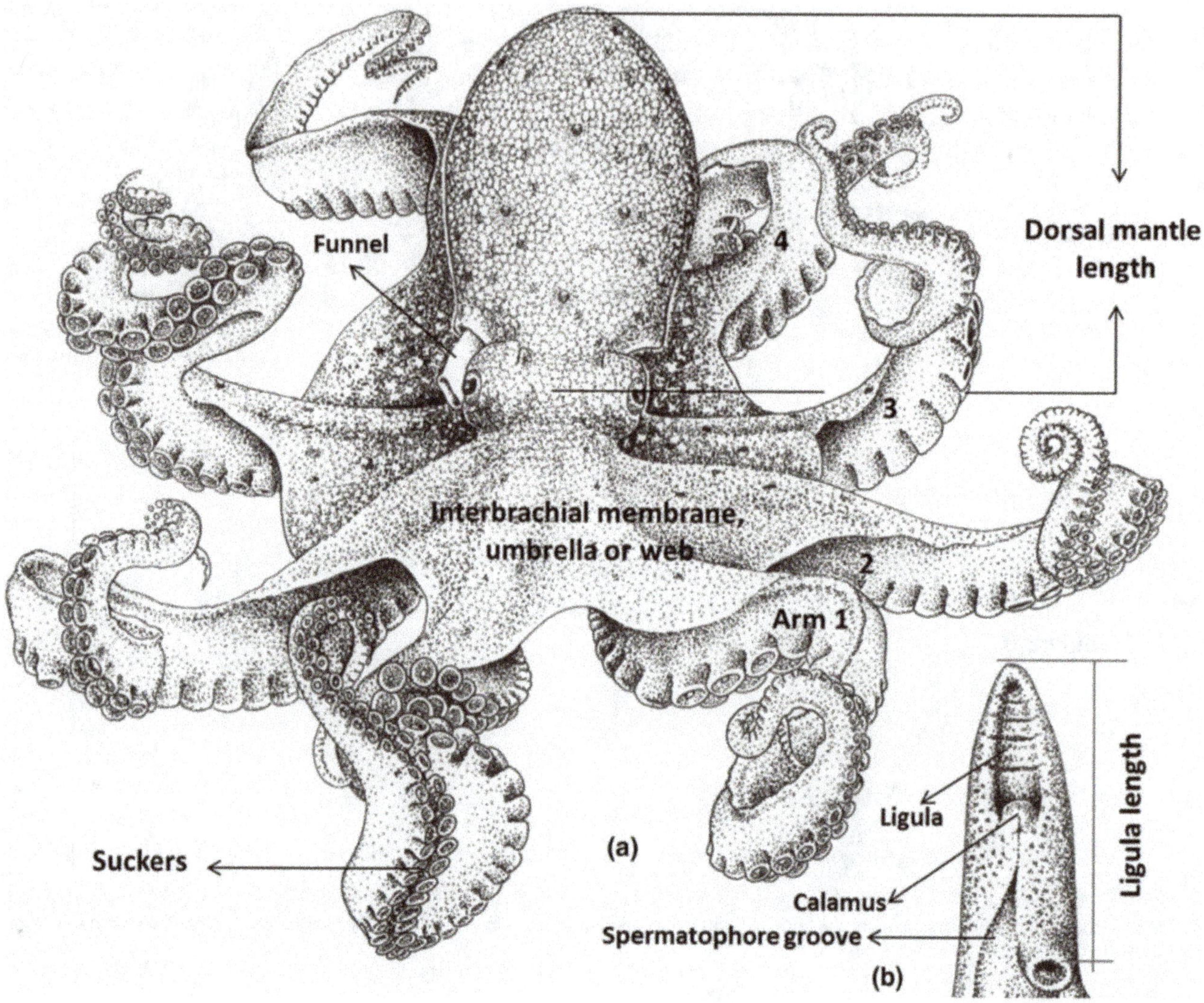

Fig. 3.7 Main measurements and terms in Octopoda Incirrata. **a** Body; **b** hectocotilized arm. (Drawings from Guerra 1992)

(Fig. 1.6). The central or "hand" portion of the club may have suckers and/or hooks. The distal, terminal section of the club, often characterized by suckers of reduced size is the dactylus.

The ventral, subconical tube through which the water is expelled from the mantle cavity during locomotion and respiration, and that also serve to expelled ink, reproductive and waste products, is the funnel. In Sepioidea, Myopsida, and Oegopsida, the funnel is located within a depression in the posterior-ventral surface of the head called funnel groove. However, in Octopodiformes, it is embedded in the tissues of the head, leaving only the apical region free. The funnel groove of Oegopsid squids has a series of structures with taxonomic value. Thus, in some genera (e.g. *Todorodes, Illex*), there are transverse, membranous folds of skin that form a pocket in the anterior end of the funnel groove, called foveola. Other genera, like Ommastrephes, have also small shallow pockets lateral to foveola in the funnel groove. The muscles that support the lateral attachment of the funnel to the head, called funnel-adductor muscle, are generally well developed. In many groups of cephalopods, within the funnel, there is a semilunar muscular flap in the dorsal surface near the distal opening of the funnel—the funnel valve—and also a glandular structure—the funnel organ -, which adopts different forms; the configuration of the funnel organ has taxonomic importance, especially in Cranchiidae and Octopodidae.

The lower lateral margins of the funnel may be fused to the mantle (e.g. Cranchiidae) or be connected to it by a cartilage: the funnel-locking cartilage. The cartilage portion found in the funnel of Sepioidea, Myopsida, and Oegopsida presents a varied morphology, and it is also a character of taxonomic importance. There is also a funnel-locking cartilage in the Argonautoidea superfamily, but the rest of the Octopodiformes lack this structure. The cartilaginous ridge, knob, or swelling on each side of the ventro-lateral, internal surface of mantle that locks into the funnel component is called mantle-locking cartilage. Both structures funnel and mantle-locking cartilages form the locking apparatus which is essential for locomotion.

The mantle of cephalopods is basically a muscular sac. The dorsal part of the mantle cavity is small, while the ventral part is larger and lodges the viscera. Cephalopod muscles are arranged in three dimensions in closely packed blocks, which allow rapid and abrupt contractions. The contraction and relaxation of the different types of muscle fibres of the mantle allow the expulsion and entry of water into the mantle cavity. The best-known peripheral nervous system is that of the giant axons, which in three steps from the magnocellular lobe and the paleovisceral lobe of the brain innervate the mantle musculature. These axons have a diameter between 0.5 and 1 mm (thousand times greater than the axons of mammals). Its reaction potential is so high that the nerve transmission runs at high speed, allowing the extremely rapid, complete, and instantaneous reaction of the pallial musculature to give rise to the incomparable hydrodynamic invention of the jet propulsion.

The mantle musculature in some Oegopsida (e.g. Cranchiidae) and pelagic octopuses (e.g. *Japetella diaphana,* Fig. 3.4) has been reduced and has a high water content. Many of these species have gelatinous consistency, medusoid aspect, and the walls of the mantle are translucent so that they allow the internal organs to be seen.

The members of the family Lepidoteuthidae have a distinct dermal cushions present on the mantle. These dermal cushions, which are thickening of the skin with abundant vacuoles and connective tissue, are relatively large, diamond, or hexagonal-shaped structures that cover the whole circumference of the mantle and in overlapping arrangement.

Most cephalopods have a pair of fins of varying shapes and sizes. They are located in the back of the mantle in the Myopsida and Oegopsida (Figs. 3.3 and 3.6), in its middle zone in the Octopoda Cirrata (Fig. 3.4) or in its lateral borders in Sepioidea (Fig. 3.2). Octopoda Incirata has no fins. This pair of muscular flaps is used for locomotion, steering and stabilization.

The mantle of many Myopsida and Oegopsida has a posterior narrow extension or tail, in which length may be very long (Fig. 3.3). The end of the fins and the beginning of the tail often overlap. This posterior extension of the body is often very long in paralarval stages. Some species (e.g. *Alloteuthis subulata* or *A. africana*) show a lengthening of the tail as the males mature sexually and constitute a secondary sexual character.

3.4.1.3 Integumental System: The Skin and Elements Contributing to Colour and Body Patterns

The epidermis contains three main kinds of cells: epithelial columnar cells, gland cells, and sensory cells. Immediately bellow the epidermis, there is a layer (dermis) that possesses a series of sacs with pigment—the chromatophores, which are typically only red, yellow, or brown and determine colour changes in camouflage (Fig. 3.8). Other colours are attainable by using a second layer of structures in the cephalopod skin called iridophores and leucophores, which are located in the dermis. Iridophores are stacks of very thin cells that are capable of reflecting light back at different wavelengths and possibly different polarities. Cuttlefish and octopuses possess an additional type of reflector cells called leucophores. They are cells that scatter full spectrum light so that they appear white. By combining reflection from the iridophores and leucophores with the correct patterning of chromatophores, the cephalopod can create a very convincing copy of the surrounding conditions. The rest of the dermis consists of an outer tunic with collagen fibres, the musculature, a layer with nerve fibres and blood vessels, and, finally, an inner tunic. In Sepioidea and Incirrata Octopodiformes, there is a complex musculature that changes their skin from smooth and flat to rugose and three-dimensional. The organs responsible for this physical change are the skin papillae. Skin texture is an important contribution to body pattering. The photophores, which are bioluminescence cells, are also located in the skin and in different regions of the body, for instance, around the eyes, in the ventral part of the mantle, arms, tentacles, and even inside the mantle cavity over the ink sac.

3.4.2 Functional Anatomy

3.4.2.1 The Shell

At present, the only representatives of this class of the phylum Mollusca with external shell are *Nautilus and Allonautilus*. The shell of these cephalopods is divided into chambers bounded by transverse septa, the latter occupying the animal. Through the septa, there is a tissue cord tube-like form or siphuncle, which intervenes in the control of the buoyancy of the animal, regulating the relative volume of gases and liquids present in the chambers of the shell.

The rest of the cephalopods present an internal shell, as it occurs in cuttlefish, squids, or it is totally vestigial, or it does not exist as such (Incirrata). *Spirula* has a flattened spiral

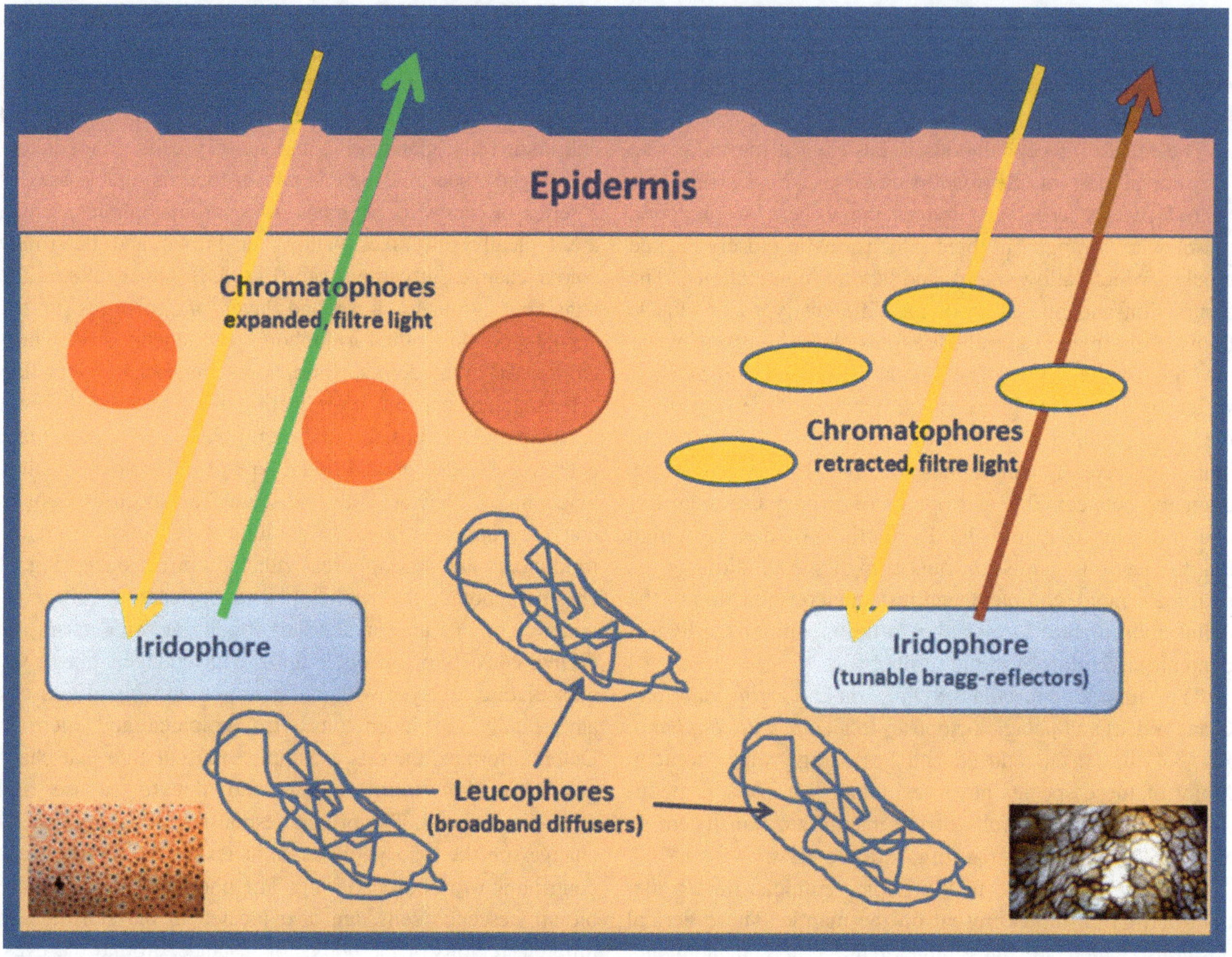

Fig. 3.8 Diagram showing the elements that contribute to colour body patterns and their arrangement in the skin

internal shell that does not intervene in the protection of the animal, although it contributes to maintaining the body shape and acts as a hydrostatic skeleton. The cuttlebone of the cuttlefishes (*Sepia* spp) is an intricate structure composed of a dorsal shield and ventrally placed chamber complex. It is composed of calcium carbonate in its aragonite polymorph mixed with a small amount of organic matter, a complex of β-chitin and protein. In ventral plan view, the chamber complex consists of the posterior siphuncular zone, which is characterized by a series of striae corresponding each to the posterior end of one chamber, and the septum of the last-formed chamber. In dorso-ventral vertical section, each chamber is composed of a complex arrangement of horizontal septa and membranes and vertical pillars and membranes, intervening in the control of the buoyancy of the animal by regulating the amount of gas and liquid present in such chambers.

In the Myopsida and Oegopsida squids, the shell, also called gladius or pen, is reduced to a chitinous sheet with a central axis and two lateral expansions; the pen contributes to maintain the rigidity of the body in longitudinal sense during the convulsive contraction phase of jet swimming, but it has lost its protective function. A number of pelagic from achieve neutral buoyancy by a reduction of the protein content of their tissues and the accumulation of a low-density solution of ammonium chloride either the coelomic space (e.g. Cranchiidae) or in the vacuoles within the musculature and connective tissue (e.g. *Architeuthis dux*).

Cirrate octopuses possess a well-developed internal shell that supports their muscular swimming fins. This is in contrast to the more familiar, finless, incirrate octopuses, in which the shell remnant is either present as a pair of stylets or absent altogether.

3.4.2.2 Respiratory and Circulatory Systems

Respiratory exchange with the environment occurs through well-vascularized gills suspended in the mantle cavity. *Nautilus and Allonautilus* species have two pairs of gills, but in all Coleoidea there is only a single pair (Fig. 3.9). Due to the particular orientation of the gills within the mantle

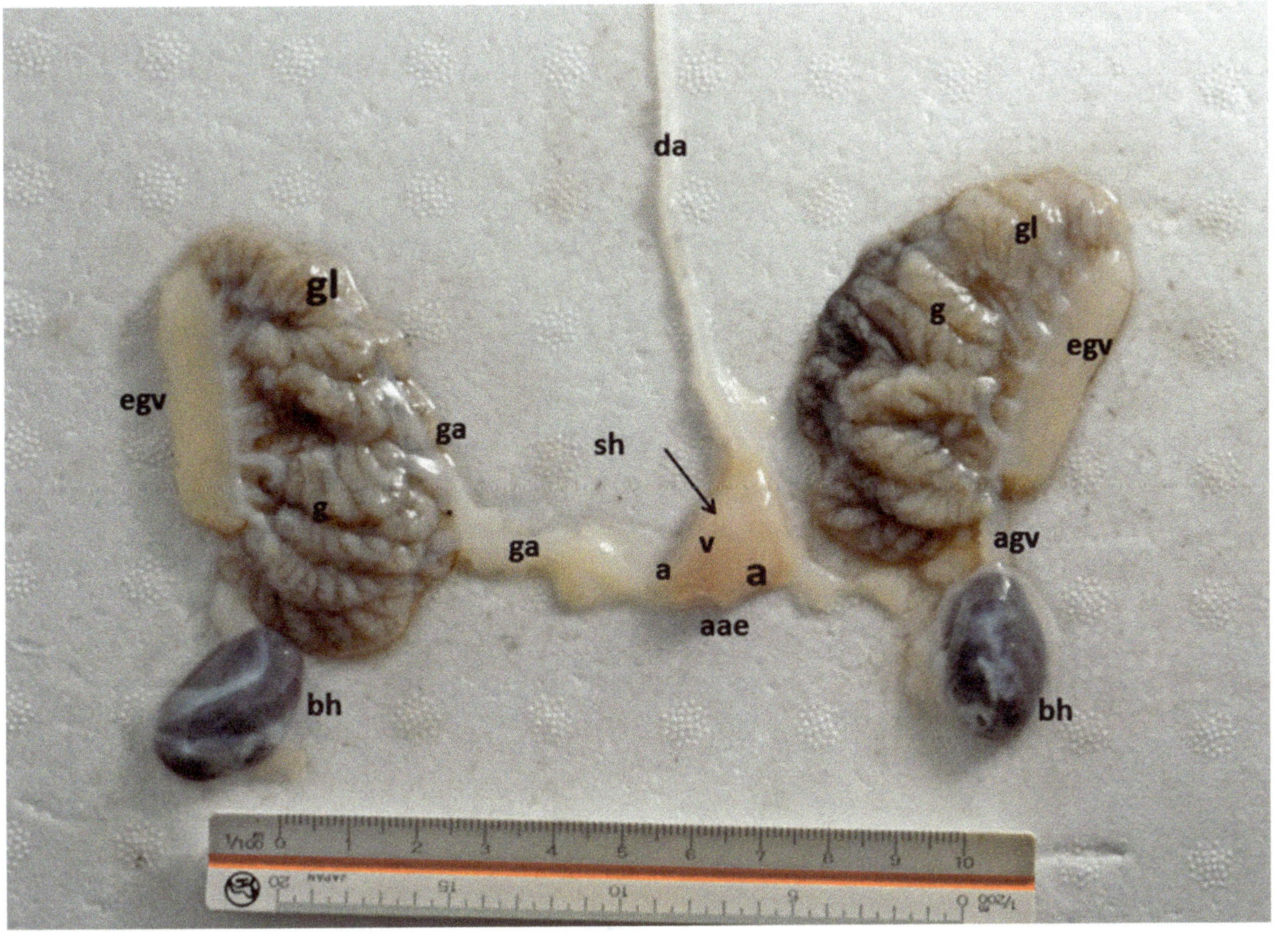

Fig. 3.9 Respiratory and circulatory system of *Octopus vulgaris* (partial); a: auricle; aae: abdominal aorta exit; agv: afferent gill vessel; bh: branchial or gill heart; da: dorsal aorta; agv; efferent gill vessel; g: gill or branchia; gl: gill lamellae; sh: systemic heart; v: ventricle

cavity, water flows between the lamellae of each gill in the opposite direction of the flow of blood through the tissue. This originates a countercurrent system that maximizes the exchange of gas.

Unlike all other molluscs, cephalopods have a closed circulatory system. This means that blood flows through a series of vessels to return to the heart, rather than bathing organs in the blood fluid as in open circulatory systems.

The core of the cephalopod circulatory system is a series of three beating hearts. This trio of hearts connects to a high pressure system of veins, arteries, and capillaries—unique among all molluscs. Two of the hearts are branchial hearts (Fig. 3.9), which pump blood through the gills for respiration and gas exchange. The third heart is a systemic heart (Fig. 3.9), receiving the blood that drains from the gills and pumping that oxygenated blood to the body system. Each of the three hearts is innervated by a variety of nerves, though it appears that the cardiac ganglion—a cluster of nerves—acts as the controlling pacemaker of the hearts. The two branchial hearts beat simultaneously, followed by the contraction of the systemic heart to supply the body with blood. Blood drains to the branchial hearts by the major veins, known as the anterior and lateral vena cava or vena cava cephalica.

The vessels within the gills are known as afferent branchial vessels, which drain back to the main ventricle of the systemic heart. Blood is then pumped from the systemic heart to the body via the main cephalic artery.

Oxygenate cephalopod blood is a blue colour due to the presence of copper-containing respiratory pigment haemocyanin in solution in the blood, because cephalopods lack of erythrocytes. The oxygen carrying capacity of the haemocyanin is less efficient that the vertebrate haemoglobin. Cephalopods exhibit the highest rates of aerobic metabolism among the marine invertebrates. However, it is very variable, depending of some environmental factors such as water temperature, but also on the performance of their haemocyanins (Pörtner et al. 1994). Accordingly with oxygen affinity, cephalopods can be divided into three groups: octopuses and some sluggish squids, with relatively low oxygen capacity; fast-swimming squids; and *Sepia* species.

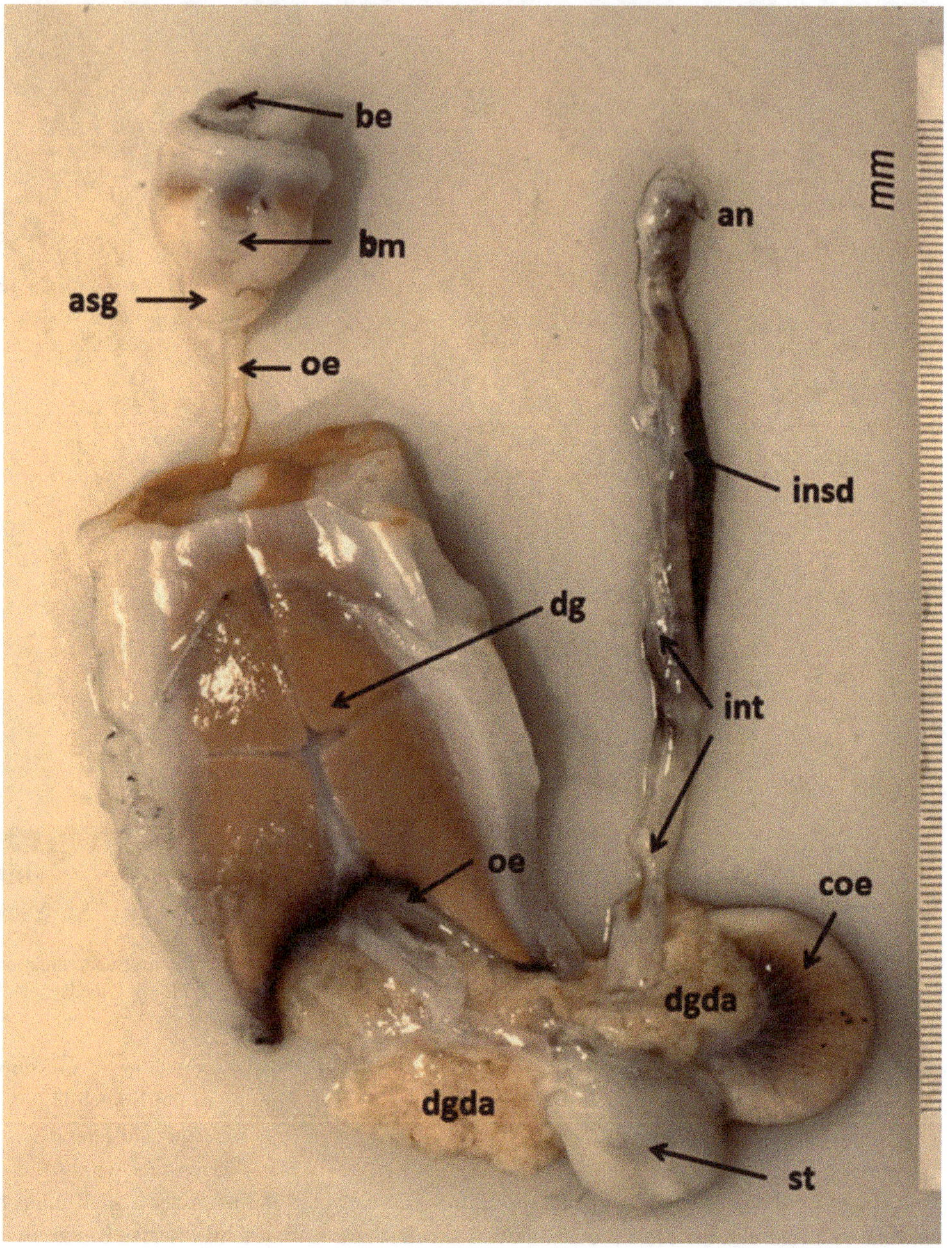

Fig. 3.10 *Sepia officinalis* digestive system; an: anus; asg: anterior salivary glands; be: beak or mandibles; bm: buccal mass; cae: caecum; dg: digestive gland (bilobulate); dgda: digestive gland duct appendages; int: intestine; insd: Ink sac duct; oe: oesophagus; st: stomach

3.4.2.3 Digestive System

The digestive system of the cephalopods (Figs. 3.10, 3.11 and 3.12) opens in the mouth. Located at the base of the arms and tentacles (circumoral appendages), the mouth is the opening of the buccal mass, which contains the beaks, radula, various glands, and the pharynx. Surrounding the mouth, the inner and outer lips possess numerous ridges or papillae. The beaks are two chitinous mandibles bound in powerful muscles. The dorsal beak is referred as "upper" beak, and it inserts within the "lower" beak to tear tissue with a scissors-like cutting action. A pair of glands of the digestive system is associated with the buccal mass, the sublingual and the anterior salivary glands. The function of these glands is poorly known but thought to be primarily in mucous production. The radula, which is a chitinous and ribbon-like band, is placed on the floor of the oral cavity; it contributes to scraping the food in order to fragment it into smaller pieces. The radula can be of various types and its structure varies depending on the group. Many *Octopus* species are able drilling shells of crustaceans and shells of other mollusks. These drilling activities are carried out by a salivary papilla that lies just below the radula. The papilla is muscular, and its anterior face is covered with very small teeth. It is now possible to say that the salivary papilla can function as an accessory radula. Some cephalopod species (e.g. *Spirula spirula*) lack of radula. Some cephalopods,

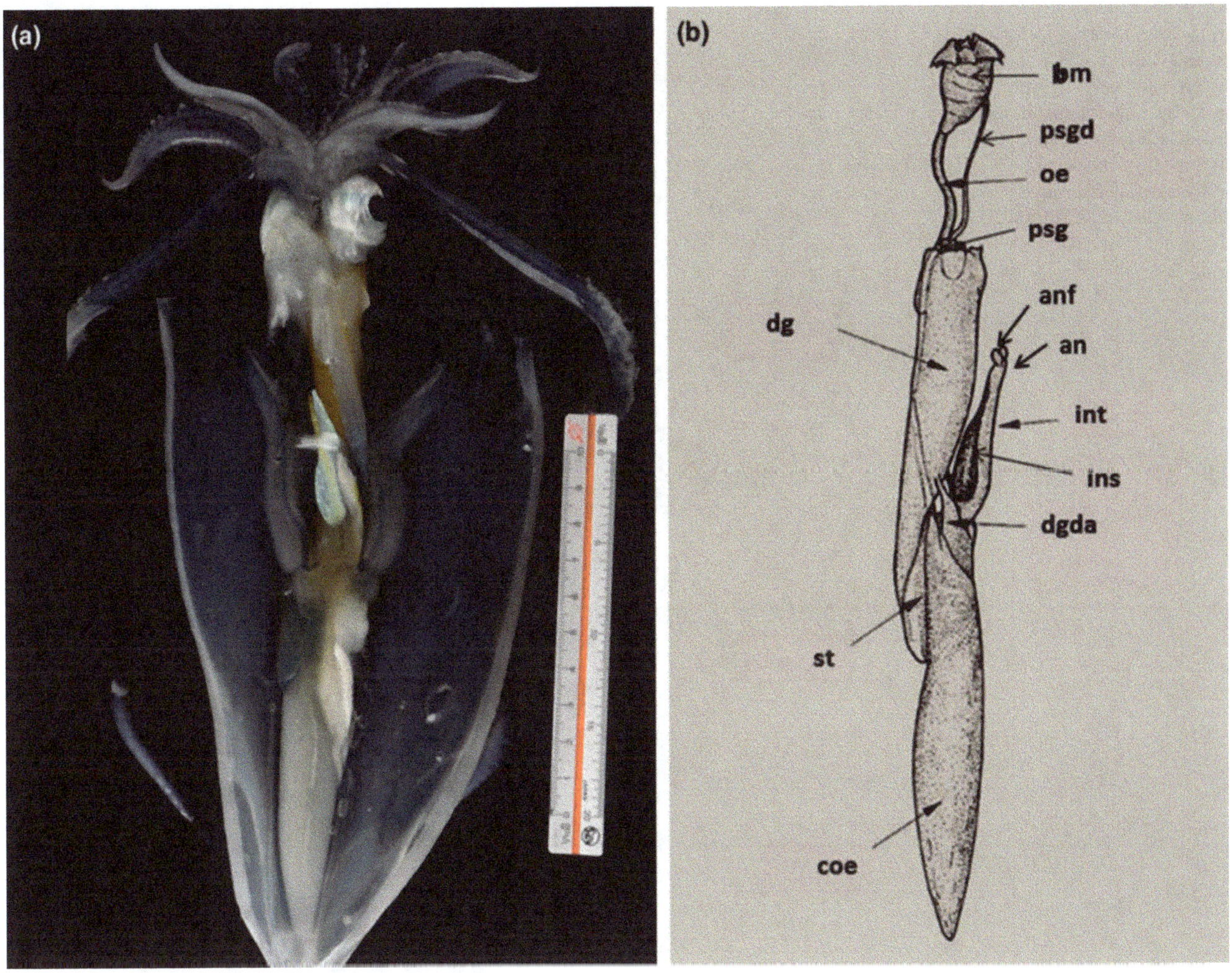

Fig. 3.11 *Loligo vulgaris* digestive system; **a** female cut from the ventral side of the mantle: **b** diagram showing the main parts of the digestive system; an: anus; anf: anal flaps; bm: buccal mass; cae: caecum; dg: digestive gland; dgda: digestive gland duct appendages; int: intestine; ins: ink sac; insd: Ink sac duct; oe: oesophagus; psg: posterior salivary glands; psgd: posterior salivary gland duct; st: stomach

such as *Sepia*, *Octopus*, inject neurotoxins into their prey in order to immobilize them and facilitate their ingestion; these are secreted by the posterior salivary glands. The blue-ringed octopus of the Pacific, *Hapalochlaena maculosa*, produces toxins that can be deadly to man.

The portion of the digestive tract between the buccal mass and the stomach is the oesophagus. The lumen of the oesophagus is narrow and slightly dilatable, which is because it passes through the brain and cranial cartilage. This is why cephalopods may chop their prey into small pieces with their beaks and then force the pieces down the throat with the radula. Often, a portion of the oesophagus is enlarged to form a crop. This expansion or diverticulum of the oesophagus serves for storing food. It is present in *Nautilus* and most Octopodiformes. When there is no crop (Fig. 3.12), the oesophagus opens in the stomach. The stomach is a cavity generally lined with cuticular ridges to grind-up food with the aid of digestive enzymes. The stomach may be greatly expandable in size and serve as a storage area, in species lacking a crop, until food can be fully processed. The caecum is a major organ of this system that is a primary site of absorption. It joins the stomach "upstream" and the intestine "downstream". Present in some Decapodiformes, the caecal sac is a thin-walled posterior portion of the caecum that lacks the internal, ciliated leaflets characteristic of the anterior portion of the caecum (Fig. 3.11b).

The digestive enzymes enter the caecum in the ducts from the digestive gland (Fig. 3.12), which is the primary organ in cephalopods that secretes digestive enzymes. The ducts leading from the digestive gland have outpockets, which are covered with glandular epithelium, and they are called digestive gland duct appendages. Digestive gland is also important in absorption, excretion, and detoxification of heavy metal accumulations.

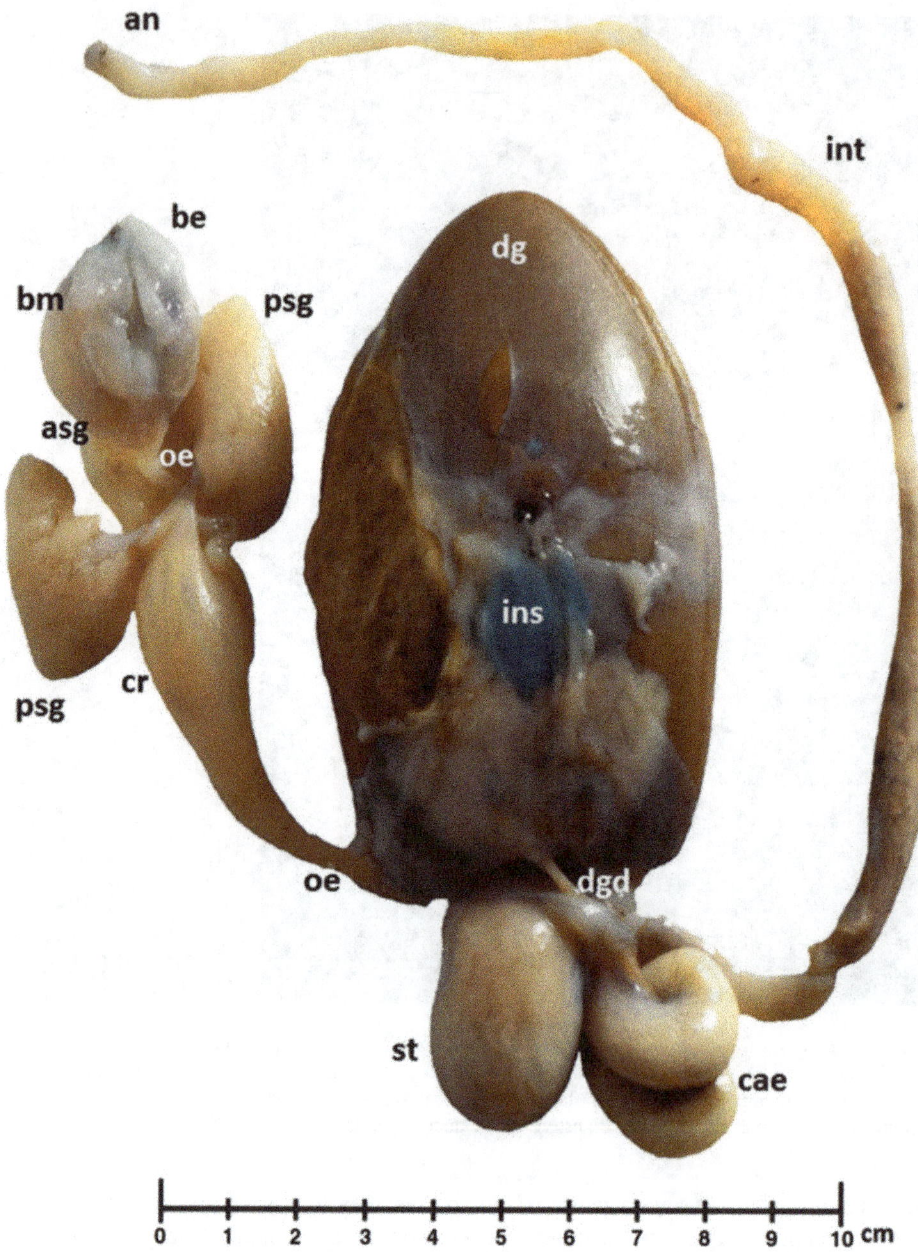

Fig. 3.12 *Octopus vulgaris* digestive system; an: anus; asg: anterior salivary glands; bm: buccal mass; cae: caecum; cr: crop; dg: digestive gland; dgd: digestive gland duct; int: intestine; ins: ink sac; oe: oesophagus; psg: posterior salivary glands; st: stomach

After the caecum begins the intestine, which opens into the anus, situated in the anterior ventral part of the mantle cavity, near the funnel. As a whole, the cephalopod digestive tract has a U-shape. A pair of muscular palps that arise at the sides of the anus in most Coleoidea are called anal flaps (Fig. 3.11).

A notable anatomical feature of the digestive tract of cephalopods is the ink sac. With the exception of nocturnal and very deep-water cephalopods, all Coleoidea which dwell in light conditions have an ink sac. The ink sac is a muscular bag which originated as an extension of the hind gut (Fig. 3.11b). It lies beneath the gut and opens into the anus, into which its contents—almost pure melanin—can be squirted; its proximity to the base of the funnel means that the ink can be distributed by ejected water as the cephalopod uses its jet propulsion. The ejected cloud of melanin forms a lump approximately the size and shape of the cephalopod, fixing the predator's attention while the cephalopod itself makes a hasty escape.

All cephalopods actively catch and eat live prey, and a very range of prey item has been recorded. The diet is probably determined as much by prey availability as predator preference. Hunting is essentially visual; however, chemical cues also probably have a role. Feeding strategies are very different. Once trapped, generally using tentacles or arms, the prey is drawn in towards the mouth which is generally paralysed by the saliva of the posterior salivary glands and bitten into the beaks. As above commented, bite-sized of flesh are shallowed. Nevertheless, hard pieces of their prey are also found in the stomach contents, which can be used for preliminary prey's identification. However, to identify prey in cephalopod stomach contents the most accurate is to use molecular techniques. It is well known that cephalopods have high requirements for protein and relatively low requirements for high-quality lipids: the cephalopod diet must consist of over 60% protein and 4% lipids.

After ingestion, the already fragmented meal enters in digestive tract. The characteristic fast growth rate of cephalopods (3–10% body weight d^{-1}) sets high requirements for digestion and assimilation. The digestion is a complex process. It starts externally at the prey, where salivary enzymes are injected after perforation by the beaks or salivary papilla. Although the exact biochemical mechanisms in different species are not fully known, it is considered that pre-digestion is probably limited to loosening muscle attachments. Partially digested food is then ingested and enters the crop, in octopus, or goes to the stomach, in cuttlefish and squid, where digestive enzymes from the digestive gland initiate digestion. Enzyme-bound soluble nutrients pass from the crop to the stomach in octopus or directly to the stomach in cuttlefish and squid, where fibrillar proteins and other macromolecules are degraded until a semi-liquid mass of partly digested food (chyme) is formed. The chyme is then separated by the caecum to be transported to the digestive gland or to form faecal pellets. Once in the digestive gland, nutrients are dissolved and absorbed by pinocytosis in the digestive gland cells, where intracellular digestion occurs. This process can take from 4 to 8 h, depending on the size of the meal, animal, and temperature. The high rate of consumption leads to interesting speculations about the fuelling by cannibalism that is relatively frequent in many cephalopods, especially in the long migrations undertaken by many shoaling squid species.

3.4.2.4 Excretory System

Because protein is a major constituent of the cephalopod diet, large amounts of ammonia (NH_4^+) are produced as waste. This waste is excreted in solution by several routes. Excretion from the blood system takes place in a well-differentiated renal system surrounding the venous return to the systemic heart. Filtered nitrogenous waste (primary urine) is produced by ultrafiltration from the blood in the pericardial cavity of the branchial hearts, each of which is connected by a narrow canal to the brachial heart appendages (Fig. 3.13). The canal delivers the excreta to a bladder-like renal sac and also resorbs excess water from the filtrate. Several outgrowths of the lateral vena cava (renal appendages) project into the renal sac, continuously inflating and deflating as the branchial hearts beat. This action helps

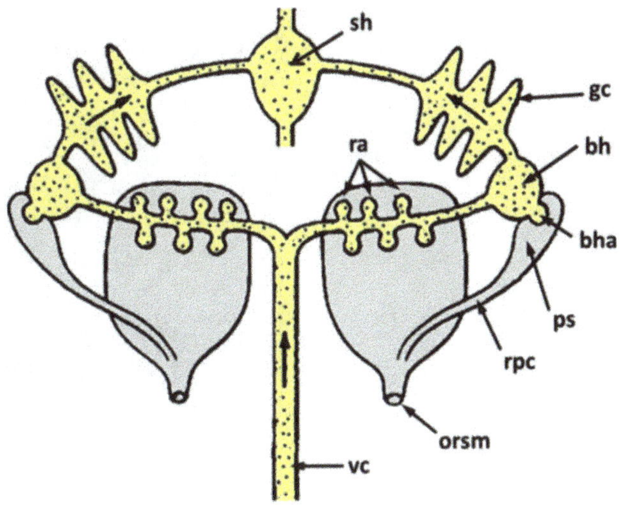

Fig. 3.13 Schematic representation of the excretory (renal) complex and associated circulatory system in *Octopus*. Arrows show the direction of the blood flux; bh: brachial heart; bha: brachial heart appendages; orsm: opening of renal sac to mantle cavity; ps: pericardical sac; ra: renal appendages; rpc: renopericardial sac; rs: renal sac; sh: systemic heart; vc: vena cava. Modified from Martin AW and Harrison FM. Excretion. In Wilbur and Yonge, C.M. (eds.) *Physiology of Mollusca*, Vol. II. Academic Press, New York, 1966

to pump the secreted waste into the sacs, to be released into the mantle cavity through a pore (the renal papilla). The main extra-renal organs involved in ammonia excretion are the gills. In this case, the waste is directly excreted from tits epithelium to the seawater. The rate of release is lowest in the shelled cephalopods *Nautilus* and *Sepia* as a result of their using nitrogen to fill their shells with gas to increase buoyancy. Other cephalopods use ammonium in a similar way, storing the ions (as ammonium chloride) to reduce their overall density and increase buoyancy. A remarkable feature of the renal system of cephalopods is its infestation by dicyemid mesozoans, which relationship with the host is apparently symbiotic.

3.4.2.5 Reproductive System and Reproduction

Sexes in cephalopods are separate. The reproductive system of the females consists of an ovary, which leads to one or two oviducts, the oviductal gland (single or paired), and the Decapodiformes of the nidamental and accessory nidamental glands (Figs. 3.14 and 3.15) The ovary is located at the back of the mantle cavity, and in it the oocytes are formed. The function of nidamental glands is to produce the outer coat for eggs. The accessory gland has many of the structural features of a secretory organ. The basic structural unit is a tubule composed of a single layer of epithelial cells containing ordered arrays of rough endoplasmic reticulum and a lumenal surface covered with microvilli, cilia, and structural specialization presumed to be involved in secretion. The lumen of each tubule is filled with a dense population of

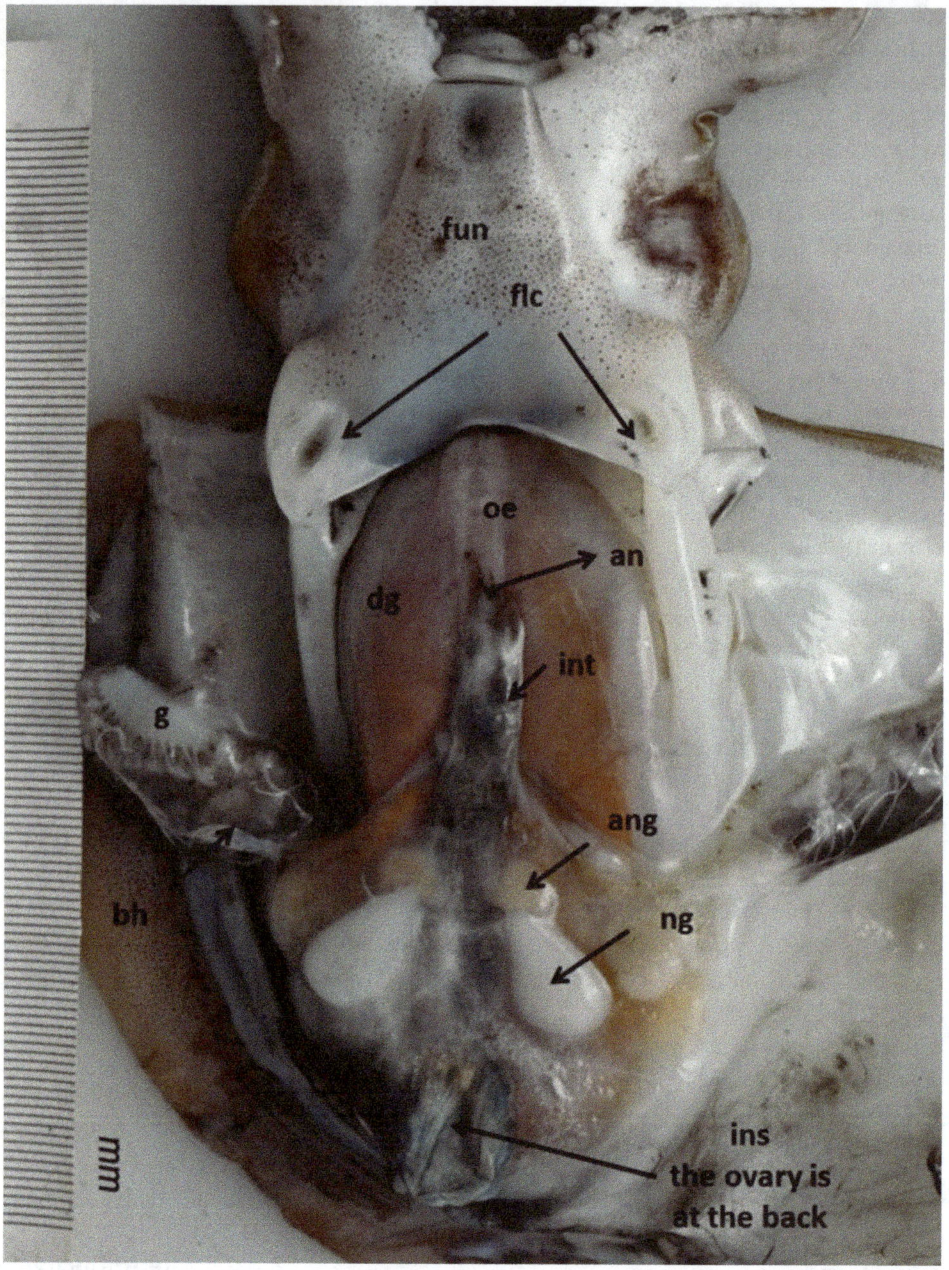

Fig. 3.14 *Sepia officinalis female reproductive* system; an: anus; ang: accessory nidamental glands; bh: branchial heart; fun: funnel; flc: funnel-locking cartilage apparatus; g: gill; ins: ink sac; int: intestine; ng: nidamental glands; oe: oesophagus

bacteria. During sexual maturation of the squid, the accessory gland changes in colour from white to mottled red (Fig. 3.15a). The accessory gland of the sexually mature squid has a mixture of red, white, and yellow tubules; in each case, the colour of the tubule is due to the bacterial population occupying the tubule. Since the red colour of the gland is due to the pigmentation of the bacteria, the bacteria must be responsive to the sexual state of the host, possible through a change in the nature of the material secreted into the tubule lumen.

Semen can be stored in different parts of the female's body: a sperm receptacle located on the buccal mass, a pouch under the eye, specialized structures found in the skin of some females Decapodiformes or as pockets of the oviducal glands seminal or spermatheca in *Octopus* species (Fig. 3.16b), a lateral split located in the anterior ventral part of the mantle, within the mantle, etc. The extruded, exploded, evaginated spermatophore/s often in form of round bulb is called spermatangium (pl. spermatangia).

In males, the spermatozoa produced by the testis are packed and surrounded by membranes, forming the spermatophore (Figs. 3.17b and 3.18b). Therefore, a spermatophore is a tubular structure manufactured by male for packaging sperm, capable of holding millions of spermatozoa. A spermatophore is composed by the sperm cord, the cement body, and the ejaculatory apparatus. It is transferred and attached to the

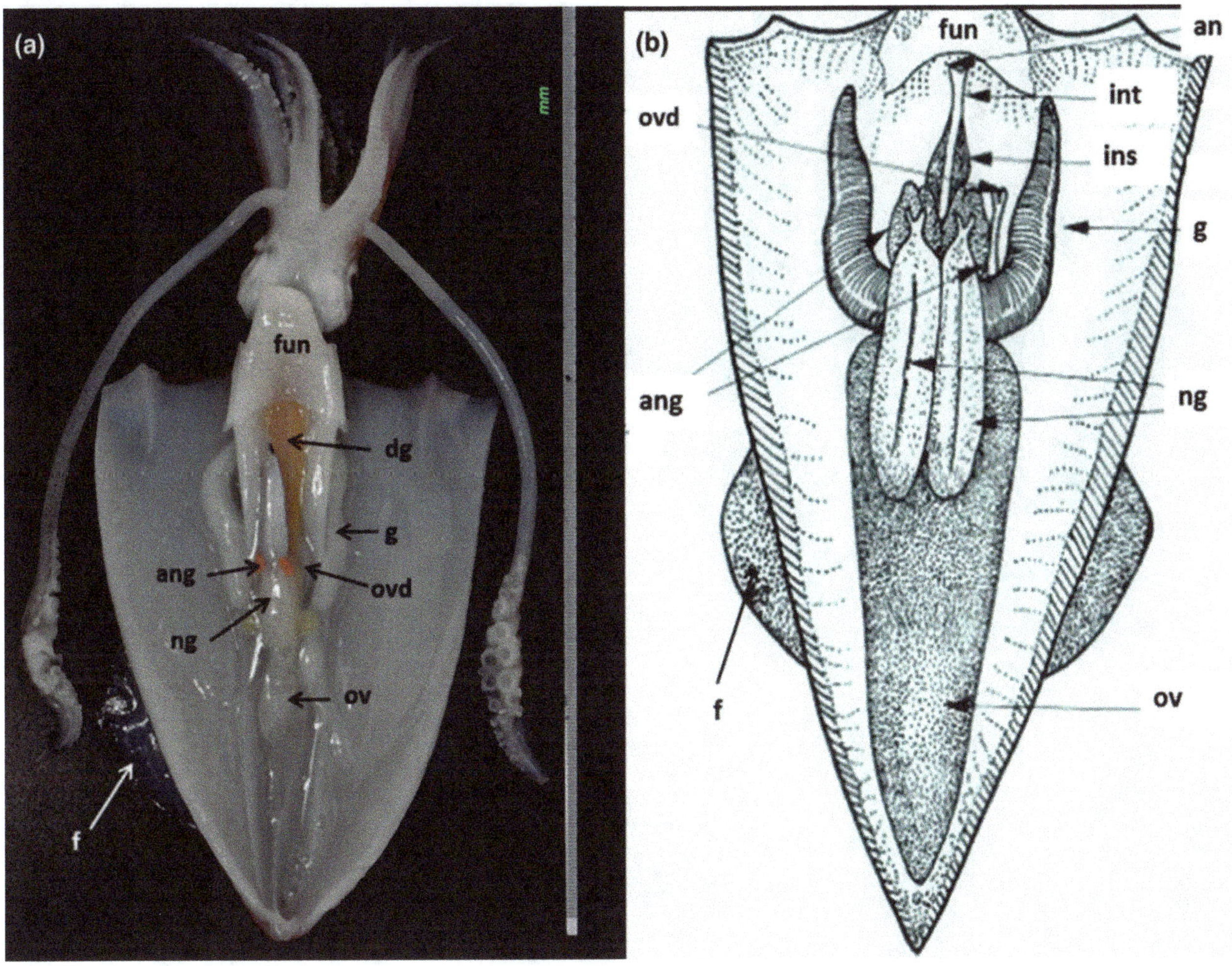

Fig. 3.15 *Loligo vulgaris* female reproductive system; **a** general view; **b** diagram showing main parts; an: anus; ang: accessory nidamental glands; bh: branchial heart; dg: digestive gland; f: fin; fun: funnel; in: intestine; ins: ink sac; g: gill; int: intestine; ng: nidamental glands; oe: oesophagus; ov: ovary; ovd: oviduct (single in Ommastrephidae, and other Oegopsida are in pair)

female after fertilization begins, and it forms the spermatangium after the spermatophoric reaction occurs and the spermatophore has everted. After the spermatozoa are formed, they pass to the spermatophoric organ through the vas deferens. The spermatophoric organ is composed by distinct structures different in Decapodiformes (Figs. 3.17 and 3.18) than in Octopodiformes (Fig. 3.18). In *Octopus* species, it is formed by the seminal vesicle and the prostate, which are the structures engaged in forming the spermatophore sheaths. Ripe spermatophores are stored in the spermatophoric sac or Needham's sac. This sac opens into de mantle cavity or directly into the water through the terminal organ, which by some authors incorrectly denominate penis. Although the terminal organ of some Oegopsida (e.g. *Architethis dux*) can be extremely long (up to 80% of mantle length), its functioning is not that of a true penis. This because spermatophore is transferred by the male generally using a modified arm called a hectocotylus. In some species of *Octopus*, the terminal organ widens into a diverticulum (Fig. 3.19b).

Sexual maturation is under the control of hormone(s) released from the small bodies called optic glands located on the optical tract, which connecting optic lobes to the brain. At the onset of sexual maturity, there is a rapid gonad growth, yolk formation in the ova, and ripening of nidamental and accessory glands. In most of the coastal and epipelagic species, reproduction is seasonal and afterwards both males and females die shortly after spawning or after a variable time taking care of the eggs during the embryonic development (e.g. *Octopus vulgaris*). The causes of the senescence and universal mortality that become after reproductive events are not still understood, although they seem to be related with physical changes in the optic gland and its secretions. Nevertheless, variations of this pattern of monocyclic reproduction and short lifespan are found or suspected in deep-water benthic octopuses and a range of other species.

Cephalopod mating usually includes a courtship that often involves elaborate colour and body pattern changes. Most females then lay large yolky eggs in clusters on the

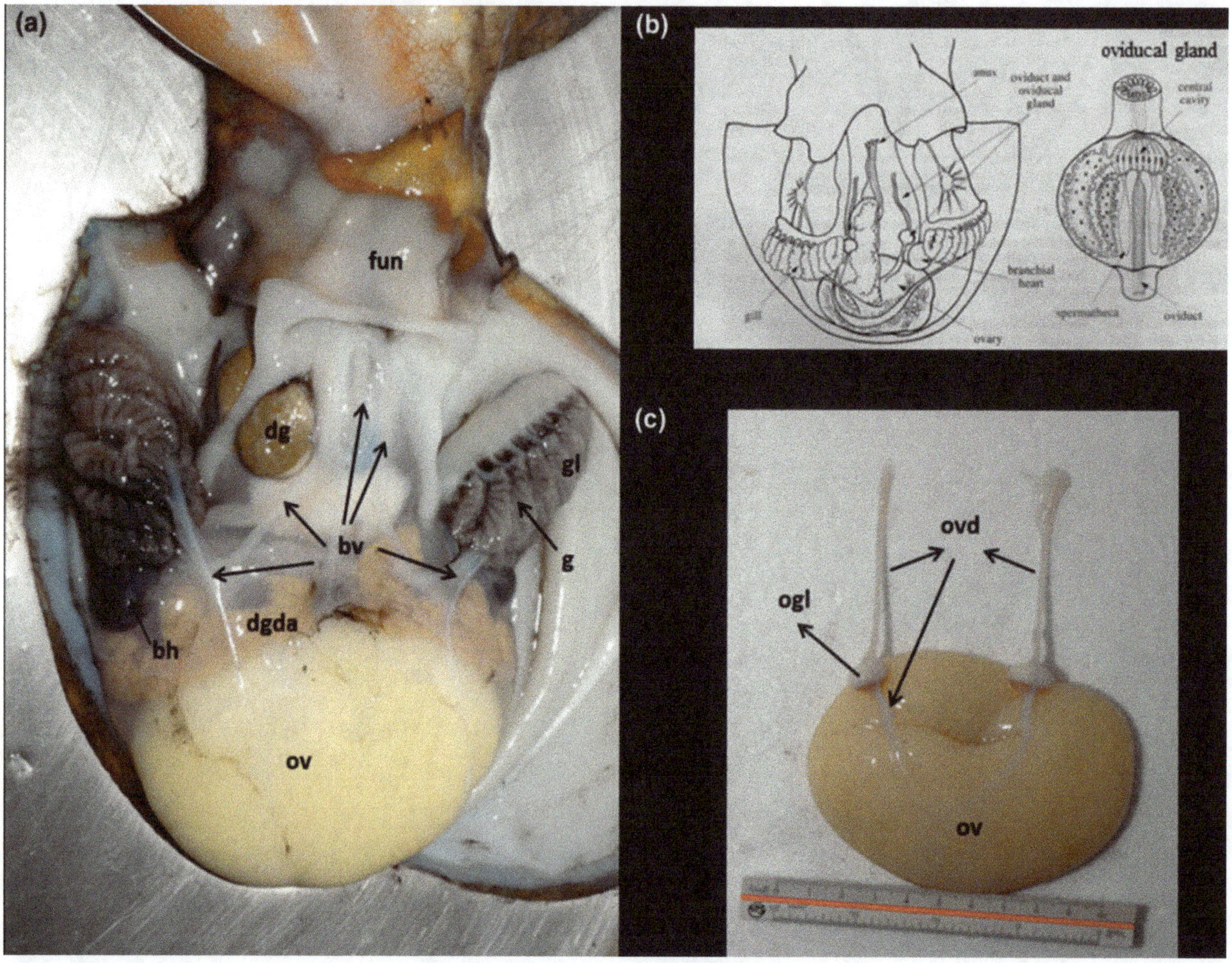

Fig. 3.16 *Octopus vulgaris* female reproductive system; **a** general view; **b** diagram showing main parts and a section of the oviducal glands; **c** main parts; bh: branchial heart; bv: blood vessels; fun: funnel; dg: digestive gland; g: gill; gl: gill lamellae; ov: ovary; ovd: oviducts; ogl: oviducal gland

ocean floor or on any other hard substrate. However, other (e.g. Ommastrephidae and Thysanoteuthidae) spawn neutrally buoyant egg masses that retain a specific location in the water column by floating at the interface between water layers of slightly different densities. Eggs develop by dividing unequally instead of in the spiral pattern of other molluscs. It is thought this is a derived mode of development. After a period of development within the egg, juveniles hatch out directly without the swimming larval stage common to many other molluscs.

3.4.2.6 Sensory Systems

Cephalopods (excluding *Nautilus*) are predatory, agile, swift-moving and, except few exceptions, highly visual animals that can see well under highly varying light conditions. Nevertheless, cephalopod sensory systems cover a wider range of possibilities than vision. The studies of a few nearshore species have revealed complex behaviour and remarkable capacity for learning. The kind of information collected by these sense organs, the nature of its effectors or motor apparatus, and the organization of the brain are the main factors on which its behaviour depends (Hanlon and Messenger 1996). In the previous sections, the main effectors or body organs that carry out, or "effect", the responses an animal makes to a stimulus (e.g. arms, tentacles, suckers, fins, chromatophores organs, reflecting cells, photophores, and ink sac) were show. In this section, information about the sense organs is given. The following one will deal with the organization of the brain and the peripheral nervous system, which in these organisms is very important. Table 3.1 summarizes main information on the sense organs of these peculiar marine molluscs.

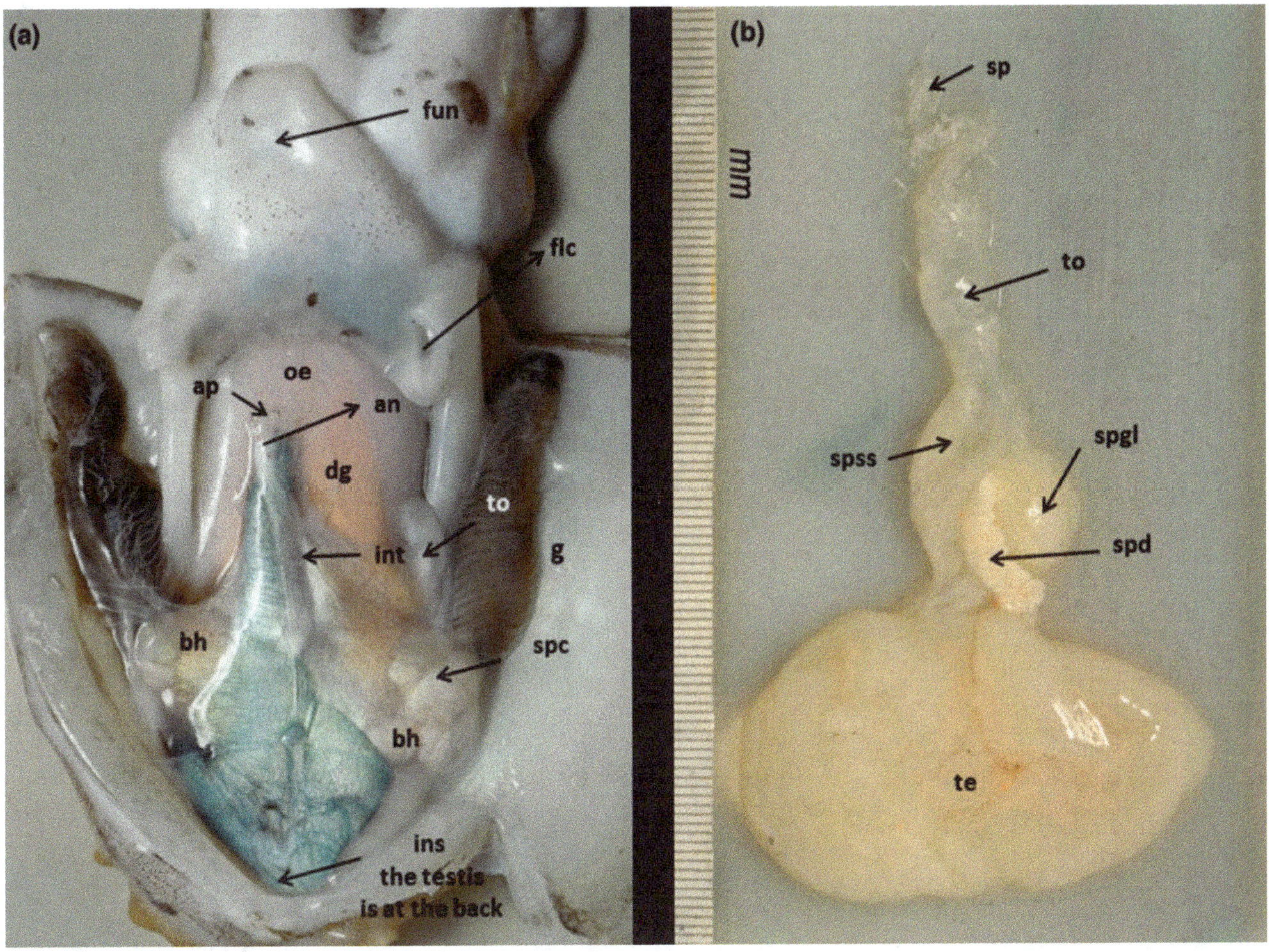

Fig. 3.17 *Sepia officinalis* male reproductive system; **a** general view; **b** main parts; an: anus; anf: anal flaps; bh: branchial heart; fun: funnel; flc: funnel-locking cartilage apparatus; g: gill; ins: ink sac; int: intestine; oe: oesophagus; sp: spermatophores; spgl: spermatophoric gland; spss: spermatophoric sac or Needham's sac; te: testis; to: terminal organ ("penis")

3.4.2.7 Nervous System

The cephalopod nervous system is divided into a central and a peripheral part. The central part includes the brain proper and the optic lobes; the large peripheral part includes the nervous system of the body and of the arms.

The brain is protected by a cartilaginous skull or cephalic cartilage. It is arranged around the oesophagus. There is a supra-oesophageal and a sub-oesophageal part, and they are laterally connected by a part that may be considered as peri-oesophageal. Each of these parts is further subdivided into a varying number of lobes. In octopods and decapods, 25 major lobes have been described; however, some are further subdivided, giving a total number of 37 and 38 lobes, respectively (Fig. 3.20). It is beyond the aim of this section to describe the structures and possible functions of all the 38 brain lobes. For and excellent and comprehensive descriptions and reviews, see Nixon and Young (2003). Table 3.2 shows the principal information about the common octopus (*Octopus vulgaris*) brain, which is the well-known central nervous system among cephalopods.

The peripheral nervous system contains twice as many nerve cells (350 million) as the central nervous system. All peripheral ganglia are lower motor centres. The largest part of the peripheral nervous system is the five brachial nerve cords; each has one large axial cord, four much smaller peripheral intramuscular cords, and as many brachial ganglia as the arm has suckers; in addition, each sucker has its own small sucker ganglion. Most of the neurons in the brachial and sucker ganglia are (lower) motor neurons that drive the muscles of the suckers, but they also analyse chemo- and mechanosensory as well as propiosensory inputs.

The most well known of the peripheral ganglia are the stellate ganglia on the inside of the mantle. These ganglia are lower motor centres for the movement of the mantle. They house the giant synapse and give rise to the stellate nerves. The giant fibre system is present in Decapodiformes only

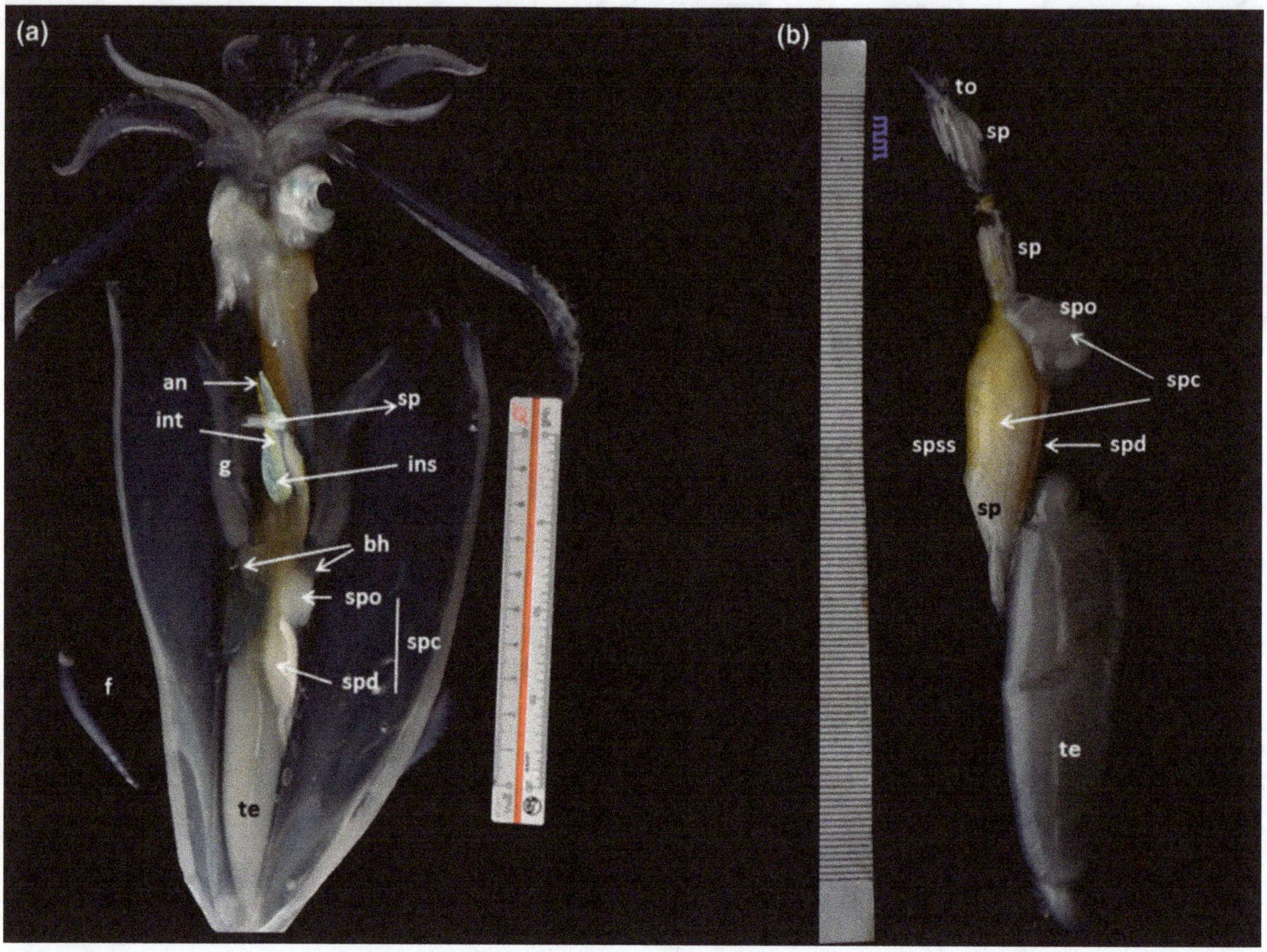

Fig. 3.18 *Loligo vulgaris* male reproductive system; **a** general view; **b** main parts; an: anus; anf: anal flaps; bh: branchial heart; f: fin; fun: funnel; g: gill; ins: ink sac; int: intestine; sp: spermatophores; spc: spermatophoric complex; spo: spermatophoric organ or gland; spss: spermatophoric sac or Needham's sac; te: testis; to: terminal organ

and is composed of a chain of three giant nerve cells on each side. The first-order giant cell lies in the ventral magnocellular lobe; its axon runs to the pallio-visceral lobe where it crosses to the contralateral side, forming a fusion (*Loligo*) or a synapse (*Sepia*) at the chiasma with its contralateral peer. From there, the second-order giant cell runs to the stellate ganglion. There, it connects via the giant synapse to the third-order giant cell (s), which drives the mantle musculature. The main function of the giant fibre system is fast escape jetting.

Other peripheral ganglia are: the inferior buccal and subradular ganglia, which control the buccal and the radula movements; the large gastric ganglion, which innervates the crop, stomach, caecum, and intestines; the fusiform, cardiac and auricular ganglia, which innervate the vena cava and the gill and systemic hearts; and the branchial (or gill) ganglia, which innervate the muscles of the gill lamellae.

3.5 Post-mortem Examination and Recognition of Tissues Abnormalities

3.5.1 Necropsy and Post-mortem Examination: Preliminary Remarks

Although there are some documents on how to necropsy some species of cephalopods, to date there was no attempt to produce a general guide. The information used to perform this section has three origins: (i) exiting partial documents (e.g. dissection technique to *Sepia officinalis* by A.V Sykes 2016); (ii) information of the excellent atlas on Salmonid diseases by Bruno et al. (2013), and (iii) our own experience.

Post-mortem examination or necropsy is the procedure of examining a body with the objective of assessing the lesions

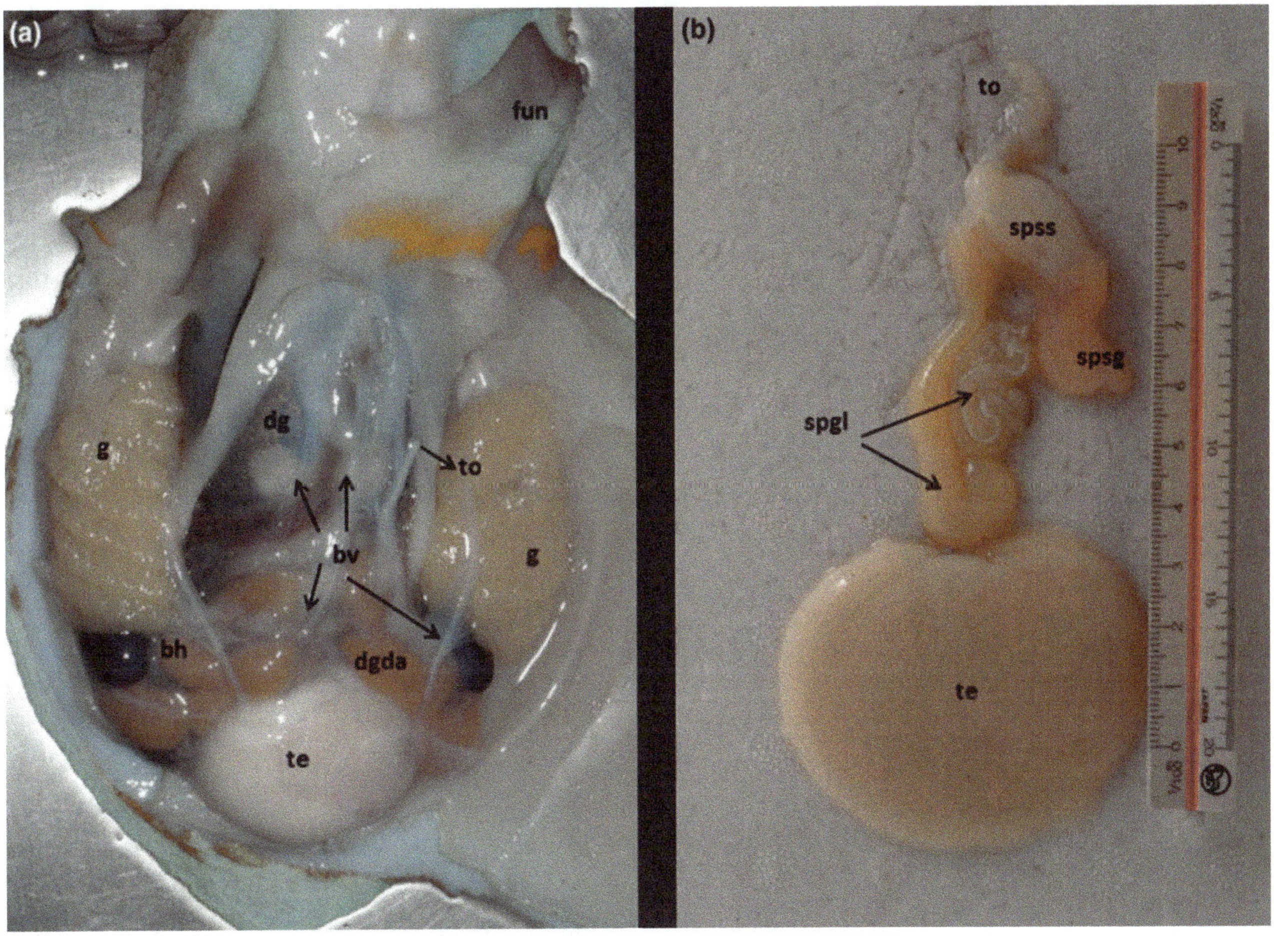

Fig. 3.19 *Octopus vulgaris* male reproductive system; **a** general view; **b** main parts; an: anus; bh: branchial heart; bv: blood vessels; d: diverticulum of the terminal organ; fun: funnel; g: gill; sp: spermatophores; spc: spermatophoric complex; spgl: spermatophoric gland; spsg: spermatophoric sac gland; spss: spermatophoric or Needham's sac; te: testis; to: terminal organ

present and the cause of death. This is achieved through a systematic approach and observation of external and internal structures, organs or tissues, assisted by the collection of samples for further analysis.

Any cephalopod sample can have two origins: wild or cultivated. As the industrial culture of these organisms is underdeveloped, it is quite unlikely that the sample comes from a farm. However, the sample could come from individuals kept in confinement in the laboratories. In order to undertake an appropriate cephalopod health assessment when the specimen is alive in their habitat, it is very useful to have data of the main parameters of the water mass (locality, water temperature, pH, salinity, and chemical and physical conditions) in which the animal has lived, as well as some characteristics of its habitat. Under farming or rearing conditions, information on changes in the standard cephalopod behaviour should be noted. Moreover, management practices as well as diet and feeding response also become of particular relevance.

When it comes to examining a group of individuals belonging to a more or less numerous population or group, records of the number (or the best possible estimation) of affected individuals within the population should be ascertained. This data, along with a detailed history of daily and total mortality, taking into account the size, sex, maturity stage, age (when possible), and origin of the stock, will allow establishing: (i) the morbidity rate and (ii) the pattern of the spread of the disease or abnormality observed.

Normally, this preliminary diagnosis made from wild animals or kept in aquaria is not definitive. This emphasizes the need of the necropsy. The description provided in this chapter describes the procedures of necropsy with particular reference to obtaining adequate samples of the most common tissues collected for histological examination. This is on the understanding that during necropsy, other samples will also be taken, e.g. for microbiological analysis, as well as blood or tissue samples for immunological or molecular studies, analyses of heavy metals concentrations, or

Table 3.1 Cephalopod sensory organs (modified from Nixon and Young 2003)

Eyes	Larger posterior chamber, lens, iris, retina, choroid, sclera, and argentea. Extraocular eye muscles. Similarity to vertebrate eyes	Rabdomeric type; rabdomera instead rod and cone cells in the retina. Generally a single visual pigment: rhodopsin. Most species blind to colours	Excellent visual ability an acuity. Polarization sensitivity
Photosensitive vesicles	Head and mantle	Compare sunlight with the one emitted by their own photophores themselves	Downwelling Camouflage
Statocysts	Paired organs in the skull. System 1: Macula–statolith–statoconia System 2: Cresta–cupula	Direction of gravity and linear acceleration. Countershading reflexes. Rotational acceleration	Balance and equilibrium. Infrasound. Countershading
"Lateral lines"	Mechanoreceptors or epidermis lines in different regions of the body	Detection of the impact of waves of pressure of the surrounding water	Detection in the dark
Suckers	Decapodiformes: Cuttlefishes and squids, with corneal rings Octopodiformes: octopuses; no corneal rings	Chemoreceptors. Mechanoreceptors. Propioreceptors	Taste, smell, touch, pressure, and position of the own body and limbs in space
Olfactory organs	In Coleoidea: a couple of small holes, one each side of the head under the eyes and near the edge of the mantle. Epithelial structures (rinophores)	Chemoreceptors	Smell
Nociceptors	In the skin, muscles, and viscera	They detect changes at chemical, thermal, and mechanical level, associated with cellular damage	Pain

statocysts to study of the damaging effects of the impacts of artificial sound sources. However, these procedures will not be covered or discussed in detail in this chapter.

3.5.2 Sample Size

The number of specimens sampled for a health assessment will vary according to the objectives of the study. For example, certification of freedom of a notifiable disease generally follows the guidelines from the Office International des Epizooties (OIE).

To obtain a 95–98% probability of detecting at least one infected cephalopod in a clinically healthy population, this translates to a minimum of 30 individuals. Conversely, for disease investigations, five to ten individuals showing abnormal behaviour or the characteristic signs of the condition will be adequate for necropsy. Despite these specifications, many times one will have to work with a single or few individuals.

Cuttlefishes, squids, or octopuses removed alive for examination should be placed into a smaller container where further observations can be made before any procedure or the removal of tissues or body fluids. The animal should be sacrificed (euthanized) by a humane method.

3.5.3 Euthanasia

The inclusion of "all live cephalopods" in Directive 2010/63/EU that regulates the use of animals for scientific purposes (European Parliament and Council of the European Union 2010) entails the identification of humane methods for killing, which is a particular challenge for neuroscience, as pointed out by the comprehensive paper of Fiorito et al. (2014).

The first point that should be taking into account is that a general anaesthesia is required for performing surgical procedures followed by recovery. Over the last century, a diverse range of substances has been used to induce general anaesthesia in cephalopods (see Andrews et al. 2013 for a review). Following Andrews et al. (2013), criteria for assessment of general anaesthesia in cephalopods include: (1) depression of ventilation and in some cases cessation, probably accompanied by reduced cardiac activity; (2) decrease in chromatophore tone (indicative of reduced drive to or from the sub-oesophageal chromatophore lobes); (3) reduced arm activity, tone, and sucker adhesion (particularly octopus); (4) loss of normal posture and righting reflex; (5) reduced or absent response to a noxious stimulus.

The Directive requires that if, for a justified reason (e.g. at the end of project, to obtain tissue for an in vitro study,

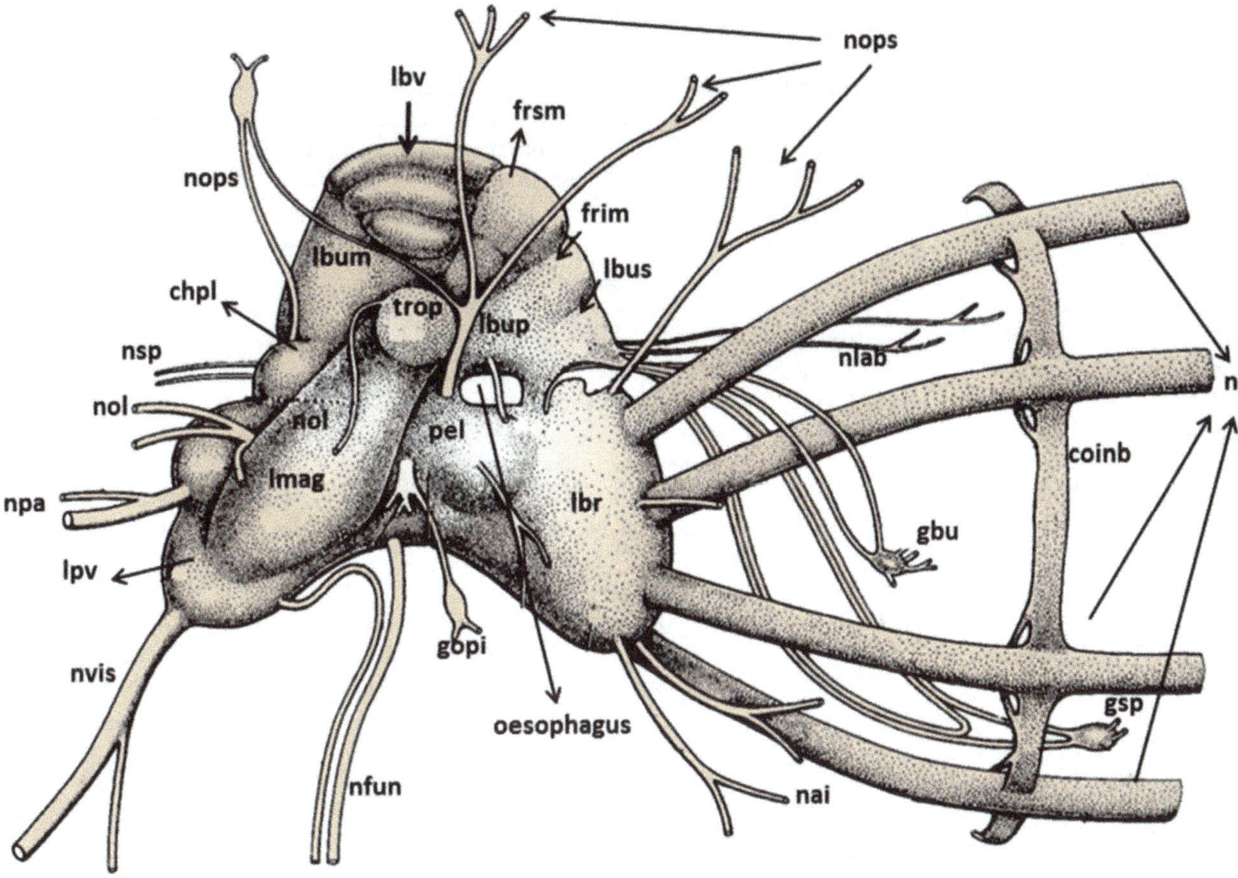

Fig. 3.20 Drawing of reconstruction of the *Octopus vulgaris* central nervous system (brain) drawn from serial sections; see from the right side (Young 1971); chpl: chromatophoric lobe; coinb: interbrachial commissure; frim: median inferior frontal lobe; frsm: median superior frontal lobe; gbu: buccal ganglia; gopi: inferior optic ganglia; gsp: posterior salivary ganglia; lbra: brachial lobe; lbum: median buccal lobe; lbup: posterior buccal lobe; lbus: superior buccal lobe; lbv: vertical lobe; lmag: magnocellular lobe; lpv: pallio-visceral lobe; nbr: brachial nerve; nlab: labial nerves; nops: superior posterior ophthalmic nerves; nol: olfactory nerve; nsp: posterior salivary nerve; nvis: visceral nerve; nfun: funnel nerve; pel: lateral pedal lobe; trop: optic tract

because a humane end point is reached), it is necessary to kill an animal, it must be done "with the minimum of pain, suffering, and distress" (Article 6). The methods to euthanize a specimen can be summarized in two main categories: (1) mechanical methods (cutting between the eyes to destroy the brain and/or decapitation); (2) chemical methods—(a) cooling: cool water containing 2% ethanol; (b) magnesium chloride $MgCl_2$ alone or in combination with eugenol; (c) chloroform; and (d) carbon dioxide. All current techniques use immersion in sea water containing the anaesthetic agent. Time of exposition will depend on the species and size of the cephalopod.

Based upon current evidence, the following method is proposed for humanely killing cephalopods such as *Sepia officinalis, Dorytheuthis pealei, Octopus vulgaris, and Eledone cirrhosa*: at least 15 min immersion in $MgCl_2$ (with a rising concentration [optimal rates remain to be determined], ending with a final concentration of at least 3.5% in the chamber used for humane killing), possibly enhanced by using a chilled solution or with the clove oil active constituent eugenol, followed by immediate mechanical destruction of the brain (Andrews et al. 2013).

It must be emphasized that the above are initial proposals, and it is likely that methods will need to be refined, possibly with the identification of species-specific protocols.

Annex IV of the Directive includes methods for confirmation of death, and these are discussed in relation to cephalopods in the paper of Andrews et al. It should also be noted that the requirement for humane killing also applies to hatchlings. In this last case, killing by direct immersion in fixative would not now be considered acceptable in the EU, although it might be possible to obtain permission to use this as a method if it could be justified to the National Citizens Alliance (NCA).

Table 3.2 Number of cells and a summary of main functions of the principal lobes of the *Octopus vulgaris* brain (modified from Nixon and Young 2003)

Masses and lobes	No of cells	Main functions
Optics lobes	128 940 000	Analysers of the visual input and regulate visual behaviour They initiate the programs by which the higher motor centres (the basal lobes) produce the various motor activities of the animal Centres for simple visual discrimination learning and also involved in the expression of the various chromatic components
Sub-oesophageal mass		*Motor centres involves in most action of the animal*
Palliovisceral	108 000	Control of muscular activity of the mantle and viscera
Chromatophore	526 000	Management of the chromatophoric's muscles
Vasomotor	1 307 000	Control of the musculature of blood vessels
Brachial	341 000	Actions of the arms and tentacles
Pedal	241 000	Idem
Supra-oesophageal mass		
Vertical	25 066 000	Lobes linked for the management of exploratory actions, learning
Subvertical	810 000	and short and long term memories
Frontal Superior	1 854 000	
Inferior	1 085 000	In addition, they are closely related to the functional system
Subfrontal	5 308 000	related to the chemotactile stimuli coming from the suckers
Subpedunculate	144 000	and the mouth, as well as visual stimuli coming from the eyes
Basal		
anterior	380 000	Control of posture and movements of head and eyes
dorsal	1 796 000	Control of defence and avoidance strategies
lateral	127 000	Control of the chromatophores and the muscles in the skin
median	245 000	Control of swimming and respiration
Buccal superior	150 000	Motor control of feeding
Peduncle	142 000	Coordinate motor activity, colour changes and ink-injection
Olfactory	136 000	Control of muscles of olfactory organs
Peri-oesophageal mass Magnocellular lobe	581 000	This lobe is particularly involved in defence and fast escape reactions The giant fibre system originates there

3.5.4 Necropsy Procedure

3.5.4.1 External Examination

The first operation to be performed is to try to eliminate the water that has remained in the specimen's paleal cavity. The most convenient is to use an absorbent paper. The specimen should be placed in a tray that prevents further contamination and which allows performing the work. Above the tray, and below the animal, an absorbent paper to remove excess water should be placed. It is ideally maintained the specimen at cool temperatures throughout the necropsy, which can be achieved by placing ice below the tray.

The most appropriate is to completely extend (arms and tentacles included) the specimen in the tray and begin the inspection by its dorsal face, the opposite of where the funnel is located. The mantle, head, and arms should be carefully examined. Any deviation from normality for the species throughout the process of the post-mortem examination should be recorded in a notebook. The provision of a reference to the relative position of the abnormality or the sample taken is an essential part of the report. When the exam of the dorsal region is finished, the same should be done with the ventral one, turning the specimen over. A thorough check of the entire body external surface (which should be done under a dissecting microscope a when necessary) is anatomical anomalies, such as the integrity of the skin and fins, changes of normal pigmentation for the species, loss of arms and/or tentacles, bifurcation of the arms, anomalies in the copulatory arms, regeneration of arms and/or suckers, erosion, ulcers, grossly visible parasites, evidence of cuttlebone deformity (*Sepia*) or muscle atrophy, but, above all, tumorous-like conditions in the arms, head, eyes, and/or the mantle. Keep in mind that in cephalopods it will not be possible to denote haemorrhages, since their blood is bluish white. The mouth and the oral cavity should be examined recording the presence of any possible, vesicles, parasites, or abnormality associated with these structures. Samples of skin and mucous can be taken for immediate analysis. Carefully remove a small piece approximately 1 cm^3 and place immediately in fixative such as 10% buffered formal saline. A gross examination of the eyes should include reference to corneal opacity, cataract, or exophthalmia which, although not necessarily pathognomonic, can indicate a minor infection or a sign of a more serious condition. To remove the eye carefully dissect the skin around the orbit using small curved scissors or a scalpel until sufficient tissue is available to grip with forceps. Pull the eye forwards in order to expose the associated muscles and then cut free the entire eye ball, but it is not advisable to try to extract the optic lobes or the ocular nerves, which should be done when working with the brain. Eye fixation can be made using Carnoy's solution instead of formalin. However, when the main interest is parasitological examination, this will usually require fixation in 70% alcohol.

For the purpose of histological examination, specimens of this small size can be preserved whole, but making a cut in the ventral region that allows the fixative to penetrate within the mantle cavity and guarantee proper fixation. For larger specimens, fresh samples of tissues (mainly skin ones) or body fluids can also be taken for initial in situ analysis, but for histological examination tissues need to be dissected using scalpel, scissors, and forceps. If the animal has a rigid internal shell (cuttlebone or gladius), it is not convenient to remove it, because that preserves the rigidity of the body and the internal organs in their natural position.

3.5.4.2 Internal Examination

To access the internal organs the mantle or paleal cavity is opened. There are several ways to approach dissection, however, the choice must prevent or reduce the likelihood of the process introducing artefacts, damaging tissues, compressing, cutting, moving, or displacing organs as well as avoiding the risk of contamination. Place the animal with the ventral side facing towards you; gently press the both lateral sides of the mantle to open a cavity; then, use the scissors with the blunted side facing the inside of the mantle to perform a cut along the mid-ventral line of the mantle that reaches its end the cut can be also performed laterally (as shown in Fig. 14 to *Sepia officinalis* and in Fig. 16 to *Octopus vulgaris*; then, make two lateral incisions at the end point of the first incision, one towards the right and another towards the left, to expose the internal organs. If during this operation a long muscle that holds the mantle internally (it occurs in the octopuses) is found, it should be cut carefully and lengthwise, preventing damage of any internal organ. Exposure of the entire body cavity is required for assessment and allows access to organs for sampling. Once the internal organs are in sight, a preliminary and general inspection should be carried out. Notes on the general appearance of the cavity may include references to the extent of tissue growth or colour changes, swelling, ascites, adhesions, and absence of encysted parasites. As experience increases, all the procedures can be performed using scissors and scalpel.

The protocol that we recommend for the examination of the internal organs starts by carefully removal each one of them. After removal, each system should be placed in a Petri dish, which might be advisable to keep in a refrigerator (4 °C) for further examination. The most convenient order for the organs removal is as follows: 1°) the reproductive system (ovary, oviducts, and oviductal glands if there were, in the case of females; testicle, spermatophoric complex, and terminal organ (penis) in males); 2°) respiratory and main parts of the circulatory system (gills, branchial hearts, systemic heart, trying to conserve their connections through the associate blood vessels, as well as the most important vessels leaving the systemic heart, at least in part of their length). The excretory system is closely linked to these other two systems and is extracted together with them. Again, place these systems in a Petri dish and keep it in a refrigerator (4 °C) for further examination; 3°) the digestive system (oesophagus, posterior salivary glands, crop if present, stomach, caecum, digestive gland duct appendages, intestine and anus). If food remains are found in any part of the digestive system, it is convenient to remove them. The digestive gland and the ink sac are part of this system. As they break with relative ease, what we recommend to avoid its rupture is to keep them together with the other parts of the system, and, once in the Petri dish or in an appropriate tray, remove them carefully avoiding its rupture; 4°) the buccal mass (lips, two mandibles or beak, anterior salivary glands, buccal muscles, and radula) is relatively easy to extract using scissors and scalpel. Generally, when the buccal bulb is removed, fragments of the oesophagus remain. After these manipulations, the cuttlebone or the gladius can be removed.

Complete removal of the viscera is practical for easier assessment under a dissecting microscope, e.g. for parasitological analysis, however inappropriate, if aseptic microbiological samples are required. For tissue sampling and depending of necessities, whole organs may be fixed from small individuals (e.g. the entire gastrointestinal tract); conversely, from larger specimens portions of ~ 1 cm^3 of each organ should be removed and fixed. Bouin's fixative has been recommended for this tissue as gonads in an advanced stage of development can be hard to cut after routine formalin fixation. The digestive may vary in colour depending of the type of diet, as well as the health status of the specimen. A sample should be collected using a sharp scalpel rather than scissors. An examination of the gastrointestinal tract, caecum, and associated tissues can be carried out once relevant microbiological sampling has been performed.

Finally, the cranium needs to be opened in order to expose and examine the brain. One of the most appropriate ways to access the brain is: (1) fix the specimen on a dish, dorsal side up;

(2) remove the skin of the head using a sharp scalpel; (3) remove the eyes, and the paired large optic lobes are located laterally and the white bodies over each optic lobe; (4) with a horizontal cut, remove the dorsal part of the cranium cartilage until the central part of the brain, a collection of very soft nerve tissue that actually surrounds the oesophagus, is visible. This mass corresponds to the supra and sub-oesophageal regions of the brain; (5) carefully remove the whole brain. The brain deterioration is rapid, and it is, therefore, important to fixing it. The two most common ways of fixing the brain are freezing and the use of fixative solutions. Each method has its advantages; (6) when all sub-oesophageal brain tissue is totally removed, the statocysts become visible. They are two cavities located at the posterior-ventral region of the cranium cartilage. Avoid damaging the thin cartilage between the brain and the statocyst cavities. When the anterior, lateral, and posterior outlines of the statocysts are visible, a block of cartilage containing the two statocysts can be cut out of the head. The statocysts can be also approaches from the ventral, which is the most appropriate way when operating with anesthetized animals. The tissue should fix for light microscopy or scanning electron microscopy. Statoliths are two white opaque structures located within the statocysts, which are using for ageing. It should be preserved dried or in ethanol 70%.

Maintaining an organized and systematic approach to the necropsy is an important aspect of the procedure, and careful observations made during this examination will provide valuable information not only immediately, but consequently during the interpretation of the histological sections.

All tissues samples must be clearly identified with a reference code when sent for processing to ensure that there is no risk of incorrect reporting.

3.6 Concluding Remarks

As members of the phylum Mollusca, the cephalopods share certain basic features of their body organization. Despite their basic molluscan physiology and biochemical design, there are many characteristics in cephalopods that raise their lifestyle and performance to levels similar to those found in vertebrates. Cephalopods are active mobile predators, swimming by means of jet propulsion and fin undulations, or rapid scrambling by strong suckered arms. As in other molluscs, the central nervous system in arranges around the oesophagus. However, sense organs, particularly eyes and organs of balance (statocysts), are highly developed. Moreover, the brain does not just have centralization of the molluscan ganglia but also contains lobes with "higher-order" functions such as storage of learned information. Most of the cephalopods have a skin display system of unmatched complexity and excellence of camouflage, which is also used for communication with predators and conspecifics. In addition, the muscular systemic heart, the branchial hearts, and contractile blood vessels contributed to a strong blood circulation within a close circulatory system. The particularities set out here, which are not the only ones, require special knowledge of the morphology and gross anatomy of these organisms, when studies on their pathologies are focused. On the other hand, this type of knowledge is crucial when considering an adequate protocol for external and internal examination. Also its sacrifice, in the case that it would be necessary, must be considered attending to their particular characteristics.

Cephalopods also play an important role in the trophic web of marine ecosystems. The importance of cephalopods as hosts for parasites, which may travel up the food chain to top predators, such as marine mammals and man, has been emphasized elsewhere.

Finally, the growing importance of cephalopods in different research's fields, aquaculture, and human consumption requires a top priority and wider knowledge of their health. This knowledge includes detailed information about the cause, mechanisms of development (pathogenesis), morphological and anatomical alterations, and their clinical manifestations.

References

Andrews PLR, Darmaillacq A-N, Dennison N, Gleadall IG, Hawkins P, Messenger JB, Osorio D, Smith VJ, Smith JM (2013) The identification and management of pain, suffering and distress in cephalopods, including anaesthesia, analgesia and humane killing. J Exp Mar Biol Ecol 447:46–64. https://doi.org/10.1016/j.jembe.2013.02.010

Arkhipkin AI, Rodhouse PGK, Pierce GJ et al (2015) World Squid Fisheries. Rev Fish Sci Aquac 23: 92–252. Taylor & Francis Group, LLC, https://doi.org/10.1080/23308249.2015.1026226

Boyle PR, Rodhouse PGK (2005) Cephalopods. Ecology and Fisheries. Blackwell, London, p 452

Bruno DW, Noguera PA, Poppe TT (2013) A colour Atlas of salmonid diseases. Springer, Heidelberg

Darmaillacq A-S, Dickel L, Mater J (eds) (2014) Cephalopod cognition. Cambridge University Press, Cambridge, UK, p 247

Fiorito G, Affuso A, Basil J et al (2014) Cephalopods in neuroscience: regulations, research and the 3Rs. Invertebr Neurosci 14(1):13–36. https://doi.org/10.1007/s10158-013-0165-x

Guerra A (1992) Mollusca, Cephalopoda. In Ramos, MA et al (eds) Fauna Ibérica, vol. 1. Museo Nacional de Ciencias Naturales. CSIC, Madrid, p 318

Hanlon RT, Messenger JB (1996) Cephalopod behaviour. Cambridge University Press, Cambridge, U.K, p 232

Iglesias J, Fuentes L, Villanueva R (eds) (2014) Cephalopod culture. Springer, Heidelberg, p 494

Jereb P, Roper CFE (eds) (2005) Cephalopods of the world. An annotated and illustrated catalogue of cephalopods species known to date. Chambered nautiluses and sepioids. FAO Species Catalogue for Fisheries Purposes, No 4, vol. 1. Rome, p 262

Jereb P, Roper CFE (eds) (2010) Cephalopods of the world. An annotated and illustrated catalogue of cephalopods species known to date. Myopsid and Oegopsid squids. FAO Species Catalogue for Fisheries Purposes, No 4, vol. 2. Rome, p 605

Jereb P, Roper CFE, Norman MD, Finn JK (eds) (2016) Cephalopods of the world. An annotated and illustrated catalogue of cephalopods species known to date. Octopods and Vampire squids by. FAO Species Catalogue for Fisheries Purposes, No 4, vol. 3. Rome, p 352

Mangold K (1989) Céphalopodes. In: Grassé PP (ed) Traité de Zoologie, vol 4. Masson, Paris, p 804

Nixon M, Young JZ (2003) The brains and lives of Cephalopods. Oxford University Press, Oxford, UK, p 392

Pörtner HO, O'Dor RK, Macmillan DL (1994) Physiology of Cephalopod Molluscs: lifestyle and performance adaptations. Gordon and Breach Publishers, Basel, Switzerland, p 214

Young JZ (1971) The anatomy of the nervous system of octopus vulgaris. Clarendon Press, Oxford, p 690

Young RE, Vecchione M, Mangold KM (2018) Cephalopoda Cuvier 1797. Octopods, squids, nautiluses, etc. Version 20 (under construction). http://tolweb.org/Cephalopoda/19386/2018.02.20 in The Tree of Life Web Project, http://tolweb.org/ Accessed Sept 8 2018

4 Functional Histology: The Tissues of Common Coleoid Cephalopods

Ramón Anadón

Abstract

The knowledge of the organization of normal tissues and the changes occurring during physiological or pathological processes is basic to interpret the relationship between structure and function. There are numerous microscopic studies focused on different cephalopod organs that are based on the use of high-resolution methods as the transmission electron microscopy. However, there is no comprehensive basic histological guide to the different tissues in common species of cephalopods. To fill this gap, we present a careful description of the normal histological organization of cephalopods. Through 35 plates including 225 photomicrographs and the accompanying text descriptions, this chapter covers the body systems of three common species of European coleoid cephalopods, the cuttlefish (*Sepia officinalis*), the squid (*Loligo vulgaris*) and the octopus (*Octopus vulgaris*). The histology of the three species is presented in parallel, emphasizing those significant between-species differences. Sections used for study and photomicrographs were mostly stained with hematoxylin–eosin (H&E), a standard light microscopy method widely accessible for most laboratories of histology and pathology. Some sections of octopus were stained the Masson's trichrome or the periodic acid–Schiff (PAS) methods.

Keywords

Cephalopods • Tissues • Comparative histology • Light microscopy • Atlas

4.1 Introduction

The microscopic anatomy or histology is based on examination of stained thin sections of the different structures of the body. The knowledge of the organization of normal tissues and the changes occurring during physiological or pathological processes is fundamental to interpret the relationship between structure and function. Most textbooks of histology are dedicated to human or mammalian tissues, and the scant books existing on comparative histology generally do not mention cephalopod tissues at all. There are numerous detailed microscopic studies focused on different cephalopod organs that are based in the use of high-resolution methods such as the transmission electron microscopy, which have been comprehensively presented in a chapter on cephalopods by Budelmann et al. (1997). For ultrastructural data, interested readers are directed to this chapter, which also includes an exhaustive list of references. However, there is no comprehensive histological guide to the different tissues in common species of cephalopods using standard light microscopy methods available in most laboratories of pathology. This chapter covers the "normal" histological organization of three representative coastal species of Coleoidea. The species studied here are two representatives of decapodiformes, the cuttlefish (*Sepia officinalis*; Sepiida) and the squid (*Loligo vulgaris*; Teuthida) and a representative of the octopodiformes, the common octopus (*Octopus vulgaris*).

The anatomy of the cephalopods has been studied for centuries (Swammerdam 1737; Cuvier 1817; Owen 1855;

R. Anadón (✉)
Department of Functional Biology, University of Santiago de Compostela, Campus Vida, Santiago de Compostela, Spain
e-mail: ramon.anadon@usc.es

C. Gestal et al. (eds.), *Handbook of Pathogens and Diseases in Cephalopods*,
https://doi.org/10.1007/978-3-030-11330-8_4

Isgrove 1909; Williams 1909; Meyer 1913; Chun 1914). In this chapter, the microscopic anatomy of main systems of the three species is summarily presented in parallel, emphasizing those between-species differences in tissue organization when significant. Photomicrographs were taken of histological sections of four octopus (two adult males and two females, one immature), two squid (a male and an immature female) and three cuttlefish (two adult males and a female).

Previous to histological methods, live specimens were deeply anaesthetized by immersion in seawater containing 1% $MgCl_2$ and 1% ethanol (10–15 min) and then euthanized in seawater with 3.5% $MgCl_2$ followed by immediate mechanical destruction of the brain. After dissection of the various organs and structures, fixation was done in Davidson fluid (formalin, alcohol and acetic acid in tap water). Tissue blocks were embedded in paraffin wax and sectioned on a rotary microtome. Dewaxed sections were routinely stained with hematoxylin–eosin (H&E). Some sections of octopus were additionally stained using the Masson's trichrome or the periodic acid–Schiff (PAS)-staining methods.

4.2 Skin (Fig. 4.1)

The skin of cephalopods has evolved to separate the internal medium from the seawater but also to provide a quick changing way adapted for intra-specific communication, camouflage, or prey attraction (Osorio 2014). The skin covers the outer surface of the body, showing highly different regional specializations, as in the suckers, and is continuous with the inner surfaces of the siphon and the pallial cavity. The skin of the cephalopods consists of a transparent epidermis formed of columnar epithelial cells and interspersed mucous cells, and a dermal layer of varying thickness formed of connective tissue that includes a number of chromatophores, iridophores and reflecting cells. Light microscopy of histological sections shows little detail of the epithelial cells, but ultrastructural studies reveal complex interdigitation of lateral cell surfaces as well as the presence of an apical microvillous layer (see Lee et al. 2014). A thick basal lamina anchors the epidermis to the dermal tissue. The epidermis of the pallial cavity mostly shows flattened epidermal cells and is deeply modified in some regions of the funnel (see below) where it may form extensive thickened glandular surfaces.

The dermis mostly consists of a connective tissue formed of fibroblasts and networks of collagen fibers included in varied amounts of ground substance that exhibit in many places conspicuous chromatophore organs and also other types of pigment cells below. The skin of octopus and cuttlefish, mainly dorsally, contains a number of muscle fascicles that allow rapid changes in the animal appearance of skin papillae and tubercles caused by erector muscles or its disappearance by contraction of depressor muscles. Collagen fibrils are abundant in the skin and muscles of cephalopods, where they form fiber bundles with various orientations. These fibers are eosinophilic in H&E stains but are better distinguished from muscle fibers with the Masson's trichrome stain, showing a similar affinity for colorants as vertebrate collagen fibers. The thickness and appearance of the dermis vary along the animal surface. In octopus and cuttlefish, the dermis is thick and endowed of various

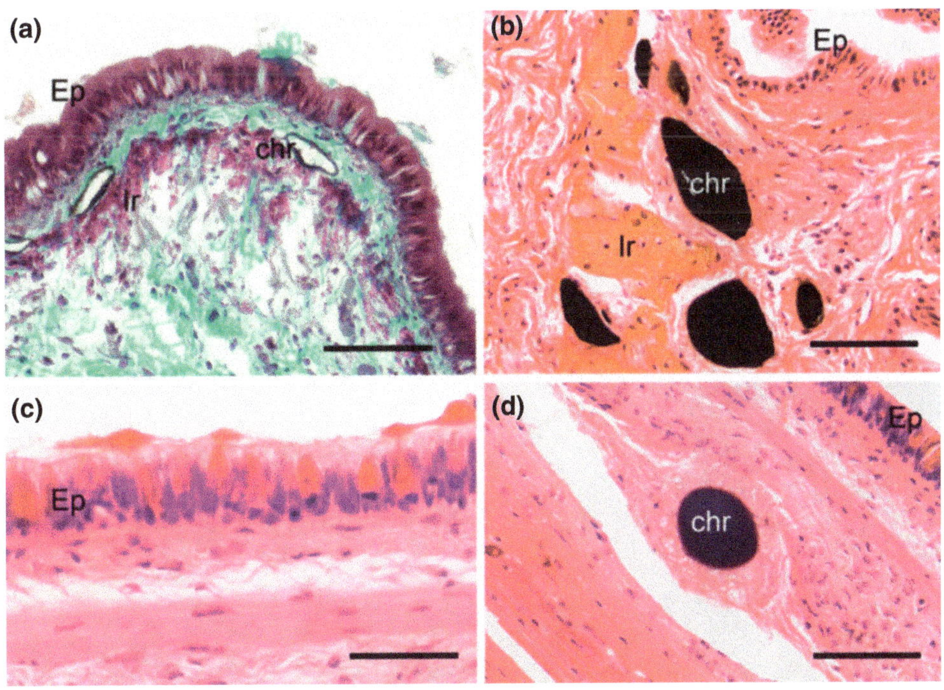

Fig. 4.1 Sections of the skin of octopus arm (**a**, **b**) and squid mantle (**c**, **d**). In **a**, note the abundant collagen stained in green and the iridophores in pink. In **c**, goblet cells and secreted mucus appear red-stained. In **d**, note muscle fibers inserted at both poles of the organ. Chr, chromatophoric organs; Ep, epidermis; Ir, iridophores (reflecting cells). **a** Masson's trichrome. **b**, **c** H&E stain. *Scale bars* **a**, **d** 100 μm; **b** 200 μm; **c** 50 μm

bundles of muscle fibers whose contraction transforms the skin from smooth to papillae or tubercles (papillary erector muscles) or the smoothening of the surface (papillary depressor muscles). This, together with fast changes in pigmentation in an instant, allows animals to adopting flexibly very different appearances for camouflage or communication (Hanlon 2007). The dermis of the inner pallial surface is thin and mostly lacks pigment cells.

4.3 Chromatophores

The chromatophore organs are complex pigment-containing structures that consist of a large elastic sac (sacculus) filled of pigment that is contained inside of a chromatophoric cell and a crown of radial muscle fibers that join this cell (Fig. 4.1d). Specialized histological methods and/or transmission electron microscopy reveal that radial muscle fibers are richly innervated by nerve fibers accompanied of glial cells, as well as the unsheathing cells around the chromatophore cell. In live animals, chromatophore organs exhibit changing size and colors that vary from black-brown in melanophores to red or yellow in other chromatophores. The contraction of radial muscle fibers extends the pigment sacculus and its relaxation concentrated pigment showing a small surface. In histological sections of anaesthetized animals, they appear contracted as black organs. The contraction and/or relaxation of different types of chromatophoric organs combined with the reflection of light by other types of pigment cells located below allow the extremely rapid changes of the coloration patterns in the skin of cephalopods (Packard 1995). A number of videos of cephalopods showing fast changes of skin pigmentation patterns are freely available in the Web.

In the skin, eyes and other tissues of cephalopods, there are different types of reflecting cells. In H&E-stained histological sections, the reflecting cells appear to contain yellowish platelets or granules that are mostly unstained (Fig. 4.1b), but granules appear brightly stained in red with Masson's trichrome method. The internal organization of reflecting cells has been thoroughly studied with transmission electron microscopy. These ultrastructural studies reveal several types of pigment cells named as iridophores, leucophores and reflecting cells with varied structural organizations of reflective structures (see Budelmann et al. 1997). Recent studies show that reflecting platelets contain condensed proteins coded by the reflectin gene family that is specific to cephalopods (Crookes et al. 2004; DeMartini et al. 2015). The regular arrangement of collagen fibers in the dermis may also contribute to the skin appearance and reflectivity.

In many species of pelagic cephalopods, but not in the octopus, squid and cuttlefish species illustrated here, the skin may bear a number of photophores, specialized organs that emit light.

4.4 Cartilaginous Tissues (Fig. 4.2)

Cephalopods use cartilaginous tissues in a few locations of the body (Cole and Hall 2009). Chondroid tissues form a part of buccal bolsters contributing to mechanical properties of the buccal mass. In squid, buccal bolsters show an onion-like organization of connective cells around a pulpous-like connective center. The cerebral ganglia are surrounded by cartilage in some respects similar to that of vertebrates, although chondrocytes exhibit thin-branched processes. Isogenic groups of chondrocytes are frequently observed. A dense perichondrium consisting of thin fibroblasts included in an abundant matrix of collagen fibers surrounds some surfaces of cranial cartilages. In the eye, the equatorial and subequatorial scleral regions exhibit a cartilaginous skeleton that reminds the scleral bones or cartilages found in many vertebrate eyes. In squid and cuttlefish, the scleral cartilage shows a single or a double layer of radial columnar chondrocytes embedded in homogeneous cartilaginous matrix. In octopus eyes, the equatorial sclera exhibits a thick cartilage-like tissue with dense accumulation of very thin and long radial cells that are well-stained with the Masson's method. These cells are embedded in scarce matrix, and the inner and outer tissue surfaces are flanked by thin muscle layers (scleral muscles). Connective tissues in the base of the octopus cranium often may show atypical appearances with very thick collagen fibers embedded in an abundant homogeneous unstained matrix containing fibroblasts and lacking blood vessels, which make them difficult to classify.

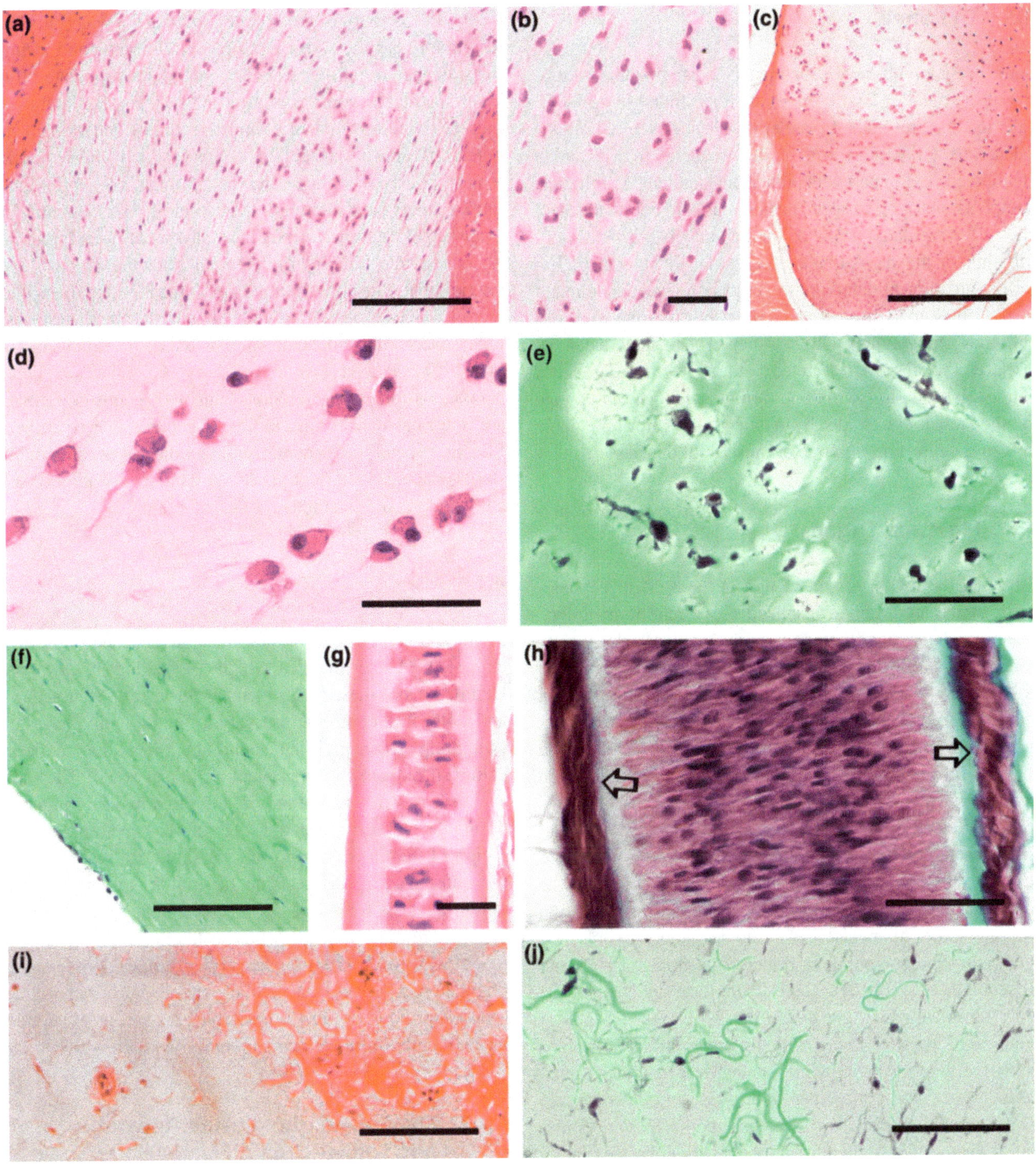

Fig. 4.2 Sections of cartilage and related skeletal tissues. **a**, **b** Chondroid tissue of a buccal bolster of squid showing an onion-like organization of connective cells around a pulpous-like connective center. **c** Section of the cranial cartilage of squid. **d** Detail of processes of chondrocytes. **e** Section of the cranial cartilage of octopus showing branched chondrocytes. **f** Dense perichondrium of a cranial cartilage. **e** Equatorial scleral cartilage of the squid with a single layer of chondrocytes. **f** A typical equatorial scleral cartilage-like tissue of the octopus eye showing dense accumulation of thin and long radial cells. The tissue is flanked by thin muscle layers (scleral muscles; outlined arrows). **i**, **j** Sections through connective tissue in the base of the octopus cranium showing thick collagen fibers in a homogeneous matrix. **a–d**, **g–i**, H&E stain; **e**, **f**, **h**, **j** Masson's trichrome. *Scale bars* **a**, **f**, **h**, **i**, **j** 100 μm; **b**, **g** 25 μm; **d**, **e** 50 μm; **c** 200 μm

4.5 The Shell

Some cephalopods have a shell that is located within a dorsal sac of the mantle. Two types of shell are found in coleoids, calcified and chitinous. In cuttlefish, the shell (cuttlebone) is calcareous (aragonite) with a dense dorsal region and a chambered ventral part with pillars and lamellae. A siphuncle complex consisting of specialized epithelium below the shell allows the regulated filling of shell chambers with gas, contributing to the regulation of the cuttlefish buoyancy. For further anatomical details of the cuttlebone, see Budelmann et al. (1997) and Checa et al. (2015). In squid, the shell is a chitinous pen (gladius), a feather-shaped plate, included in the dorsal epithelial sac and secreted by the shell gland. The squid pen is thickened in the midline forming a rachis. In octopus, the shell relicts surrounded by mantle muscles are appreciable only at the insertion of retractor muscles of the funnel.

4.6 Muscular Organs

Muscular tissues form a major part of the body of cephalopods, which are highly specialized active marine predators. The musculature of cephalopods, as in other mollusks, mostly consists of muscle fibers with contractile material organized in oblique band or oblique striation, which is hardly visible in normal histological sections as those shown here. These fibers are very thin and long cylindrical cells with the contractile material forming an external tubular region around a central cytoplasmic core that can be mitochondria-poor ("white" muscle fibers) or mitochondria-rich ("red" muscle cells) (Mommsen et al. 1981). Fibers bear a single elongated nucleus. Ultrastructural and functional descriptions of the organization of these fibers including the oblique organization of contractile filaments, dense bodies and sarcoplasmic reticulum can be found in Budelmann et al. (1997) and Rosenbluth et al. (2010). These fibers form the basis of the body muscles, which are most often observed in bands or bundles of parallel fibers with different orientations (see below). Based on their biomechanical features, these muscular masses form muscular hydrostats, muscular organs which lack typical systems of skeletal support (Kier and Smith 1985). In addition to the muscle fibers with oblique striation that form most of the cephalopod muscles, thin cross-striated muscle fibers with myofilaments aligned in register have been reported in transverse muscles of tentacles of cuttlefish and squid and in intrinsic eye muscles (Kier 1985).

4.7 The Mantle and Its Muscle Layers (Fig. 4.3)

The mantle forms the muscle walls of the large pallial cavity enclosing the gills and the visceral mass. In squid and cuttlefish, lateral extensions joined to the mantle form the fins. Contractile activity of the mantle provides the water flux for respiration and the water jerks for rapid escape and swimming of the animal, whereas fin contractions mediate "flying." The mantle consists of a complex tubule-like lamina of muscle tissue covered of connective tunics and skin in its outer and inner surface. In octopus, the mantle muscle mainly consists of inner and outer layers of longitudinal muscle fibers sandwiching a thick central region of circular (transverse) muscle fibers. Thin layers of radial muscle fibers separate bundles of fibers in both the circular and longitudinal muscles. In the squid mantle, the muscular region mainly consists of thick bands of circular muscle fibers alternating with thin circular bands of radial muscle fibers. These layers are covered by the inner and outer connective tunics, and oblique lattices of connective fibers are intercalated with muscle fibers. These connective fibers fold or expand with mantle contractions to accommodate strain gradients (Kurth et al. 2014). The organization of the cuttlefish mantle is similar to that of squid.

4.7.1 Fins

Squid and cuttlefish have muscular fins attached to the lateral side of the mantle, which is lacking in octopus. Undulations of these fins, together with mantle contractions and water jets, contribute actively to the different phases of swimming. The lateral fins extend along most the mantle in cuttlefish but only in the apical region in squid. They are attached over the mantle musculature to a region originated during development from the shell sac. The central muscular region of the fin is covered of skin similar to that covering the outer mantle surface. The fin musculature forms two opposite bands separated by a connective layer. In each band, there are bundles of muscle fibers with longitudinal (deep region), transverse (superficial) and dorso-ventral orientation arranged in a regular pattern. An intramuscular array of crossed connective fibers probably provides support during gentle fin movements (Johnsen and Kier 1993).

4.7.2 The Funnel, the Closure Apparatus and Funnel Organ (Fig. 4.4)

The siphon or funnel is a foot-derived muscular organ that projects from the margin of the mantle between the ventral mantle corners into a conical tube, the siphon that leads from the mantle cavity to the exterior. The extended funnel ventral region allows the free entrance of water in the pallial cavity between the it and the ventral mantle during pallial dilatation, and make the function of a valve (siphonal valves) during mantle contraction, forcing the flow of water through the siphon (water jerks). The muscles of the squid funnel valves are formed of thick inner and outer bands of longitudinal fibers and circular (transverse) fibers,

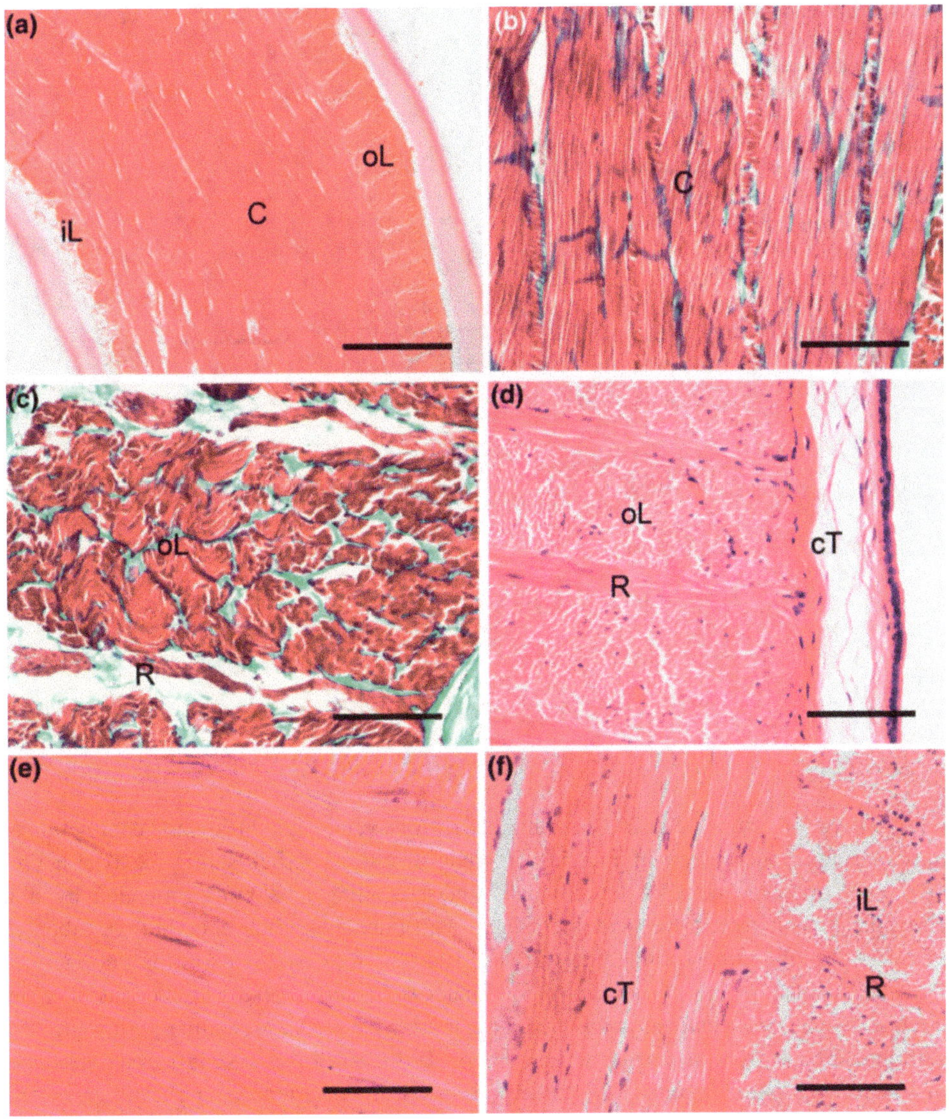

Fig. 4.3 Muscle fibers of the mantle of octopus (**a–c**) and squid (**d–f**). **a** Panoramic view of a transversal section showing bundles of longitudinal fibers in the inner and outer side of the thick central region with circular muscle fibers. **b** Detail of the central region showing thin layers of radial fibers separating thick bundles of circular fibers. Note also the net of collagen fibers (green stained) among muscle bundles. **c** Section through the outer bundles of longitudinal fibers showing the net of collagen tissue and thin bands of radial muscle separating circular bundles. **d** Outer region of the squid mantle musculature showing circular and radial muscles. **e** Detail of muscle fibers running in parallel. **f** Inner region of the squid mantle musculature showing bundles of radial, circular and longitudinal fibers and fascias of dense connective tissue. cT, connective tissue; C, circular muscle; iL, inner longitudinal muscle; oL, outer longitudinal muscle; R, radial muscle. In all figures excepting E, the outer surface is at the right. **a**, **d–f** H&E stain. **b**, **c** Masson's trichrome. *Scale bars* **a** 500 μm; **d**, **f** 100 μm; **b**, **c**, **e** 50 μm

respectively, with thin bands of radial fibers interspersed. The muscles are covered of connective tunics that are continuous with the perichondrium of the funnel cartilage. In squid and cuttlefish, this funnel cartilage is covered of a thin skin and forms a socket for the complementary bouton-like cartilaginous protrusion of the mantle. Thus, the funnel articular cartilage is part of the paired closure apparatus joining the siphonal valves and mantle.

The epidermis of the inner surface of the funnel of squid (and other cephalopods) forms an extensive and very thick intraepithelial gland. It consists of a superficial layer of small epithelial cells of cuboid cylindrical appearance that covers a large mass of tall mucous glandular cells that show nuclei in basal regions and enlarged secretory regions in upper regions. The basal cytoplasm of glandular cells is associated with the fibro-vascular tunic of the epithelial gland. It is thought that the secretion of this gland adds to ink-jets and contributes to minimize water turbulences and facilitate the dynamic of the ink clouds ejected in the water during escape behavior (Derby 2014).

4.7.3 The Arms and Tentacles (Figs. 4.5 and 4.6)

Cephalopods bear a characteristic crown of highly mobile elongated fleshy appendages (eight arms and, in squid and cuttlefish, two tentacles). These appendages are arranged around the mouth and are essential for feeding. These cephalopod appendages, together with the siphon, are derived from the embryonic foot. The arms are thicker basally and taper toward the tip. Transverse sections of the arm shaft show a large cylindrical mass of muscle fibers and connective tissue around an axis formed of a ganglionic nerve cord (see below). The large central circular or ovoidal

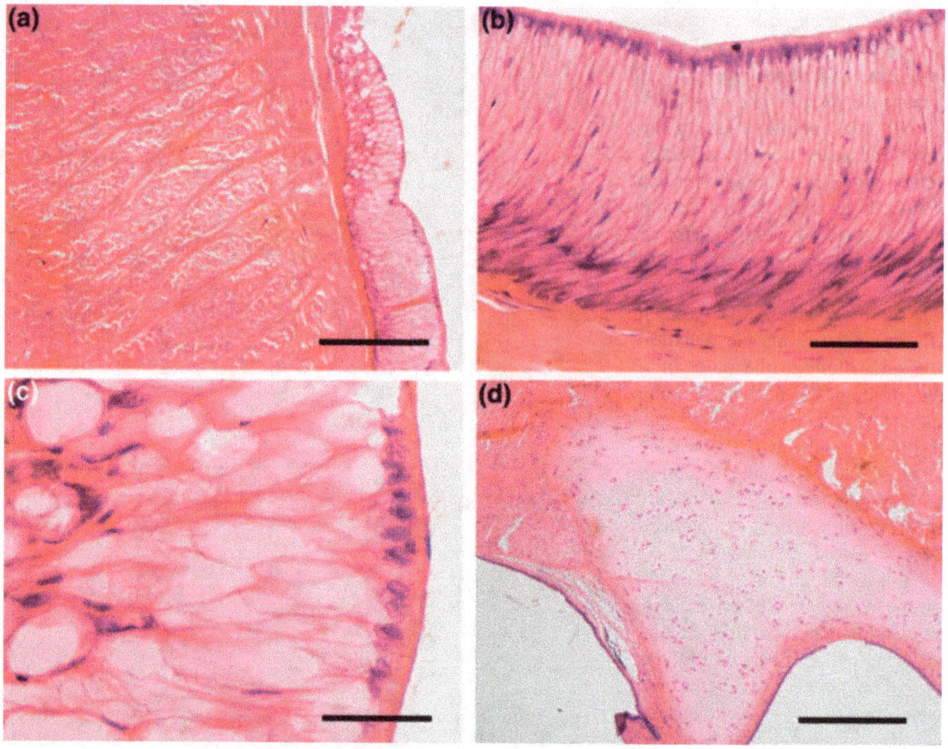

Fig. 4.4 **a** Section of the squid funnel showing the thick muscle layers and the funnel organ. **b**, **c** Photomicrographs of the funnel organ showing details of the thick glandular epithelium. Note the large mucous cells basally located and the small non-glandular cells apically. **d** Section of the funnel passing through the funnel cartilage forming part of the closure organ. H&E stain. *Scale bars* **a** 500 μm; **b** 100 μm; **c** 50 μm

muscle mass of octopus consists of a number of transverse muscular fibers organized in bundles crossed in various directions oriented more or less radially and extending peripherally as muscle trabeculae intercalated with bundles of compact longitudinal muscle fibers arranged in four sectors. This central region is surrounded by thinner bands of oblique (helical) muscle fibers and longitudinal muscle fibers surrounded by a layer of circular muscle fibers. Trabeculae of connective tissue accompany bundles of muscles. For further details of the octopus arm organization, see Kier and Stella (2007). Along the inner side surface (facing toward the mouth), they bear numerous suckers on thin peduncles (decapods) or sessile suckers (two alternate rows in octopus). Muscular bands join these stalked of sessile suckers to the shaft musculature. The shaft is also connected to protective membranes, lateral flaps flanking the sucker region and swimming keels by muscle bands. These lateral membranes contribute to the hydrodynamic properties of squid facilitating arm cohesion and forward or backward swimming and steering. During squid swimming, the arms are pressed together and enclose the tentacles. The fourth ventral pair of arms of cuttlefish bears prominent lateral flaps.

The pair of tentacles found in squid and cuttlefish are modified 4th pair appendages inserted in a pocket between the arm pairs III and IV (the fifth ventral arm of decapods is named as arm IV). Tentacles consist of a long, highly protractible shaft ending in a dilation or club armed with suckers and a terminal region. They are able of considerable fast extension and contraction and are used for prey capture. The shaft shows the axial nerve cord with thick nerve fibers (see below) surrounded by a large mass of crossed bands of transverse muscle fibers, whereas bands of longitudinal muscles in the periphery are small and separated by transverse muscle bands. Thin circular and helical layers of muscle fibers surround the large central muscular mass. Interestingly, the transverse and circular muscle fibers of the tentacular shaft are thin and cross-striated. Unlike oblique-striated fibers, ultrastructural observations reveal that the contractile material is organized in short sarcomeres with thick myosin myofilaments of only about 1 μm long, but this is inappreciable with the conventional light microscopy methods used here. The functional properties of these cross-striated fibers differ dramatically from those of oblique-striated fibers and exhibit contraction curves about ten times faster than the other arm muscles. For additional information on the functional organization of muscles of cephalopod arms and tentacles, see Kier and Curtin (2002) and Kier (2016).

The suckers are muscular suction cups on arms and tentacles used in feeding and other functions. The arms and suckers grow continuously, and new suckers are added to the growing apex. The size of suckers decreases toward the arm tip. In octopus, the suckers are symmetrical protrusions and consist of a muscular cup-shaped acetabulum joined to a flattened distal ring, the infundibulum, which is the surface that attaches to the substrate. Suckers are attached to the arm

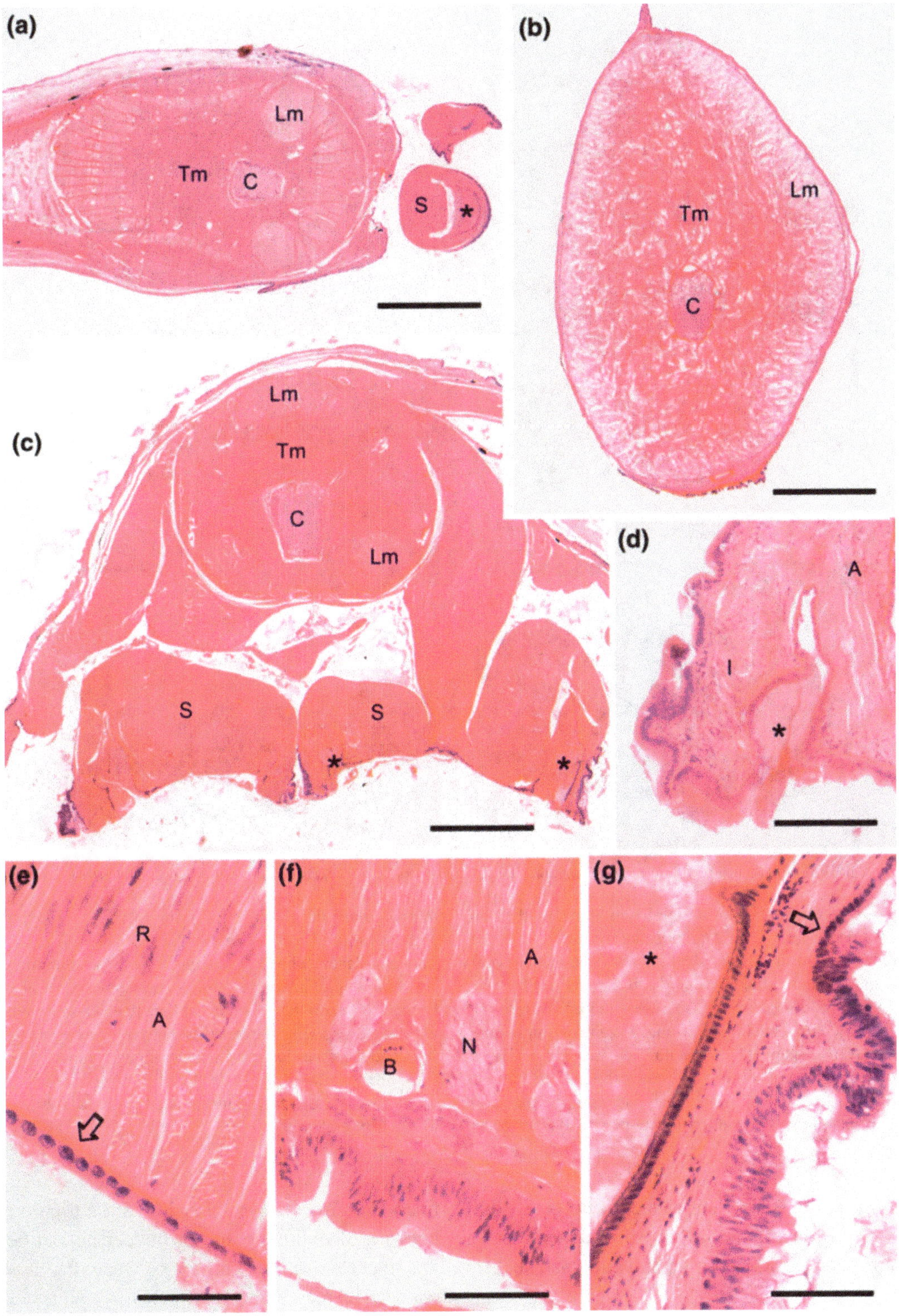

Fig. 4.5 Transverse sections of a squid arm (**a**), tentacle (**b**) and tentacle club (**c**) showing their different appearances. In **a** and **c,** suckers (S) are visible. Note in C the long pedicle joining the suckers to the club and lateral protective membranes. C, nerve cord; Lm, longitudinal muscle; Tm, transverse muscle. **d** Detail of the base of the acetabulum (A) separated by a groove from the infundibulum (I) of a club sucker. **e** Detail of the acetabulum outer surface showing the insertion of radial muscle fibers (R) in the fascia (outlined arrow) that is just below the epidermis with cuboid cells. **f** Detail of the central region of the acetabulum showing the insertion of pedicular muscles in the fascia below a thickened epithelium. N, nerves; B, blood vessel. **g** Detail of the border between the acetabulum (A) and infundibulum (I) showing the secretory epithelium producing the ring teeth (star) at left, and the sharp transition between skin zones (outlined arrow). Stars in **a**, **c**, **d**, **g** indicate the ring teeth. H&E stain. *Scale bars* **a**, **b** 1.2 mm; **c** 1 mm; **d** 200 μm; **e** 50 μm; **f**, **g**, 100 μm

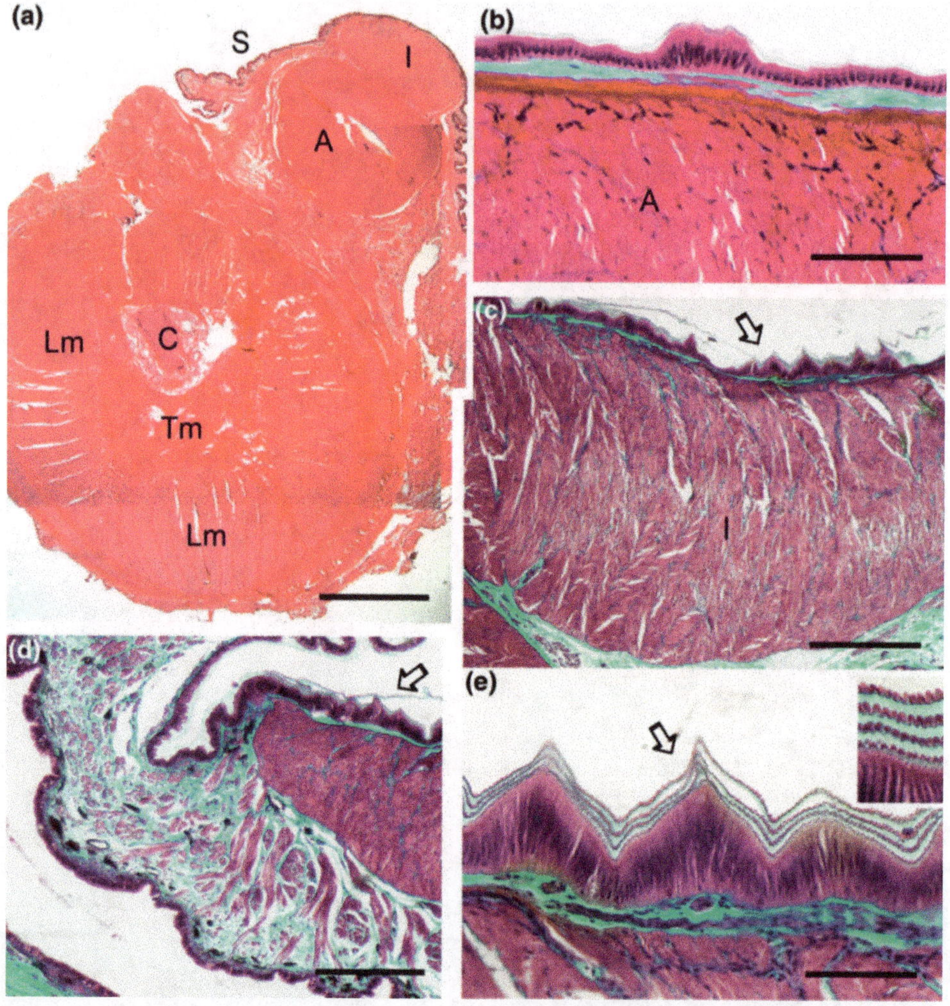

Fig. 4.6 **a** Transverse sections of an octopus arm showing the core muscles around the nerve cord (C) and the non-stalked base of a sucker (S). The sucker is sectioned marginally showing the thick muscle walls of the acetabulum (A) and infundibulum (I). **b** Lateral wall of the acetabulum showing the complex fascia between the epithelium and muscles. Only a very thin cuticle covers the acetabular epithelium, which shows occasional papillae. **c** Section of the infundibulum showing the papillae of the epithelium (outlined arrow). Muscle bands with different orientation (radial, meridional and circular) are also appreciable. The acetabulum is at the left low corner. **d** Border of the infundibulum showing the transition of the papillae to the normal skin with chromatophores. Note the thick dermis traversed by thin muscle fiber bundles which are in contrast with thick infundibular muscle wall. **e** Detail of infundibular epithelial papillae covered of a cuticular layer formed of two different types of lamellae. The inset shows a detail of the cuticle showing the relation between apical borders of epithelial cells and the inner lamella with small pegs. Superficial lamellae appear to be seeded out easily (note detached lamellae in **c** and **d**). A, H&E stain. **b–e**, Masson's trichrome. *Scale bars* **a** 1.2 mm; **b** 100 μm; **c**, **d** 200 μm; **e** 50 μm

or tentacle club via a stalk. The attachment is a short cylindrical basal region in octopus (sessile suckers), but a conical and elongated pedicle in squid and cuttlefish suckers (stalked).

Histological sections of octopus suckers show the acetabulum and infundibulum formed of the thick-walled intrinsic sucker musculature, which is separated from other external tissues by a continuous connective fascia. In the acetabulum (sucker chamber), most muscle fibers extend radially between the outer and inner connective membranes or fasciae, but bundles of meridional (oriented toward the communication with the infundibulum) and circular muscle fibers are also visible. After Masson's trichrome staining, a network of oblique collagen trabeculae can be observed in this muscle wall extending between the inner and outer connective membranes and accompanying radial fibers. At the junction with the infundibulum, there are sphincters with numerous circular muscle fibers. In the thick muscle wall of the infundibulum, there are radial, meridional and circular muscle fibers.

In the acetabulum, a poorly specialized cuboidal epithelium bearing scarce small papillae covers the inner connective layer. Instead, the inner surface of the infundibulum is covered by a papillary epidermis consisting of tall epithelial cells arranged in conical papillae or denticles. The epithelial surface is covered of a thick cuticular layer formed of thin alternate laminae of small pegs and amorphous material, which exhibit different staining affinities with the Masson's trichrome stain. Pegs and amorphous material are secreted by tall epithelial cells, and the presence of alternate layers suggests a cyclical renewal of the adhesive surface. At the rim around the papillary surface of the infundibulum, over the end of the thick muscular wall, the papillae and pegs disappear and the surface of the epidermis is only covered of amorphous cuticular material. This cuticle disappears at the transition with the normal epidermis. The suckers are highly specialized for anchoring to a number of substrates and preys. Combined actions of the acetabular and infundibular muscles together with the properties of the infundibular surface provide the basis for the adhesion. For details on the structure and adhesion mechanisms of octopus suckers, see Tramacere et al. (2013, 2014). Below the acetabulum, a musculo-connective region connects the arm and sucker. Numerous muscle bundles of the acetabulo-brachial extrinsic musculature allow the directional extension and retraction of the sucker. A detailed description of the extrinsic acetabulo-brachial muscles of octopus suckers along the arm, arm muscles, and interbrachial muscles is found in Guérin (1908).

In squid and cuttlefish arms and tentacles, the stalked suckers exhibit striking differences with those of octopus. Vertical sections of the sucker show a pedicular muscle that enters through the central roof of the acetabulum and inserts in a thick connective fascia just below the epithelium of the roof, which is unlike the octopus acetabulum (Guérin 1908). The thickened muscle walls of the acetabulum surround this pedicular insertion, being separated by connective tissue. The junction between the infundibulum and acetabulum is wide, unlike in octopus suckers. Moreover, the epithelium of the inner surface of the infundibulum secretes a thick hard annular material known as sucker ring teeth, which lacks in octopus suckers. The ring teeth perform grappling functions during prey capture. Recent studies reveal that the characteristic and mechanically robust ring teeth are formed of a new family of proteins named suckerins, and lack chitin. Suckerins self-assemble into a unique type of supramolecular protein network mechanically reinforced by β-sheets and are embedded in an amorphous matrix (Guerette et al. 2014; Ding et al. 2014; Hiew et al. 2016). In the outer rim of the infundibulum, there is a toothed cuticular epithelium of tall cells covered of cuticular material that is probably related with sensory neurons. It is followed of a region of folded and thickened epidermis with mucous glandular cells. The external skin of the sucker is mostly formed of a smooth cuboidal or flattened epithelium directly attached to the connective fascia surrounding sucker muscles, without any loose connective tissue separating it from the sucker muscles, which is unlike the complex skin and muscle bundles of the basis of suckers found in octopus. The suckers of decapod arms and tentacles are generally asymmetric. In the tentacular club, numerous and simple small suckers lacking distinction between the acetabulum and infundibulum are found adjacent to the large suckers.

4.8 The Digestive System (Figs. 4.7, 4.8, 4.9, 4.10, 4.11, 4.12, 4.13 and 4.14)

Cephalopods are highly evolved carnivorous mollusks that pursue and capture prey as crustaceans, fish or other cephalopods using arms and tentacles. Their digestive system (gut) is highly developed and consists of the alimentary canal formed of specialized compartments united by tubular parts. In the coleoids studied in this atlas, the alimentary canal starts in a mouth opening in the large buccal mass. It bears two mandibles or beaks and a radula moved by a complex muscular system and distal parts of salivary glands. The mouth is surrounded by lips (buccal funnel) and the arm apparatus. The arms capture and present prey to feed. A feature of cephalopods is that the esophagus runs through the brain, so the prey must be reduced to fragments by the buccal mass before swallowing. Below the buccal mass, the esophagus allows food to pass to a stomach that is united to a large digestive gland and a caecum, and a thick short intestine continues the system to the anus. Specialized salivary glands accompany the esophagus, their conducts coursing to the buccal mass. Anatomical differences in the digestive system are noted among the three species illustrated here (see Boucaud-Camou and Boucher-Rodoni 1983). For instance, in octopus a crop separates the esophagus into proximal and distal parts, and in cuttlefish, the digestive gland is paired.

4.8.1 The Buccal Mass (Buccal Bulb, Pharynx)

The buccal mass is a complex structure surrounded by the buccal and peristomial membranes or lips that comprises a pair of strong, chitinous beaks moved by large muscles, a radular apparatus associated with the buccal cavity, the intrinsic mandibular and radular musculature and nerves, salivary glands and papilla. For a detailed description of the complex anatomy of the buccal mass of squid, including muscles, jaws, radula and glands, the reader is directed to

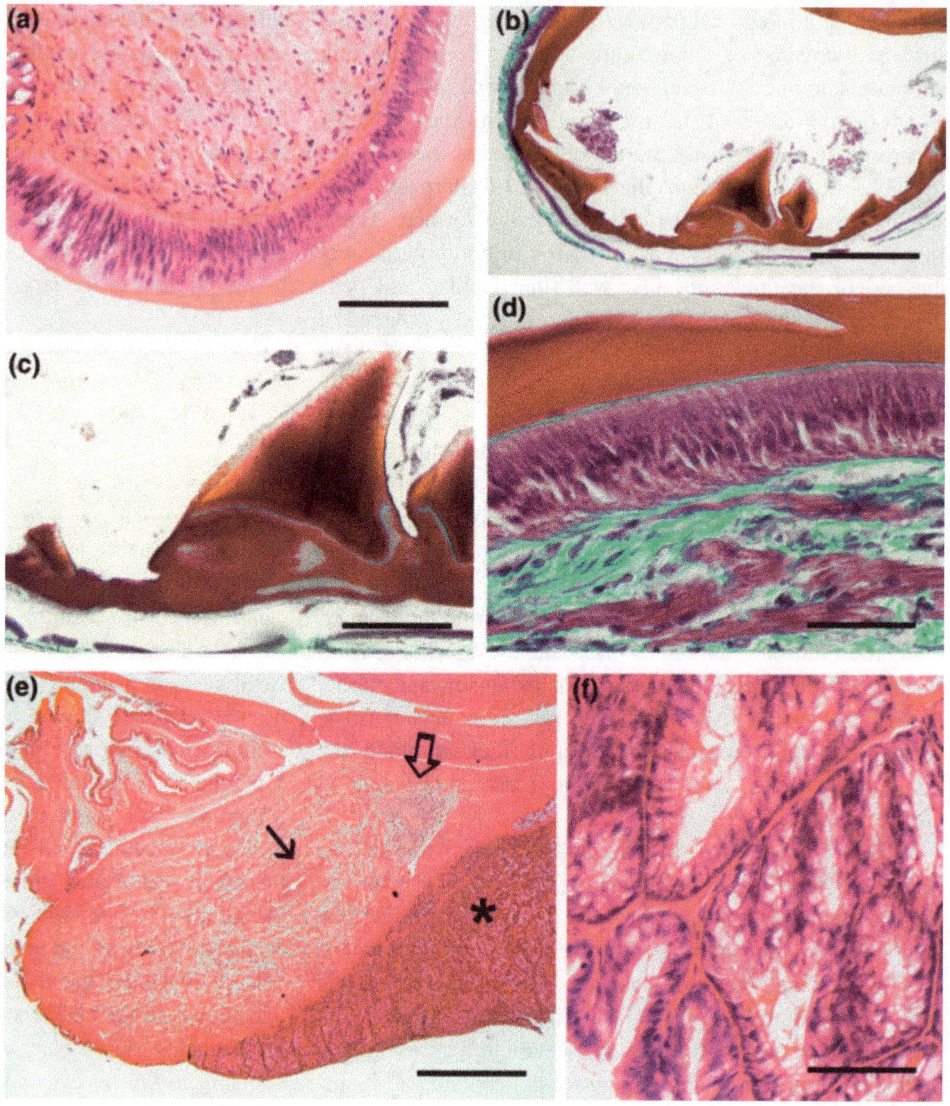

Fig. 4.7 MA1. Sections of the buccal mass of cuttlefish and octopus. **a** Section through the base of a beak wing showing the thick epithelium of beccublasts and the growth of the beak thickness away from this initial region. **b** Section of a portion of the invaginated radular sac of octopus showing the lamina with radular teeth. **c** Detail of a radular tooth united to the lamina. **d** Section showing the tall odontoblasts sinthesizing radular structures. **e** Section of the buccal mass of an octopus passing through the salivary papilla and the large submandibular salivary gland (star). The arrow points to the salivary duct and the outlined arrow to the subradular ganglion. **f** Detail of the mucous secretory epithelium of the submandibular gland. **a**, **e**, **f** H&E stain; **b**–**d** Masson's trichrome. *Scale bars* **a** 100 µm; **b** 0.5 mm; **c** 200 µm; **d**, **f** 50 µm; **e** 1.2 mm

Williams (1909). The functional organization of beak muscles of octopus was studied by Uyeno and Kier (2005). In the following, we only describe the histology of some most characteristic structures including beaks, radula and salivary glands.

4.8.2 Beaks

The mandibles, beaks, or jaws resemble a parrot's beak inverted. The upper mandible is longer, straighter, and more compressed than the lower which is strongly convex and closes outside the upper jaw (Williams 1909). Each mandible is formed of two wide and transparent soft chitinous basal plates or wings, which extend apically in a progressively much harder tip or rostrum that forms the cutting edge, where they are generally brownish-black. In histological sections, adult beaks appear frequently broken or separated from the epithelium. The beaks are formed by and lye on a specialized beak-forming epithelium consisting of tall epithelial cells that secrete chitin and proteins, often called beccublasts (Dilly and Nixon 1976). The beccublasts are very tall at the basis of the beak and decrease progressively in height toward apical regions, whereas the beak plate is thin near the basal border and increases considerably its thickness toward the rostrum. The jaws grow constantly by additions to their margins and to their unexposed surfaces. Away from the alar border, the sections of the beak plate (at least in cuttlefish) show two different regions, the distal one that is continuous with that early appearing at the basis and an inner one over beccublasts that shows a different staining with general histological methods. A recent biochemical study in octopus has shown that the hydration, hardening and protein composition of the beak changes from

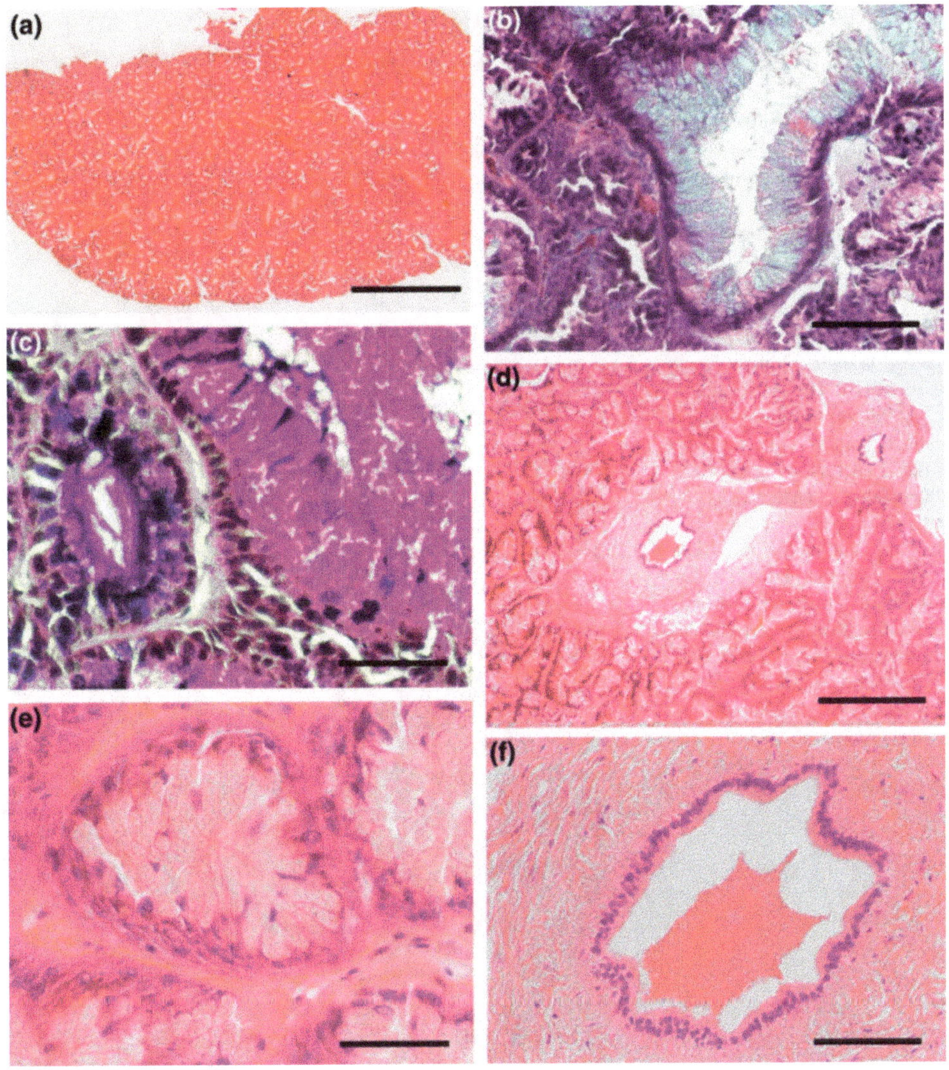

Fig. 4.8 D1. Sections of the anterior salivary gland of octopus (**a**–**c**) and the posterior salivary gland of cuttlefish (**d**–**f**). **a** Panoramic view showing the branched secretory tubules. **b** and **c** Secretory portions mainly consist of mucous gland cells that stain pale blue (**b**) or pink (**c**) with the Masson's trichrome and the PAS method, respectively. **d** Panoramic view of the cuttlefish glandular tissue showing its branched tubular organization. **e** Detail of the mucous cells of glandular tubules. **f** Section of a glandular duct showing the tall epithelium and the thick musculo-connective wall. **a**, **d**–**f** H&E; **b** Masson's trichrome; **c** PAS method. *Scale bars* **a** 1 mm; **b**, **c**, **e** 50 μm; **f** 100 μm; **d** 500 μm

the base to the apex. In soft basal parts, there are proteins belonging to the chitin-binding protein family joined to chitin, whereas in harder apical parts appear proteins of the highly modular histidine-rich protein family (Tan et al. 2015). Mandibular muscles are inserted on the basement connective lamina of the beccublast epithelium (Dilly and Nixon 1976).

4.8.3 The Radular Apparatus

The radular apparatus is an eversible buccal structure comprised of the radula and various associated structures. The cephalopod radula consists of a long chitinous membrane with regularly attached teeth arranged in transverse rows, which is better appreciated in dissected and macerated radulas (Messenger and Young 1999). It is lodged in a radular canal that emerges from the radular sac located in the median line. Radular teeth are formed by a set of elongate cells with apical microvilli, the odontoblasts. These cells are organized in two layers, the outer cells producing the radular membrane and the bases of the teeth, and the inner ones producing the cusps. The membrane extends laterally in the hyaline shield covering the cavity in which the retracted radula is lodged. The odontoblasts also secrete the hyaline shield. A subradular connective lamina is intercalated between odontoblasts and muscles. Histological sections of octopus show some details of the radula as the composite origin of teeth, the tall cuticle-secreting odontoblasts and the connective tissue of the subradular membrane. A pair of large protractor muscles (bolster rods), together with the retractor muscles, moves the radula away of and toward the sac allowing to rake food into the pharynx. The radular muscles are innervated by the inferior buccal ganglion (Young 1971). For further details of the anatomy of the radular complex of squid and octopus, the reader is directed to the studies of Williams (1909) and Messenger and Young (1999).

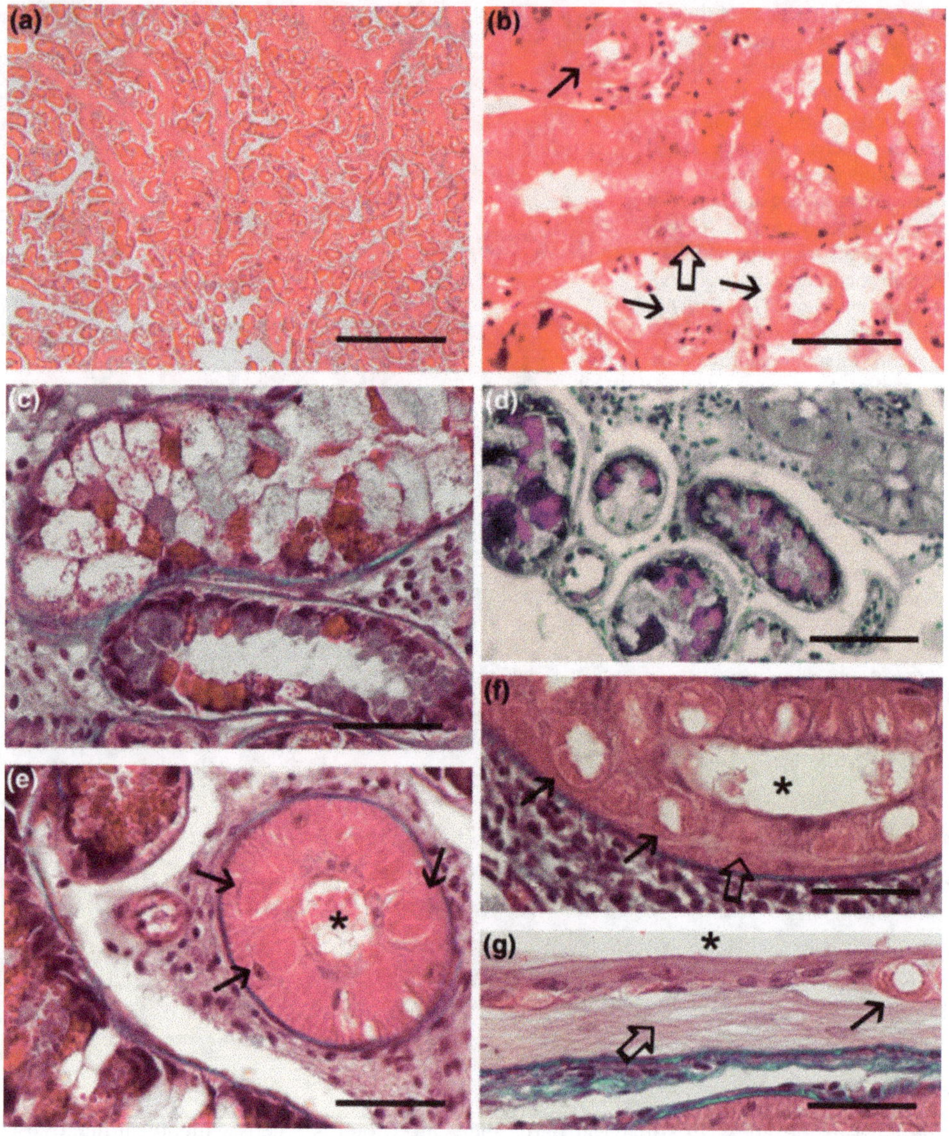

Fig. 4.9 D2. Sections of the posterior salivary (venom) gland of octopus. **a** Panoramic view showing the loose organization of branched glandular tubules and striated ducts. **b** Section showing the transition of the striated duct to the glandular tubule (outlined arrow). Numerous small blood vessels are also observed (thin arrows). **c** Glandular region showing cells with pale secretion granules and cells with brightly stained granules. Masson's trichrome. **d** The PAS method stains in purple some glandular cells. **e** Transverse section of a striated duct showing the characteristic "cistern cells" (thin arrows). **f, g** Longitudinal sections of a striated duct (**f**) and one side of a larger duct showing cistern cells (thin arrows) and nerve fibers into the epithelium (outlined arrows). In **e–g,** stars indicate the duct lumen. **a, b** H&E; **c, e–g** Masson's trichrome; **d** PAS method. *Scale bars* **a** 1 mm; **b, c, e–g** 50 μm; **d** 100 μm

4.8.4 The Salivary Glands (Figs. 4.8 and 4.9)

Three types of salivary glands secrete different substances in the buccal mass region contributing to the first phases of feeding including killing preys. These are the submandibular gland and the paired anterior and posterior salivary glands.

The submandibular gland consists of a series of invaginated glandular tubules separated by connective-vascular septa that form a rather compact mass around a central canal lined by the same type of epithelium. In section of octopus glands stained with H&E, the glandular tubules show differentiated apical and basal (terminal) regions. The apical part consists of a columnar epithelium formed of large mucous (goblet) glandular cells with basal nuclei and cytoplasm mostly filled of pale granules and, among goblet cells, slender supporting epithelial cells with the nucleus in subapical location. In the basal part of glandular tubules, goblet cells are replaced by shorter glandular cells filled of eosinophilic granules in the supranuclear cytoplasm. Supporting cells are also found among glandular cells. In cuttlefish, the submandibular gland also exhibits goblet cells and granular eosinophilic cells, together with supporting cells, but goblet cells do not form a massive layer.

4.8.5 Anterior Salivary Gland

In octopus, the paired anterior salivary glands are located just behind the buccal mass. These glands produce abundant mucus. In H&E-stained histological sections, the gland appears as a compact mass formed of numerous epithelio-glandular tubules with a thin connective-vascular layer

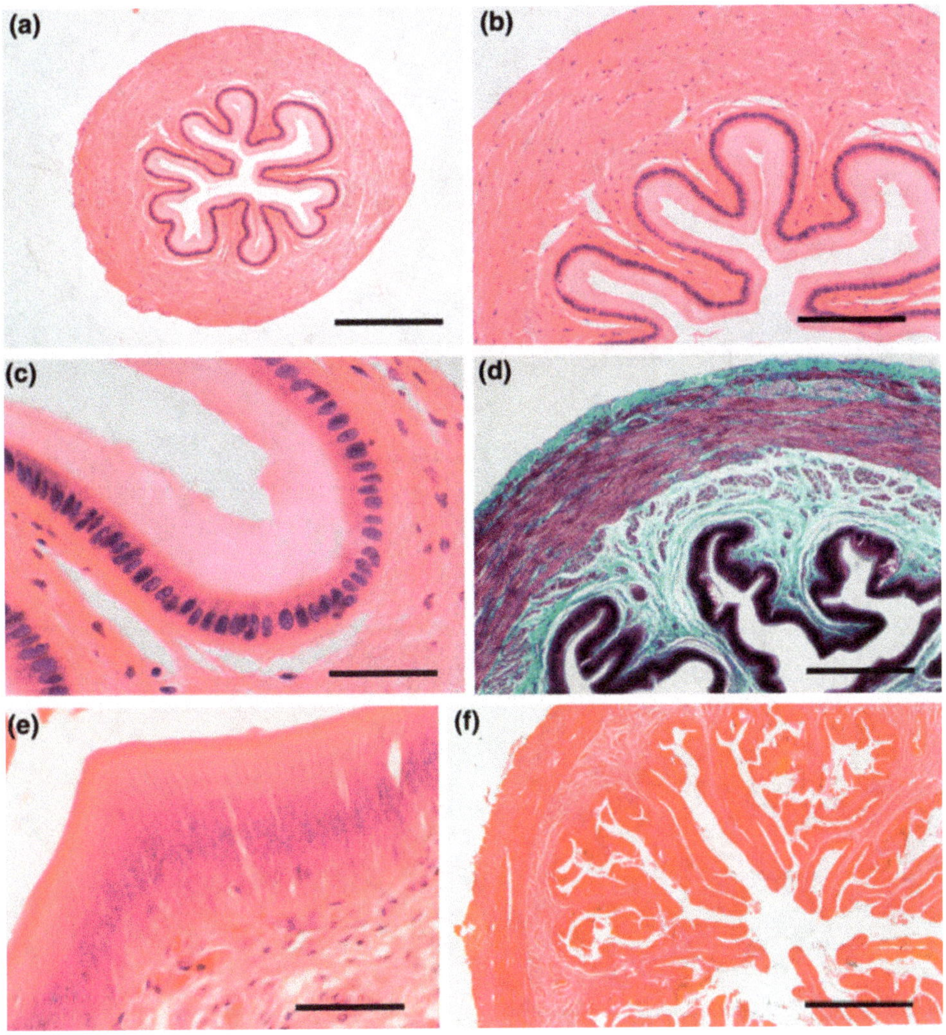

Fig. 4.10 D3. Transverse sections of esophagus and crop. **a** Section of the squid esophagus showing the thick muscle layers surrounding the folded mucosa. **b**, **c** Details of the muscular wall and the low prismatic epithelium showing a thick cuticle-like layer. **d** Esophagus of octopus stained with the Masson's trichrome. Note the abundant connective tissue and scarcity of muscle fibers in the submucosa and mucosal folds more complex than in squid. **e** Detail of the mucosa of octopus esophagus showing the tall cylindrical epithelium and the thin cuticle. **f** Section of the crop of octopus showing the long and complex folds of mucosa. **a–c**, **e–f** H&E stain. *Scale bars* A, 0.5 mm; **b**, **d** 200 µm; **c**, **e** 50 µm; **f** 1.2 mm

surrounding them. Two types of tubules can be distinguished attending to the appearance of glandular cells. Proximal (toward the ends) parts of tubules show columnar cells with basal rounded nuclei surrounded by basophilic cytoplasm and apical cytoplasm filled of small basophilic granules. Distal tubules are coarser and show a higher glandular epithelium with numerous condensed small nuclei basally and a wide cytoplasm mass filled of eosinophilic granules in which lateral limits between cells are hardly appreciable under light microscopy. The thickest intraglandular ducts show the same type of glandular epithelium.

4.8.6 Posterior Salivary Glands (Poisonous Gland, Venom Gland)

The posterior salivary glands of coleoids lie dorsal to the mantle cavity behind the cranium. These glands secrete mixtures of proteins and other substances that are toxic for other animals (Ruder et al. 2013). In cuttlefish, the posterior salivary gland is a massive branched tubular gland with abundant dense connective-vascular tissue among the glandular tubules. Unlike octopus, these glandular tubules show a homogeneous appearance along the gland. The epithelial wall consists of tall columnar glandular cells with basophilic basal cytoplasm including the nucleus and a wide apical region filled of small pale granules, possibly mucous. Among these cells, there are also thin supporting cells with condensed nuclei located subapically. The main duct of the posterior salivary gland of cuttlefish is lined by a short columnar non-glandular epithelium with abundant cell nuclei located at middle heights. This duct is surrounded by abundant circular muscle fibers.

In octopus, the posterior salivary gland consists of branched tubules embedded in a translucent matrix, with two types of tubules, secretory (A) and striated (B), which are continuous. The spaces among tubules are filled of loose connective-vascular tissue. The distal A tubules are clearly

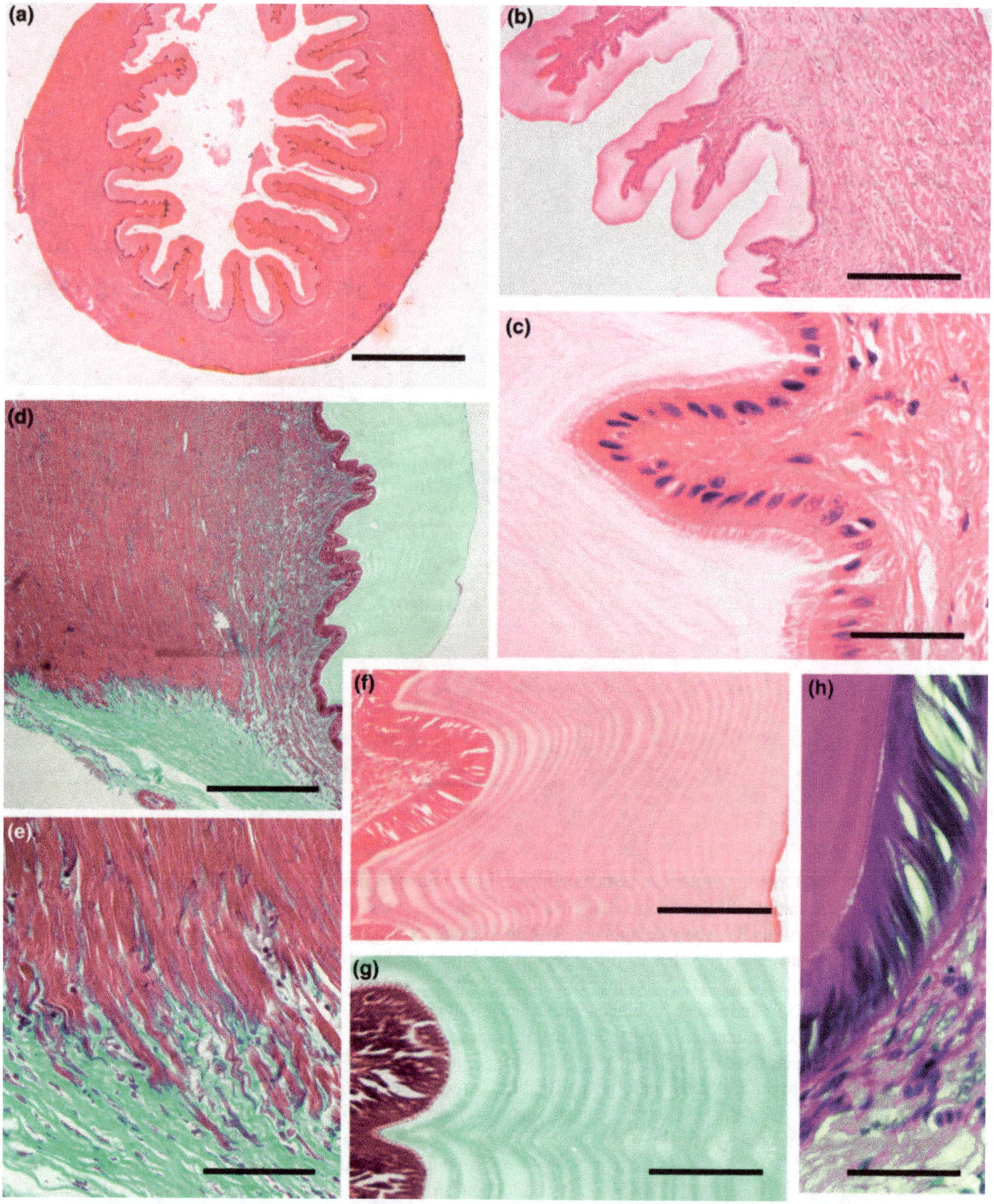

Fig. 4.11 Transverse sections of stomach. **a–c** Sections of squid stomach showing the muscular wall, the pleated mucosa and the thick cuticle. In **c,** note long microvillous appendages in the surface of epithelial cells. **d–h** Sections through one of the paired central pads of the octopus stomach showing the insertion of the much thickened muscle layers in the thick collagenous fascia joining both sides (**d** and **e**). Note also in **d** the thick submucosa and the small epithelial folds. **f–h** Details of the differential staining showing the multilayered cuticle. **a–c** and **f** H&E staining, **d**, **e**, **g** Masson's trichrome, **h** PAS method. *Scale bars* **a** 1 mm; **b** 500 μm; **c**, **g**, **h** 50 μm; **d** 0.7 mm; **f** 100 μm

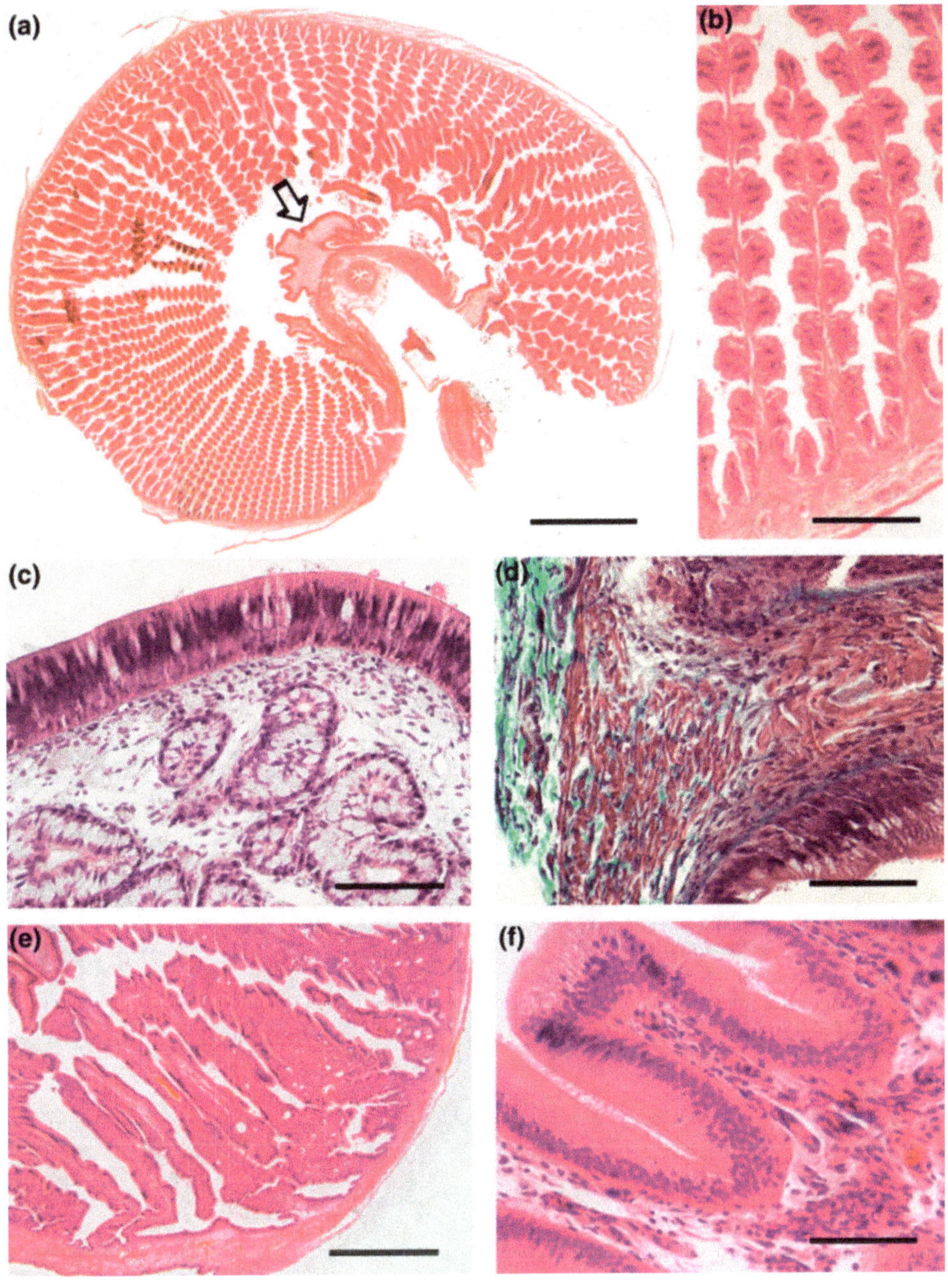

Fig. 4.12 Sections of the caecum of octopus (**a**–**d**) and cuttlefish (**e**, **f**). **a** Panoramic view of a transverse section showing the spiral organization of primary and secondary caecal leafs around the columella (outlined arrow). Note the counterclockwise diminution of the size of leafs and the alternate arrangement of long and short lamellae. **b** Detail of lamellae of the caecum showing the lateral leaflets mostly consisting of high ciliated epithelium. **c** Section passing through the apex of a primary lamella showing the mucous tubular glands and the tall epithelium. **d** Detail of the base of a leaf showing muscle fibers entering in the axis. **e** Section of the caecum of cuttlefish showing leafs with leaflets. **f** Detail of the tall ciliated epithelium covering the leaflets. **a**, **b** and **e**, **f** H&E; **c**, **d** Masson's trichrome. *Scale bars* **a**, **e** 500 μm; **b** 200 μm; **c**, **d**, **f** 100 μm

glandular and show at least two types of glandular cells whose cytoplasm appears either bluish (basophilic) or orange (strongly eosinophilic) with the H&E-staining method. Distal A tubules mostly consist of eosinophilic columnar gland cells that are short or very short in the thin terminal regions, whereas more proximally the epithelium consists of mixed basophilic and eosinophilic cells. The glandular epithelium is continuous with the striated tubules, with a sharp transition between them. In the striated tubules, three types of cell were reported using electron microscopy, striated cells, cistern cells and lumen-lining cells (Matus 1971). The striated cells show a wide basal eosinophilic cytoplasm of striated appearance with nuclei inside. The cytoplasmic striations are better observed in transverse sections of these tubules. Ultrastructural studies in octopus reveal numerous basal infoldings of these cells containing mitochondria and canaliculi, as well as an apical brush border, which reminds the striated ducts of mammalian salivary glands. Cistern cells are rather conspicuous in light microscopy sections, because of their spherical shape, striated cytoplasm and hollow apical region. These cells are surrounded apically by flattened supporting (lining) cells with nuclei located apically. This glandular portion is thought to be involved in active ion transport and excretion. In tangential sections to the two types of tubules, it can be appreciated the presence of a layer of flattened thin muscle fibers surrounding the epithelial tubules,

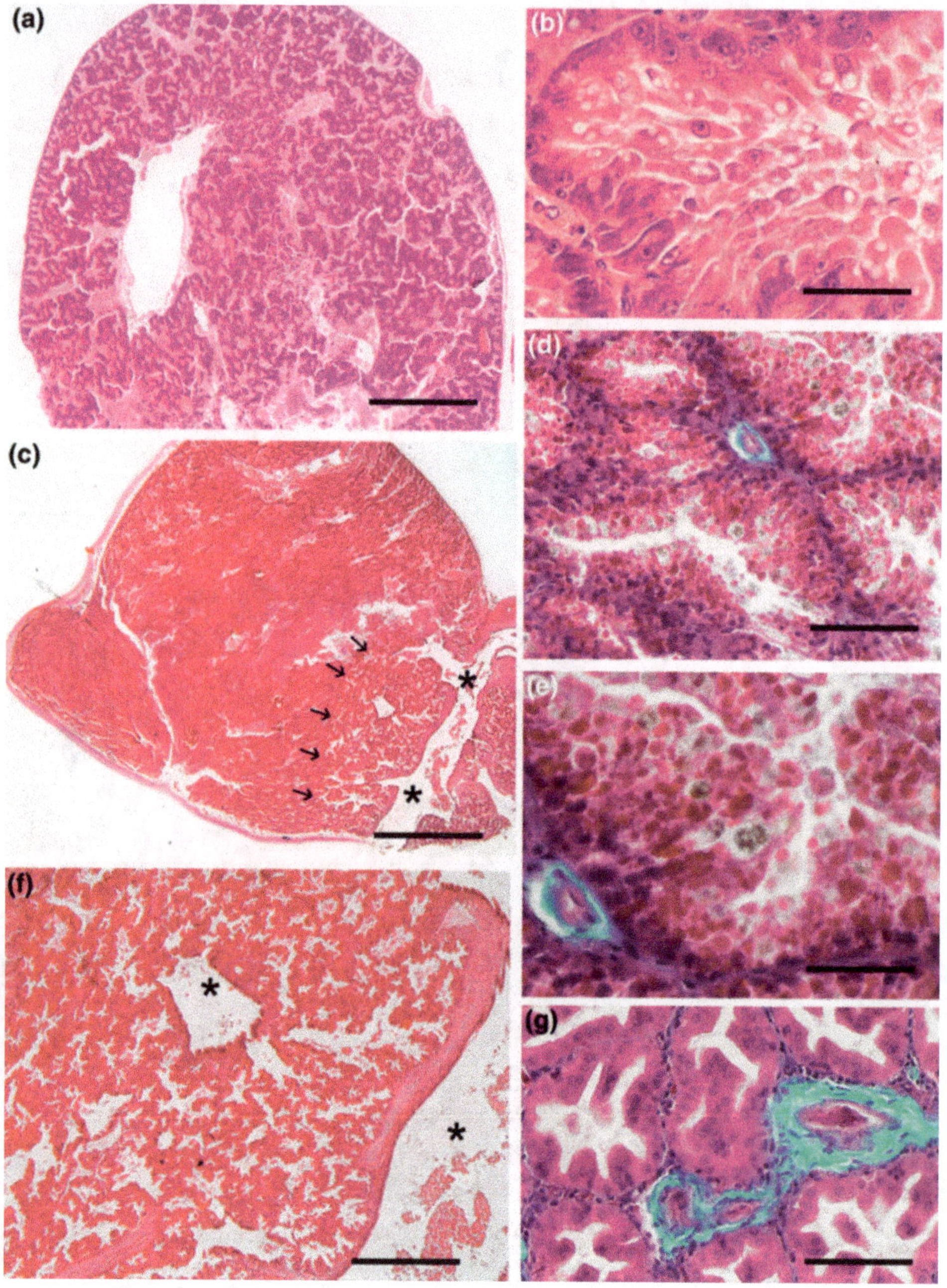

Fig. 4.13 Sections of the digestive gland of squid (**a**, **b**) and octopus (**c–g**). **a** panoramic view showing branched glandular tubules open to a large conduct. **b** Section showing the complex appearance of the digestive gland cells, which appear to form extensions of cytoplasm toward the central region. **c** Panoramic view showing the two sectors of the octopus digestive gland, main and accessory (limit indicated by arrows). In the low right corner, the accessory gland tubules are open to the branched duct of the gland (asterisks). **d–e** Portions of the main digestive gland stained with Masson's trichrome showing the complex appearance of gland cell cytoplasm, with granules of various appearances. Note also the vasculo-connective cords among acinar units. **f** Section of the accessory digestive gland showing the branched system of tubules converging on larger ducts. **g** Detail of the secretory units of the accessory digestive gland showing the complex star-shaped aspect of the inner cavity and the homogeneous appearance of gland cell cytoplasm. Note the vasculo-connective cords. **a–c** and **f** H&E; **d**, **e**, **g** Masson's trichrome. *Scale bars* **a** 0.8 mm; **b**, **e**, **g** 50 μm; **c** 1.2 mm; **d** 100 μm; **f** 300 μm

which reminds the myoepithelial cells in mammalian glands. The gland receives rich nerve supply from the superior buccal lobe whose integrity is necessary to poison a crab after catching it (Young 1965). Nerve bundles enter the wall of proximal striated tubules and can be observed coursing along the basal region of the epithelium (Matus 1971).

4.8.7 Esophagus and Crop (Fig. 4.10)

The pharynx is continuous with the esophagus that, at the level of the cranium, is surrounded by the brain masses, and that is accompanied by large vessels. In cuttlefish and squid, the esophagus shows a pleated mucosa and submucosa surrounded by muscular layers. The epithelium consists of columnar cells covered of a thick cuticle layer. The mucosa lays over a thick submucosa and three muscle layers with different fiber orientations. The inner muscular layer is thin and consists of longitudinally oriented muscle fibers, whereas the outer layer is thicker and consists of circular muscle. In octopus, the folds of the wall of esophagus are long and thick, and its epithelium is much thicker than in squid and cuttlefish, showing taller and thinner cells. The octopus esophagus only exhibits a thin cuticular layer.

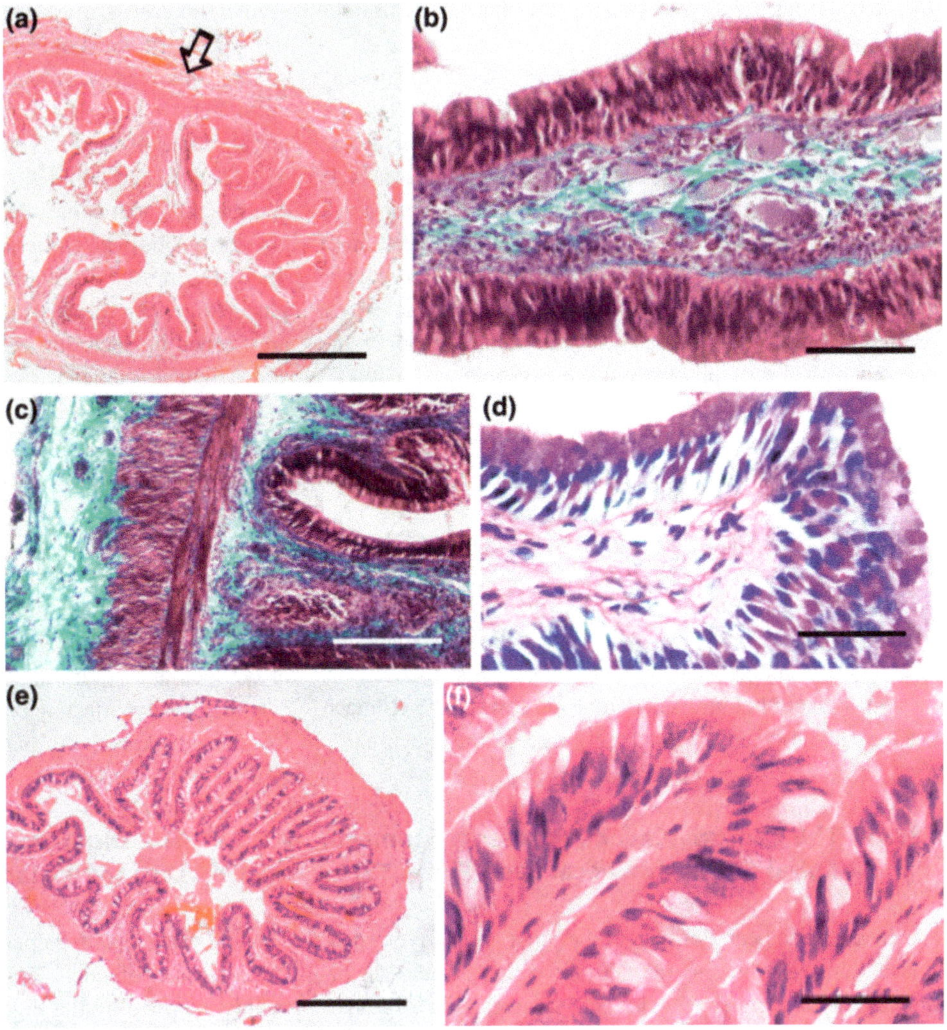

Fig. 4.14 Transverse sections of the octopus (**a–d**) and squid intestine (**e–f**). **a** Panoramic view showing the folds of the mucosa including the two pairs of typhlosoles flanking the bilateral plane of symmetry (outlined arrow). **b** Detail of a fold of the mucosa showing the rich vasculo-connective submucosa. **c** Detail showing the layers of circular and longitudinal muscle fibers between the submucosa and the outer connective layers. **d** The PAS method stains numerous mucous goblet cells in the intestine mucosa. **e** Section of the squid intestine. Note the lack of typhlosolis. **f** Detail of a fold of the mucosa. Note the scarce submucosa. **a**, **e**, **f** H&E; **b**, **c** Masson's trichrome; **d** PAS. *Scale bars* **a** 0.8 mm; **b**, **d**, **f** 50 µm; **c** 100 µm; **e** 500 µm

The submucosa is thick and the three muscular layers are looser arranged than in the other two species.

In octopus, but not in cuttlefish and squid, a dilated crop follows the postcranial esophagus. The crop histology is similar to that of the octopus esophagus, but the folds of the inner wall are longer and often branched. It is covered of a similar thick epithelium with thin cuticle, without glandular cells, but the submucosa and muscle layers are thicker than in the esophagus. Thus, the octopus crop forms a very expandable part of the esophagus. Peristaltic movements of the crop have been reported "in vivo" with ultrasound sonographic scannings.

4.8.8 Stomach (Fig. 4.11)

The void stomach of squid and cuttlefish shows a deeply folded inner surface, whereas the outer surface is rather smooth. The folds of the stomach wall consist of a mucosa covered by a very thick chitinous cuticular layer and the submucosa. Unlike the esophagus, the epithelium of the squid and cuttlefish stomach shows a tortuous profile and consists of a single type of cell. The short columnar epithelial cells have their nuclei at intermediate levels and apical and basal cytoplasm with different appearances. The basal cytoplasm has a striated appearance, which is typical of transporting epithelia. The apical cytoplasm is homogeneous and is covered of a conspicuous microvillous-like layer (brush border) and the thick cuticle. These cells secrete a chitinous cuticle that is PAS positive and consists of a number of thin lamellae parallel to the epithelium surface. The submucosa contains both connective and muscular tissues and is continuous with the inner layer of the muscular tunica, which consists of longitudinal muscle fibers. The thicker outer layer of the muscle tunica consists of circular muscle fibers. The outer surface is covered of thin and pleated epithelium that lays over connective tissue. The organization of the different layers allows the dilation of the stomach during feeding and suggests that the chitinous cuticle is highly flexible.

In octopus, the stomach is a very muscular grinding organ, reminding one of the gizzards of a bird (Isgrove 1909). Its central region consists of paired thick dorsal and ventral pads formed from outer to inner of a thick muscle layer and a columnar epithelium covered of a very thick cuticle. The lateral walls of this central region are thinner and lack muscle layers but exhibit thick collagenous dense connective layers to which the lateral wall muscles are inserted. Transitional regions join this central part of the stomach with the esophagus and the vestibule.

4.8.9 Vestibule

The vestibule is a dilatable small chamber that forms the link between the stomach, spiral caecum and intestine. The mucosa of the vestibule of cuttlefish consists of tall columnar cells with cilia in the apical surface and long glandular (goblet) cells interspersed with columnar cells. In octopus, the vestibule epithelium is cuticularized toward the stomach and the cuticle disappears suddenly next to the caecum.

4.8.10 The Caecum (Cecum, Accessory Stomach, Spiral Stomach, Caecal Sac) (Fig. 4.12)

The caecum has been considered the main absorptive organ. It is a thin-walled large sac spirally coiled around a columella that is connected with the stomach, the digestive gland and the intestine. The partially digested food passes from the stomach to the caecum and is filtered in it, discarding gross particles that pass directly to the intestine and allowing food to enter the digestive glands through the hepato-pancreatic ducts. The caecum has a complex internal structure that consists of numerous leafs and leaflets covered of ciliated epithelium extending from the outer surface and converging toward the columella without reaching it. In octopus, the outer border of the caecum forms three types of leafs, long (primary), intermediate (secondary) and short. Primary leafs alternate with secondary ones, and both types of leaf are flanked on both sides by very short unfolded lamellae allowing a regular organization. The primary and secondary leafs exhibit short lateral leaflets coursing longitudinally along leafs and giving them a comb-like appearance in cross section. The axis of leafs and leaflets is thin and continuous with the tissue of the border of the sac. The leaflets exhibit a clear alternate arrangement in squid and cuttlefish, but not in octopus where is irregular and leaflets often are opposite. In the octopus caecum, too, there is a clear gradient in the thickness of leafs/leaflets, largely diminishing toward the tip of the spiral. A thick ciliary epithelium covers the crests and valleys of leaflets, and also the region of the columella (typhlosole) that lacks leafs. A large number of goblet cells are scattered in the ciliary epithelium mainly in secondary crests. Similar goblet cells are observed in the folds of epithelium lining the columella. The folds of the columella and leafs of the caecum have a central axis with highly vascularized connective tissue (or chorion). Along the elongated apical border of primary folds, there are rows of simple acinar mucous glands called caecal glands that open directly into the lumen. These caecal glands are formed by secreting cells with a basal flattened nucleus and a light vacuolated cytoplasm. In the columella of the octopus caecum, there is abundant loose connective tissue, as well as dense connective tissue surrounding the hepato-pancreatic ducts.

In squid, the caecum is less coiled than in octopus although the appearance of leafs and leaflets is similar. As in octopus, the thick folded epithelium near the columella (typhlosole) contains numerous goblet cells. In cuttlefish, caecal leafs are poorly organized by comparison with those of octopus and squid, and have a thick connective axis. In cases of heavy infestation by coccidia (*Aggregata*), caecal folds are thickened and partially disorganized.

4.8.11 The Digestive Gland and Accessory Digestive Gland (Fig. 4.13)

The digestive gland (hepatopancreas, midgut gland) is the largest gland of cephalopods. The digestive enzymes are mainly supplied by the digestive gland in alternating phases of synthesis and release. It consists of a highly branched system of glandular tubules covered of a thick epithelium of uniform appearance. Basal conducts have a prominent lumen, but most tubules show a reduced lumen. The epithelium mainly consists of large columnar cells with basal nuclei, an apical region with a brush border and central regions with numerous large rounded pale granules (lipid droplets, lysosomes) and protein spherules (“boules”). The tubules are separated by thin vasculo-connective septa containing some muscle fibers. Electron microscopic studies suggest the presence of two main types of cell, basal (replacement) cells and chief (columnar) cells (Budelmann et al. 1997), but this is hardly distinguishable with light microscopy. Chief cells are polymorphic and may exhibit different appearances during the digestive cycle, with secreting and absorptive periods (see Costa et al. 2014). In some phases of digestion, proteins are secreted as “boules” from the apical cytoplasm of the cells in an apocrine way or even the whole cell passes to the lumen. In these phases, basal cells with abundant basophilic material can be easily observed. Mitotic cells are found often in the epithelium, to replace the tall cells that are probably short-lived.

The histological appearance of the digestive gland varies very considerably from sample to sample, even in individuals sacrificed at the same time after a meal, which has lead to conflicting reports on its function.

Associated with the main digestive gland, the octopus has a different part of the gland that is known as the accessory digestive gland (pancreatic appendages). This posterior portion of the digestive gland is located around the digestive gland (hepato-pancreatic) duct to which opens through wide ducts and shows an appearance very different from the main glandular region. The main gland duct branches in a number of wide secondary and tertiary ducts ending in a network of closely packed tubules or alveoli with striking angled luminal profiles. This appearance is produced by the large variations in the height of the pleated epithelium of adjacent alveoli, which are separated by a thin vasculo-connective lamina. Cell limits are not resolved by light microscopy, and cell nuclei appear irregularly distributed in the eosinophilic cytoplasm. The apical cytoplasm shows numerous pale round structures that may correspond to lipidic droplets. Ultrastructural observations in octopus reveal cells with a large number of longitudinal folds of the plasma membrane, which explains the difficulty for seeing cell limits with light microscopy. Electron microscopy of these cells also reveals numerous mitochondria, small vacuoles and large lipid droplets in cytoplasm lamellae (see Budelmann et al. 1997). These cells are in contact with the chyme, from which they absorb different nutrients. In the limit with the main part of the digestive gland, tubules of the two glands entering in contact are separated by a thin connective-vascular layer. In cuttlefish and squid, pancreatic appendages are not enclosed in the digestive gland or surrounded by a common capsule, but tubules arising from the hepato-pancreatic duct are in contact with the epithelium of the renal sac.

4.8.12 Intestine (Fig. 4.14)

The intestine shows longitudinal folds protruding into the lumen. In octopus, but not in squid or cuttlefish, the presence of large paired folds (typhlosoles) in opposite (dorsal and ventral) regions delineates a bilateral symmetry plane in the intestine. The typhlosolis epithelium has tall ciliated cells with nuclei in basal or intermediate levels, and mucous cells intercalated among them that secrete neutral and acid mucopolysaccharides (proteoglycans). In other intestinal folds, the epithelium mainly consists of numerous gland cells that secrete neutral and acid mucopolysaccharides (proteoglycans) and non-ciliated epithelial cells. Toward the anus, the thickness of the epithelium diminishes, but its features are similar. This epithelium is presumably involved in absorption. The connective tissue is abundant in the submucosa, extending along the axis of epithelial folds, only occasionally branched, and surrounding the muscular layers. The organization of the muscular wall of the intestine comprises an internal layer of longitudinal muscle and an external layer of circular muscle, better observed in octopus because of its large intestine. In octopus and cuttlefish, too, numerous blood vessels are observed in connective regions. The end part of the intestine that opens to the anal pore is similar in structure to other intestinal parts.

4.8.13 Ink Sac Complex

The ink sac of cephalopods is the most characteristic gland of these animals. The ink sac originates from an evagination of the intestinal primordium. The ink sac complex consists of the ink gland, a large ink sac or reservoir, and the short ink duct (Girod 1881; Williams 1909). The glandular epithelium consists of immature proliferating cells in the inner portion, whereas the outer glandular portion consists of a series of connected chambers lined by a cubical glandular epithelium. The gland cells are very active in melanogenesis (Palumbo 2003). Submicrometric small melanin granules are secreted by gland cells and accumulate as ink in the ink sac, being ejected (ink-jet) on demand. The wall of the squid ink sac is formed of an outer sheet of connective tissue, a middle sheet of circular and longitudinal muscle fibers and an inner sheet of pavement epithelium (Williams 1909). The reservoir has an additional layer situated between the epithelium and the muscular layer. This layer is about as thick as the other layers combined and is formed of iridiocytes which reflect light and give the ink sac its silvery appearance (Williams 1909). The ink sac opens into the anal chamber, being separated by two sphincters, and the chamber opens into the mantle cavity through the anus (Girod 1881; Williams 1909). The released ink is a complex mixture receiving also contributions of the funnel organ (Derby 2014).

4.9 Blood and Circulatory System (Figs. 4.15, 4.16, 4.17 and 4.18)

Cephalopods have a closed circulatory system with arteries and veins joined by a capillary bed. Two branchial hearts pump blood to the gills (branchial circulation) and one systemic heart to the remainder body (systemic circulation), in a double circulation way that reminds the double circulation (pulmonary and systemic) of land vertebrates. The blood is a viscous fluid that mainly consists of plasma with a high content in hemocyanin, a copper-containing respiratory protein, and also contains hemocytes (amebocytes). Hemocyanin and hemocytes are produced in the branchial glands and the white body, respectively.

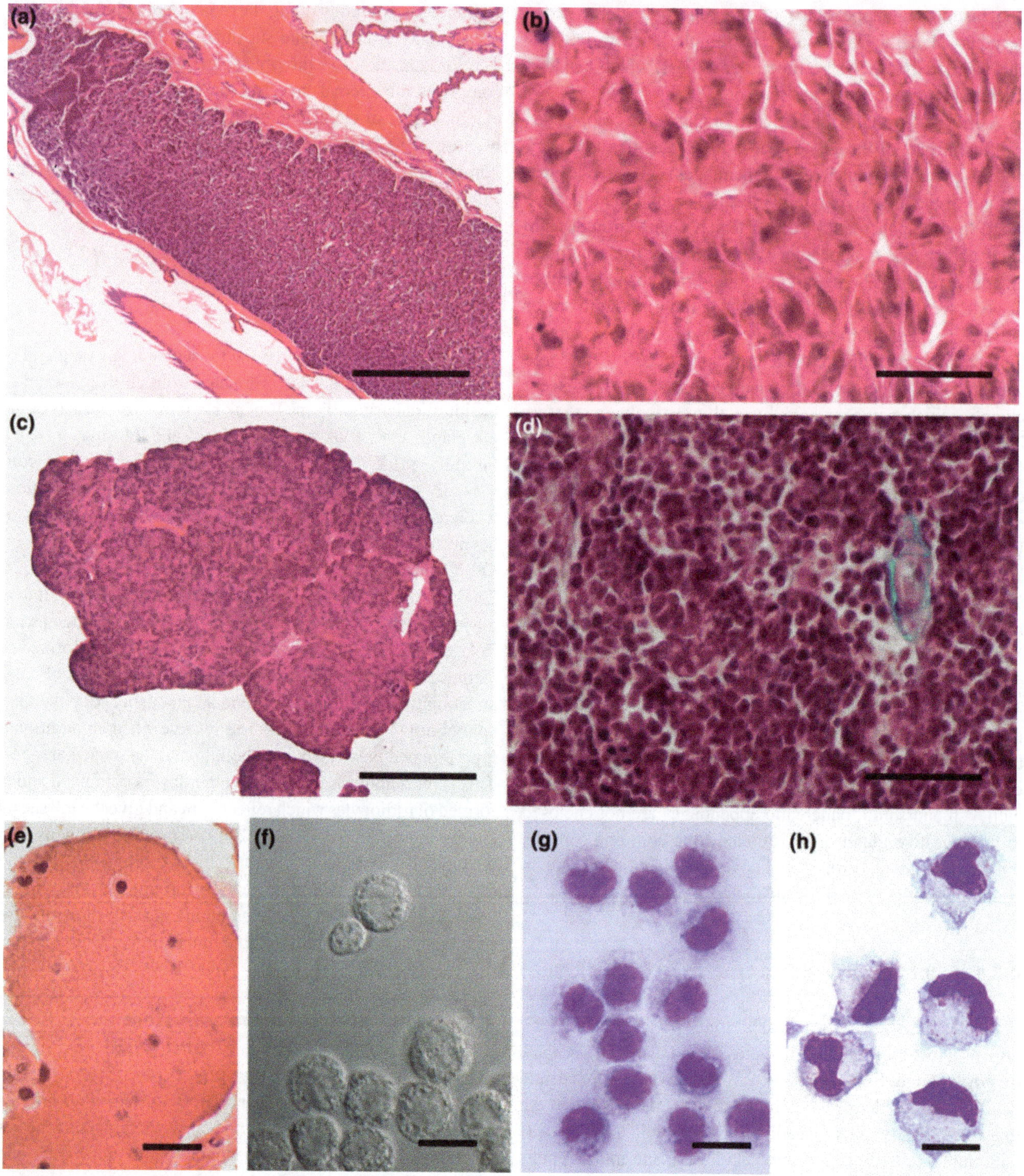

Fig. 4.15 Blood-forming organs and blood. **a** Branchial gland of cuttlefish showing a dense appearance. **b** Detail of the branchial gland showing cell cords that synthesize hemocyanin. Spaces among cords are continuous with blood vessels. **c** Lobe of the white body of cuttlefish. **d** Detail of the white body of an octopus showing the large number of blood cells (hemocytes) included in a loose connective-vascular meshwork. Note the vasculo-connective trabecula. **e** Section of an octopus vessel showing coagulated plasma containing some hemocytes. **f** Photomicrograph of live octopus hemocytes showing large cells and a small hemocyte. **g**, **h** Photomicrographs of monolayers of fixed hemocytes. **a–c**, **e** H&E stain; **d** Masson's trichrome; **f** Nomarski's differential interference contrast (DIC); **g**, **h** staining with Hemacolor® (see Castellano-Martínez et al. 2014). *Scale bars* **a** 1 mm; **b**, **d** 50 µm; **c** 1.2 mm; **e** 25 µm; **f–h** 10 µm

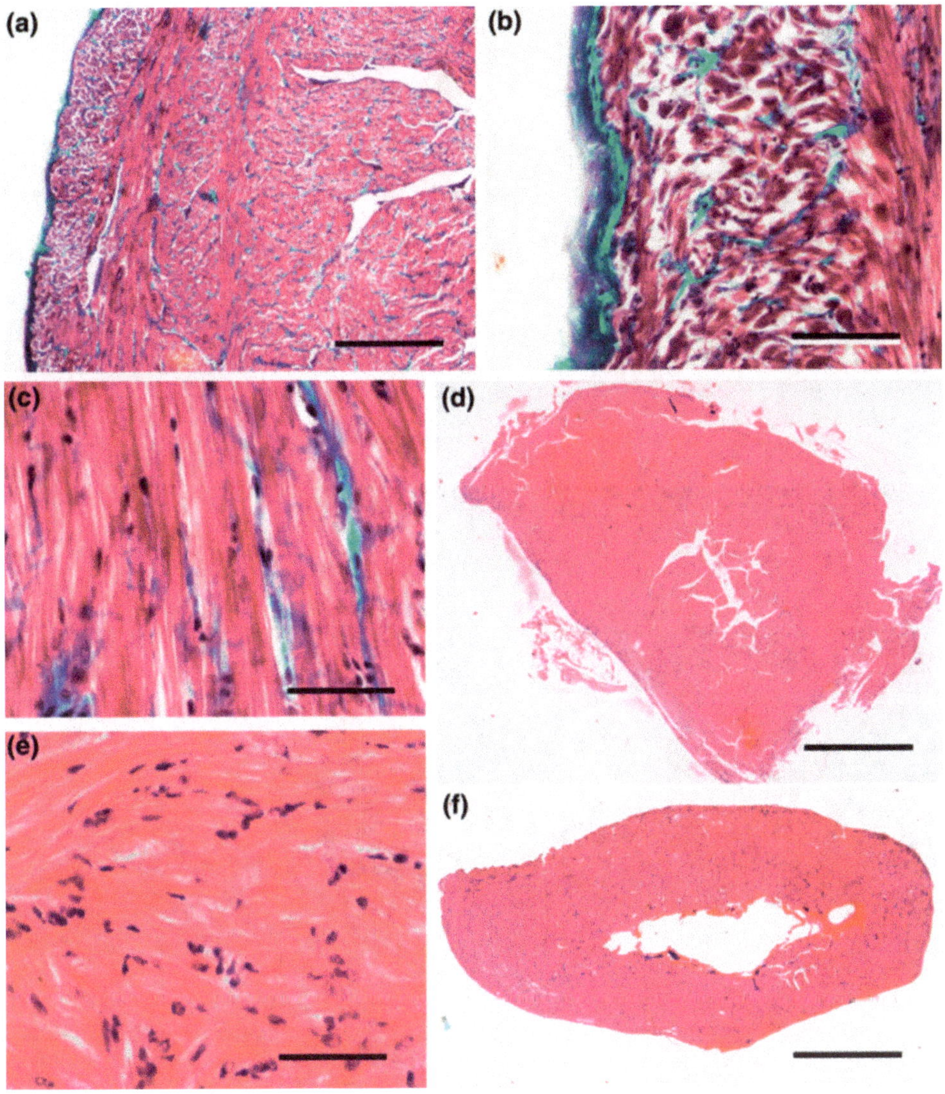

Fig. 4.16 Sections of the systemic heart of octopus (**a**–**c**). **a** Section of the heart showing the very thick myocardium with crossed orientations of fibers and the lumenal spaces at right. **b** Detail of the superficial layers of myocardium showing in cross-orientation superficial myocardial fiber layers. Note the epicardium (at the left) and the dense connective meshwork surrounding muscle fibers. **c** Longitudinal view of myocardial fibers and accompanying connective meshwork. **d** and **f** panoramic views of systemic hearts of squid (**d**) and cuttlefish (**f**) showing the very thick muscle layers. **e** Detail of the squid myocardium. **a**–**c** Masson's trichrome; **d**–**f** H&E stain. *Scale bars* **a** 0.8 mm 500 μm; **b** 100 μm; **c**, **e** 50 μm; **d**, **f** 1.2 mm

4.9.1 Branchial Gland

In Coleoids, a pair of branchial glands accompanies the branchial ligaments through the whole length of the gills. Each gland is contained in a capsule and is profusely vascularized. Under light microscopy, the branchial gland presents a dense appearance with numerous cords of basophilic cells interspersed with blood-filled capillaries. Studies using electron microscopy reveal a dense cytoplasm in these cells with numerous cisterns of rough endoplasmic reticulum. The secretory cells of branchial glands synthesize subunits of hemocyanin, a copper-containing protein that forms high-molecular-weight complexes in circulating blood of cephalopods and other mollusks. This cephalopod "hematopoietic" glands provide the plasma with an oxygen-transport protein, the most abundant protein of the blood (5–10% of blood volume), being responsible for the blue appearance of oxygenated blood. This abundant protein is also responsible for the eosinophilic staining of the content of blood vessels with the H&E stain. Capillaries of the branchial gland join to efferent vessels that are brightly red-stained with H&E.

4.9.2 White Body (Hematopoietic Organ)

There is general agreement that blood hemocytes of coleoids are mainly produced in the white bodies. White bodies are dense masses of small cells enclosed in sinuses that are organized in lobes located around the optic nerves between the optic lobe and the eye orbit. In light microscopic sections, the white body appears as a very dense mass of small cells mostly consisting of a round nucleus. A close inspection reveals islands of cells with lighter nuclei (differentiating hemocytoblasts) among areas of smaller cells with denser nuclei (mature hemocytes). Numerous mitotic cells

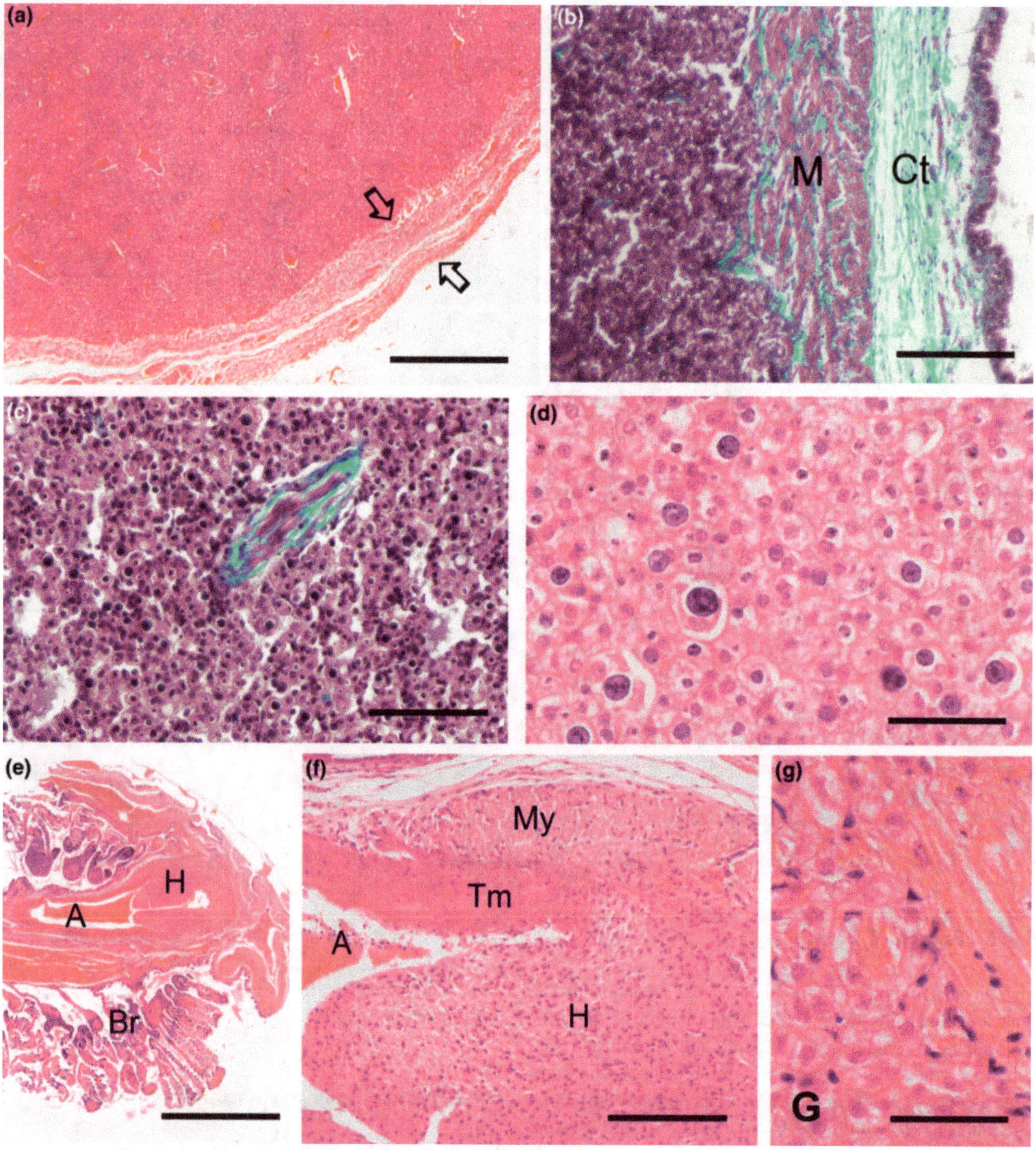

Fig. 4.17 Sections of the branchial heart of octopus (**a–d**) and squid (**e–g**). **a** Section showing the large mass of cells that appears to fill most of the heart cavity, surrounded by thin muscle and connective layers (outlined arrow). **b** Detail of the heart wall showing from outer to inner the thick coelomic epithelium, the connective (Ct) and muscular (M) layers and the inner cell mass. **c** Detail of a musculo-connective trabecula crossing the inner cell mass. **d** Detail of the inner cell mass showing cells with large spherical cytoplasmatic inclusions. **e** Section of the branchial heart (H) of a squid at the junction with the branchial arteria (A). Br, gill. **f** Detail of the junction showing the transition between the thick myocardium (My) to the arterial tunica media (Tm). **g** Detail of the cardiac muscle. **a**, **d–g** H&E stain; **b–c**, Masson's trichrome. *Scale bars* **a** 0.8 mm; **b**, **f** 200 μm; **c** 100 μm; **d**, **g** 50 μm; **e** 1.2 mm

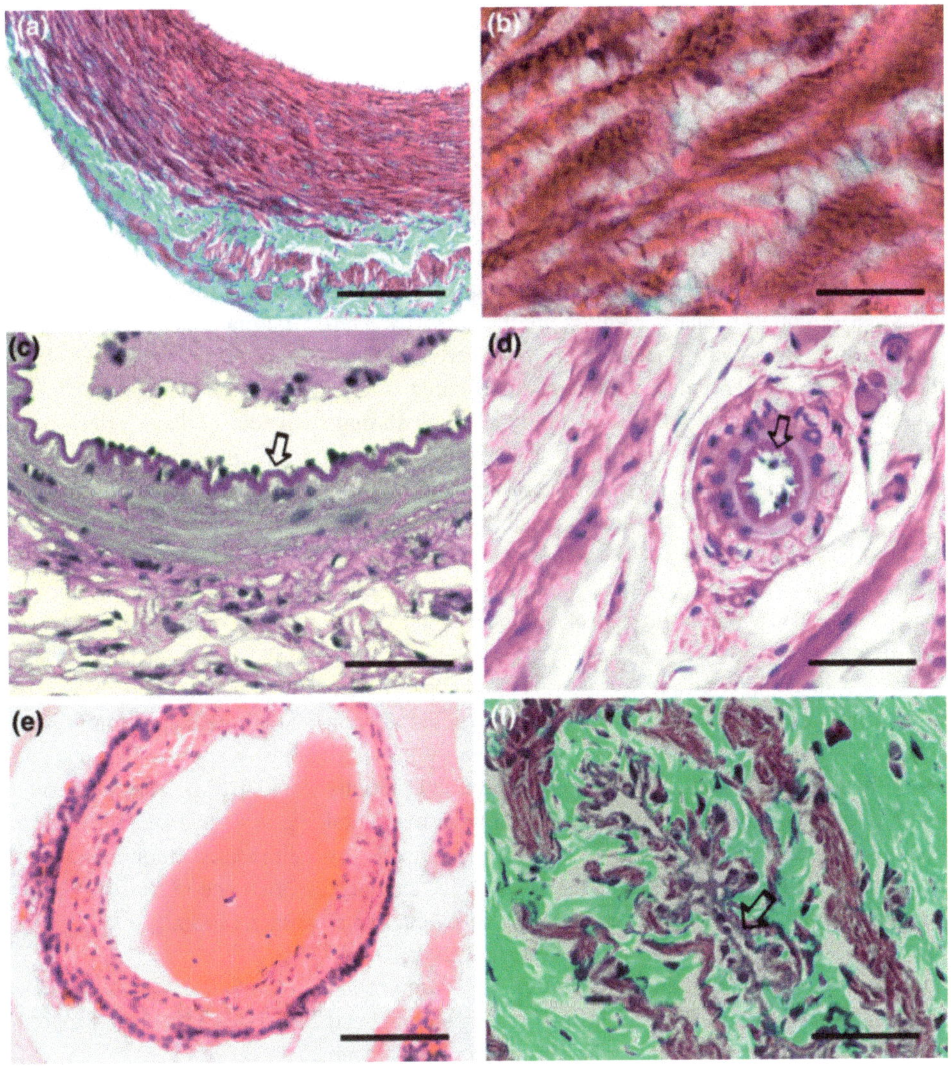

Fig. 4.18 Transverse sections of blood vessels of octopus (**a–d, f**) and squid (**e**). **a** Section of the octopus aorta showing the thick muscle wall (tunica media) surrounded by abundant collagen connective tissue (tunica adventitia). **b** Detail of the muscle layer showing muscle fibers surrounded of a dense network of thin connective fibers. **c** Section of a medium-sized arteria showing the thin tunica intima of endothelial cells on the elastic lamina stained pink with the PAS method (outlined arrow). The thin meshwork around muscle fibers is also PAS positive. **d** Section of a small arteria showing the elastic lamina separating the intima and the thin tunica media. **e** Section of an efferent branchial vessel (vena) of squid. **f** Collapsed large vena of octopus surrounded by abundant of collagen fibers but scarce muscle fibers. The outlined arrow points to the collapsed lumen. **a, b, f** Masson's trichrome; **c, d** PAS method; **e** H&E. *Scale bars* **a** 500 μm; **b** 16 μm; **c, d, f** 50 μm; **e** 100 μm

are observed in the white body, indicating it is a highly proliferating organ. As indicated above, respiratory pigments are located in the blood plasma, and no cells similar to vertebrate red blood cells are present in cephalopods.

4.9.3 Blood

The blood of coleoid cephalopods is a transparent liquid, turning blue in color when oxygenated. It is about as viscous as the vertebrate plasma, and its osmolarity is similar to that of the seawater although proportions of Na^+ and K^+ differ from seawater (lower and higher, respectively). It mostly contains plasma bearing the respiratory pigment, hemocyanin, which is mainly synthesized by the branchial glands, whereas blood is poor in cells. The efficiency of cephalopod blood as an oxygen carrier compares poorly with that the blood of vertebrates. The major circulating blood cells of cephalopods are referred to as leucocytes, amebocytes, or hemocytes. These are small ovoid cells are able to migrate to tissues. In histological sections, they are observed in scarce numbers inside blood vessels. These cells are better demonstrated in fresh hemolymph or in hemolymph smears stained with Romanovsky-type stains (Wright, Giemsa, May-Grünwall, Hemacolor, etc.), similar to blood cells of vertebrates. Flow cytometry, phagocytosis assays and enzymatic histochemistry, together with electron microscopy, have been employed to study cephalopod hemocytes. The major hemocytes identified in octopus are described as granulocytes and are phagocytic cells (Castellanos-Martínez et al. 2014). Small hemocytes are also present. Other authors have recognized haemoblast-like cells, hyalinocytes and granulocytes, hyalinocytes being the most abundant (Troncone et al. 2015). A single type of granulocyte population with variable internal complexity is described in the blood of cuttlefish (Le Pabic et al. 2014).

4.9.4 Systemic and Branchial Hearts (Figs. 4.16 and 4.17)

The systemic heart consists of a large thick-walled ventricle joined to the branchial efferent vessels through a pair of auricles. Two large arteries, the cephalic and posterior aorta, arise from the ventricle. A lacunar system extends in the walls from its inner surface to the periphery. The myocardium consists of a large mass of cardiomyocytes with abundant sarcoplasm that are united among them by intercalary discs in a way analogous to the vertebrate cardiomyocytes, as shown in electron microscopic studies (Schipp and Schäfer 1969). Blood capillaries enter through the myocardium. The myocardium of the systemic and branchial hearts is innervated by nerves from ganglia of the visceral system. Among the neurotransmitters released by cardiac nerve fibers are catecholamines or cardioactive peptides of the FMRFamide family. The heart is enclosed in a pericardial cavity that is closely related to the renal system (see below).

In coleoid cephalopods, a pair of branchial hearts that lies in the gill ligament pumps blood to the gills via the afferent branchial vessel to generate part of the circulatory pressure. These hearts are elongated and appear to be filled partially by a large mass of cells among which numerous blood branching spaces and interstices extend, recognizable by their eosinophilic staining. Most abundant cells are large polygonal or round cells that are grouped in parenchyma-like masses. These cells show a round pale nucleus and abundant cytoplasm including dark, often very large round lysosomal inclusions in the cytoplasm. These branchial heart cells are responsible of the glandular consistency of the heart and appear involved in catabolic processes eliminating hemocyanin and blood debris (Beuerlein and Schipp 1998; Beuerlein et al. 1998). In addition, blood cells enter among these cells and may attach them. No well-organized vessels are observed into this cell mass. The walls of branchial hearts consist of layers of cardiomyocytes similar in structure to these found in the systemic heart. At the output side, the transition from the heart to the branchial artery is sharp and the wall of cardiomyocytes is substituted by the thick musculo-connective layer of the arterial wall.

4.9.5 Blood Vessels (Fig. 4.18)

The vascular system of coleoids is double, closed and almost symmetrical. The anatomy of the cephalopod circulatory system, including the distribution of main arteries and veins, has been described in detail many times and the interested reader is referred to Williams (1909), Isgrove (1909) and Wells (1978). Here, only the histology of arteries and veins is described. Arteries are easily recognizable in sections by the organization of walls. Three layers or tunicae are distinguishable in the walls of large blood vessels of cephalopods, a thin intima, a thick media and a thin adventitia, analogous to that of large vertebrate vessels. The tunica intima consists of small endothelial cells attached to a thick basal lamina (inner lamina elastica) that in histological sections has a pleated appearance. The conspicuous tunica media of large arteries contain numerous circular and longitudinal muscle fibers included in an abundant connective matrix. The thickness of the media diminishes in smaller arteries. Small arteries usually appear contracted in sections. Veins resemble arteries but generally have thin walls lacking an inner lamina elastica and showing often dilated lumen filled of blood (Figs. 4.18e–f and 4.22f). Contractile veins as branchial efferents and large veins show a thin tunica media. The cephalopod organs are richly supplied of a number of small vessels forming series of different diameters, which is easily appreciable in sections of nervous tissue (Figs. 4.24b and 4.25e). The smallest (capillaries) are surrounded only by pericytes enclosing the thin, often discontinuous endothelium (see Budelmann et al. 1997). The largest vessels are often accompanied of nerves and its walls receive abundant innervation.

4.10 The Respiratory System (Fig. 4.19)

The two feathery gills of dibranchiate cephalopods protrude within the mantle cavity allowing the pass of the active respiratory water flow created by mantle movements through their folds (Wells and Wells 1982). The branchial organization is similar in cuttlefish and squid. The gill is sustained by the gill ligament that contains a large afferent vessel (branchial artery), muscles and a ganglionic nerve cord that innervates the gill. From this axis, numerous secondary branchial lamellae or primary filaments extend into the cavity and appear as finely meandering (tertiary lamellae) increasing in this way the exchange surface of the gill. Each secondary lamella receives by its proximal side collaterals of the afferent vessel that extends between the two flattened layers of epithelium (respiratory epithelium) that cover the lamella, and some perpendicular cells (pillar cells) join these epithelia. At the distal end of lamellae, blood spaces join to

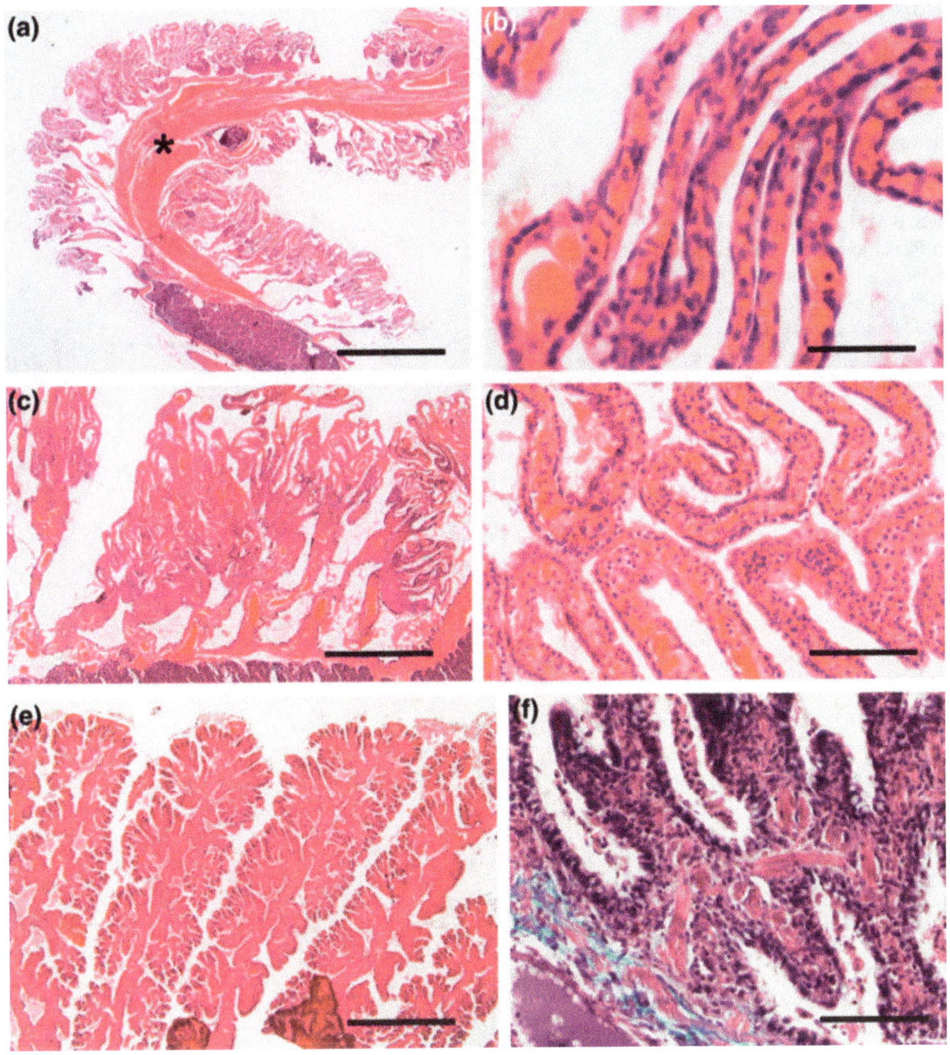

Fig. 4.19 Panoramic views and details of sections of gills of squid (**a**, **b**) and cuttlefish (**c**, **d**) and octopus (**e**, **f**). Note the similar appearance of gill primary and secondary lamellae of squid and cuttlefish, and the muscular axis of the gill (star in **a**). The branchial gland is also appreciable in **a** and **c**. **e**, **f** Panoramic view and detail of gill lamellae of octopus. Note the different branching pattern (**e**) and the thickness of the gill epithelium (**f**), by comparison with decapods. **a–e** H&E stain; **f** Masson's trichrome. *Scale bars* **a** 1 mm; **c**, **e** 500 µm; **b** 50 µm; **d**, **f** 100 µm

coarse vessels that, together, form the efferent branchial vessel. In octopus, the gills differ dramatically from those of cuttlefish and squid, because the secondary lamellae are branched and tertiary lamellae have the appearance of small trees rather than laminae. The vascularization also differs from that of the other two species (see Young and Vecchione 2002). In octopus, too, the respiratory epithelium is thicker than in these species. A thinner epithelium appears to favor the gaseous interchange in most active species. The thin branchial epithelium also allows direct elimination of substances from blood, such as ammonium and other wastes.

4.11 The Excretory System (Fig. 4.20)

The coleoids have a complex excretory system consisting of different organs with various functions. The proper excretory organs are the renal and pericardial (branchial heart) appendages, though the gills, pancreatic appendages and other structures also contribute to excretion and homeostasis of the internal milieu. The renal and pericardial appendages are gland-like structures protruding in the renal and pericardial coelomic sacs, respectively. In octopus, the renal appendages consist of highly branched structures protruding in the renal sac. They are formed of continuous sheets covered of two layers of cuboid epithelial cells separated by blood sinuses derived of the vena cava system. The epithelial cells show a central rounded nucleus and abundant cytoplasm. Ultrastructural studies reveal the complex organization of these cells, with a microvillous apical border and a lobulated basal region directly contacting blood (see Budelmann et al. 1997), which are inappreciable in conventional light microscopy sections. In octopus, the renal sac is a unique habitat for parasites and the coelomic surface of the renal appendages appears generally colonized by numerous dicyemids.

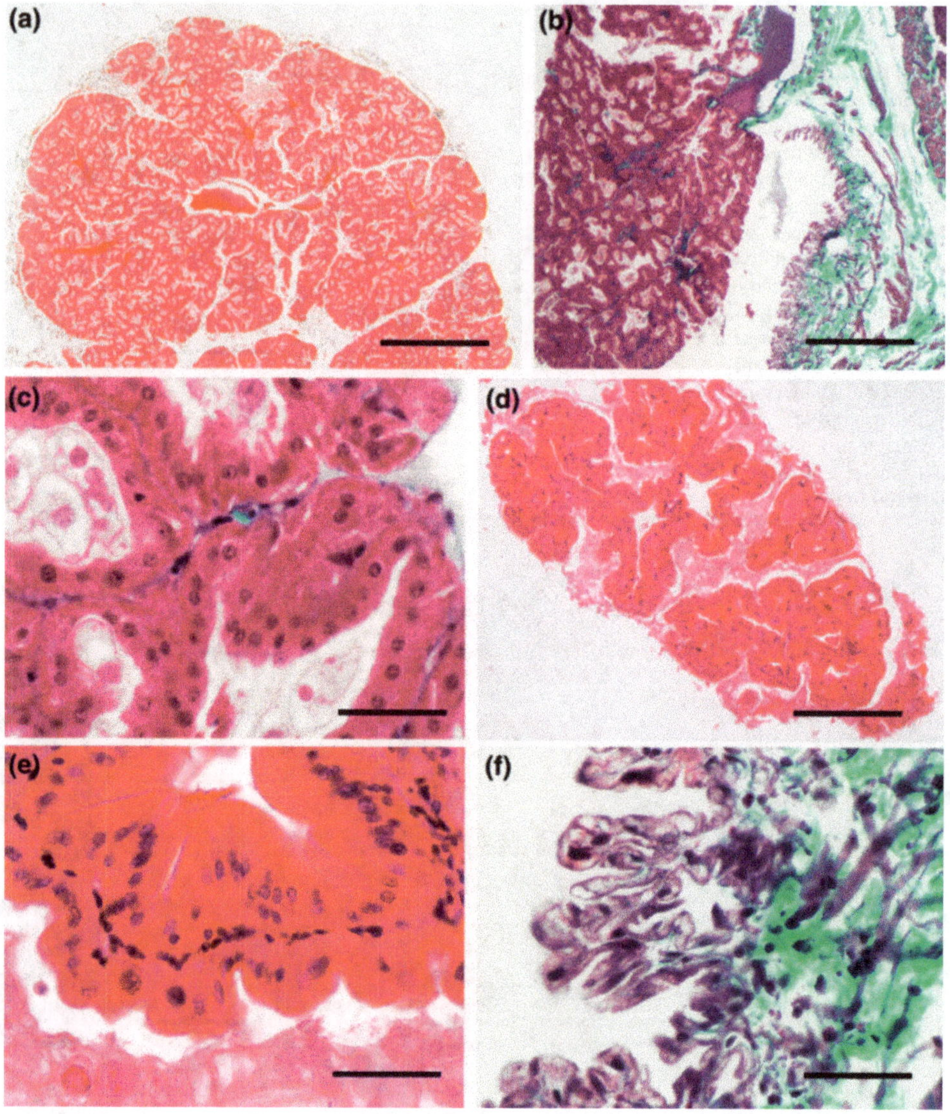

Fig. 4.20 **a** Panoramic view of the renal appendages of octopus. **b** Section showing the renal appendages associated with the pericardial surface. **c** Detail of the octorpus renal epithelium showing the luminal surface of the epithelium facing faintly stained parasites (dicyemids). **d** Renal appendages of cuttlefish. **e** Detail of the renal epithelia showing two different papillar appearances, lower facing the renal sac filled of dicyemids (bottom) and taller in the opposite surface. **f** Detail or the complex pericardial epithelium shown in **b**. **a**, **d**, **e** H&E stain; **b**, **f** Masson's trichrome. *Scale bars* **a** 0.8 mm; **b** 500 µm; **c**, **e**, **f** 50 µm; **d** 200 µm

4.12 The Visual System (Figs. 4.21 and 4.22)

The visual system of coleoid cephalopods is highly developed. It consists of a pair of big camera-type eyes connected with paired optic lobes (ganglia) through the optic nerve (Hensen 1865; Young 1971). The parts of the cephalopod eye are strikingly similar to those of vertebrate eyes, although they differ in its origin and organization, being considered a notable example of convergent evolution. The inner surface of the eye consists of a neural retina that continues anteriorly with a simple pigment epithelium extending to the lens-producing "ciliary papillae." More anteriorly, this epithelium is continuous with that of the iris. The iris lines a pupil circular (squid), horizontal (octopus), or irregular in shape (cuttlefish), and is outwardly followed by a transparent cornea. External eyelids are found in many cephalopod species as the octopus and cuttlefish. The retina is covered with connective tissues, and in the equatorial region of the eye, there is a lamina of cartilage that shows a different organization in octopus and cuttlefish/squids (Fig. 4.2). A connective fascia is also present in the posterior pole of the eye except at the exit of the optic nerve bundles. Several extra-ocular muscles (both rectus and oblique muscles) formed of muscle fiber fascicles allow eye movements with a surprising similarity with those found in vertebrate eyes, though its number and organization largely vary among cephalopod species, unlike in vertebrates.

The retina (Fig. 4.21) is a bilayered structure in the three species illustrated here, with long photoreceptor cells of a single type, with perikarya located in the deep (inner) layer and photoreceptor processes extending in the superficial (outer) layer. Note that this convention is different than that used for vertebrate eyes. In the outer layer, photoreceptor processes bear two opposite rhabdomeres (formed of long, densely packed microvilli perpendicular to the axis of the

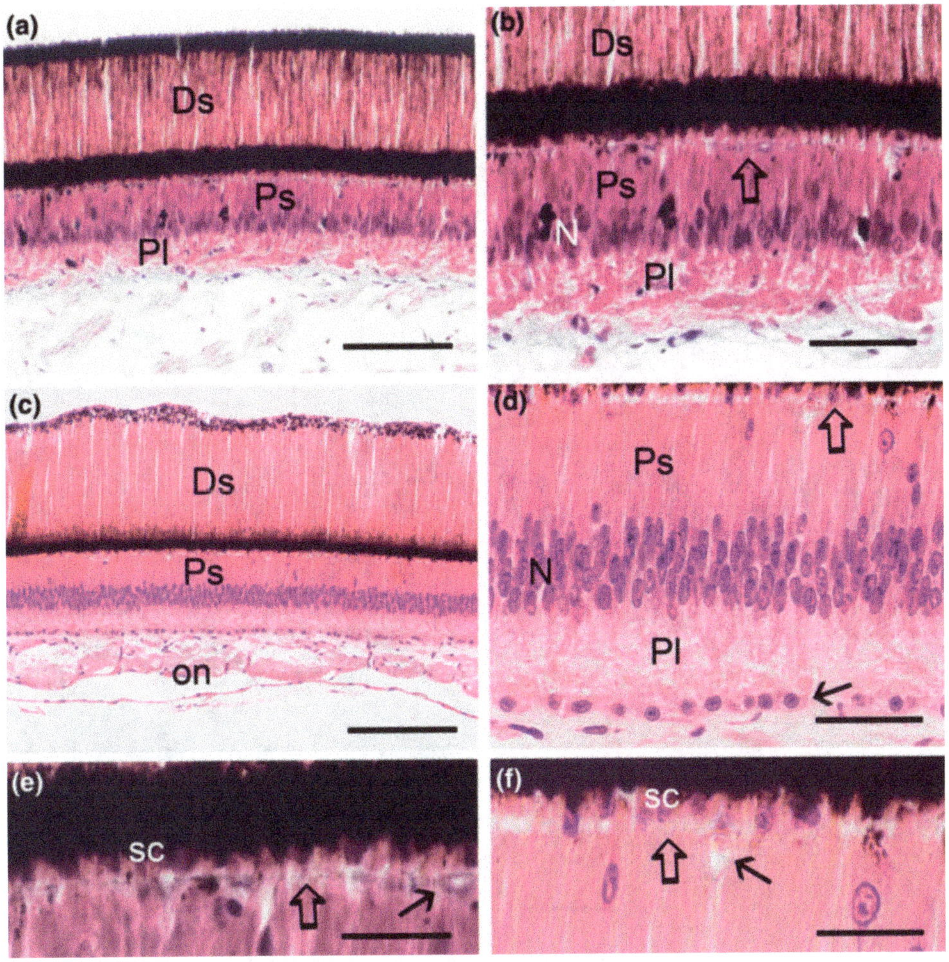

Fig. 1.21 Vertical sections through the retina of an octopus (**a**, **b**) and a squid (**c**, **d**), showing the layers of distal photoreceptive segments bearing the rhabdomeres and pigment granules (Ds), the layer of proximal photoreceptive segments (Ps) and nuclei (N) of photoreceptors, and the basal plexiform layer with axonal processes of photoreceptors and efferent fibers. Note that the distribution of pigment granules shown here is typical of light-adapted retinas. Outlined arrows in **b** and **d** point to the basal lamina separating proximal and distal segments. The thin arrow in **d** points to a defined layer of basal ("epithelial") cells below the plexiform layer in the squid retina. **e** and **f** Detail of the basal membrane (outlined arrows) separating distal and proximal segments in octopus and squid, respectively. Note capillaries in the basal lamina (thin arrows), and nuclei of supporting cells (sc) that are obscured by the accumulation of pigment granules. On, optic nerve (in **c**). **a**, **b**, **f** Masson's trichrome; **c**, **d**, **f** H&E stain. *Scale bars* **a**, **c** 200 μm; **b**, **d** 100 μm; **e**, **f** 50 μm

process bearing the visual pigment or rhodopsin), contacting laterally with rhabdomeres of adjacent photoreceptors. Using light microscopy, rhabdomeres appear as a fuzzy layer, but these structures can be resolved using transmission electron microscopy (Young 1971). This latter technique allows differentiating numerous filamentous mitochondria in the axis of the process, a well as pigment granules that cyclically migrate along the photoreceptor segment depending on light/darkness conditions. In the outer layer, there are also supporting (glial) cells with somata located basally and a long apical process extending till and forming part of the outer limiting membrane. Numerous blood capillaries are observed between the inner and outer retinal layers. The orientation of photoreceptor segments facing toward the light entering through the pupil (direct retina) is the opposite to that of vertebrate retinas (inverted retina). Inner processes of photoreceptor cells give rise to collaterals forming part of an inner plexiform layer before entering in the optic fiber bundles. Note that to observe these collaterals and their contacts with efferent axons from the optic lobes, it is necessary the use of Golgi methods or transmission electron microscopy.

The numerous optic nerves (bundles) of cephalopods do not form a single nerve as in vertebrates, but exit the eye orbit at its posterior pole and course toward the first optic center, the optic lobe, in such a way that bundles arising from the dorsal retina, course toward the ventral optic lobe, those ventral ones toward the dorsal region of the lobe and the central ones toward the central region of the lobe, i.e., inverting their relative positions along the dorso-ventral and

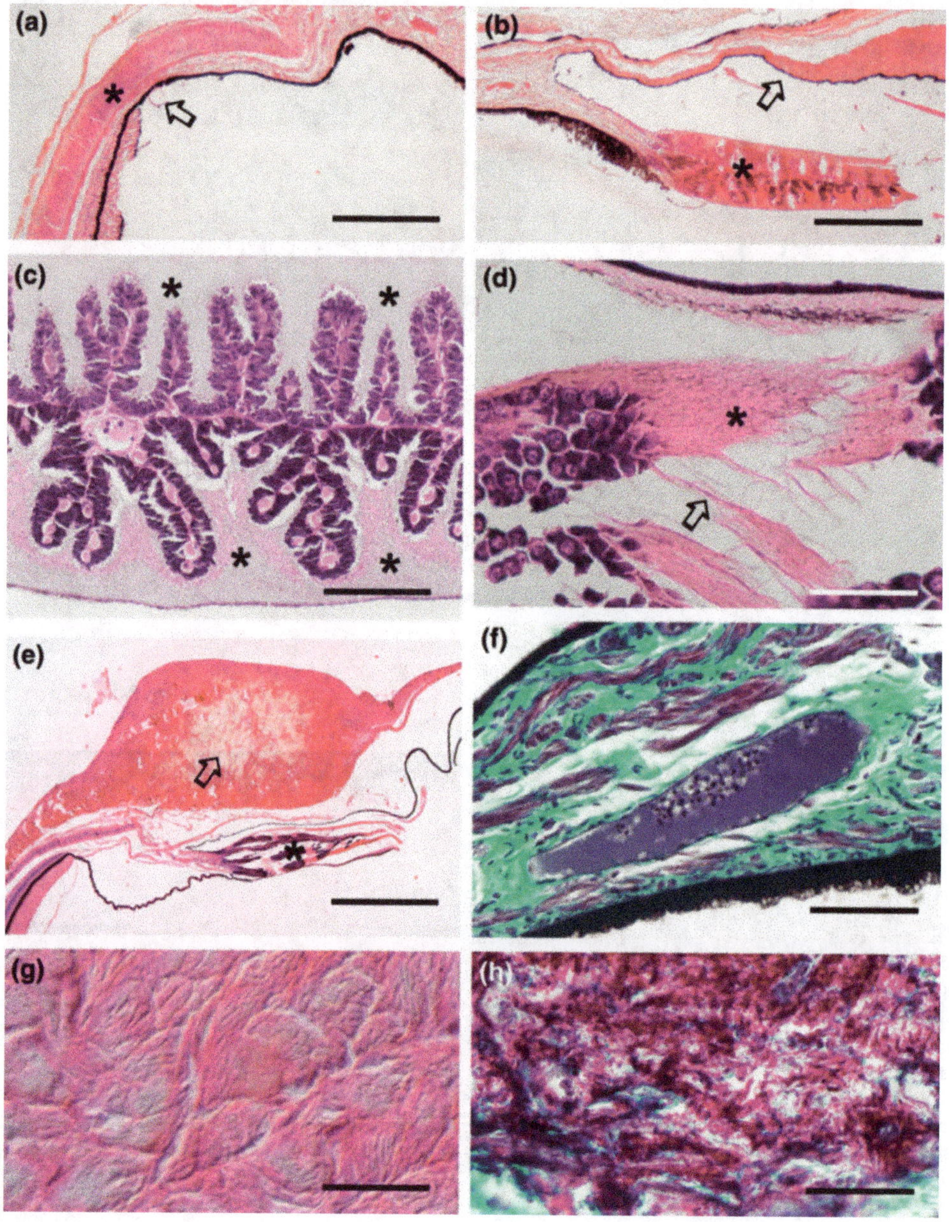

Fig. 4.22 Sections through anterior structures of cephalopod eyes. **a** Section of the octopus eye showing the transition between the retina and the ciliary region ("ora serrata"-like; outlined arrow). Star indicates the equatorial scleral cartilage. **b** Section of octopus eye showing the ciliary papillae (star) and the base of the iris (outlined arrow). **c** Transverse section of the lens-forming ciliary papillae, the upper and lower halves giving rise to the outer and inner hemilenses, respectively. The homogeneous pale material that surrounds papillae (stars) consists of innumerable cell processes of papillary cells. Note also abundant blood vessels in the axes of papillae. **d** Tangential section of a papilla showing lens cells with dense cytoplasm forming long, thin eosinophilic processes (outlined arrow, star) that form the lens. **e** Section showing the irideal angle of a squid eye, with a thick iris (outlined arrow) and ciliary papillae (star) below. **f** Proximal region of the iris of an octopus showing inner and outer pigment epithelia and a stroma with abundant collagen, small muscular bundles and blood vessels. **g**, **h** The granule-filled iridophores of octopus iris appear colorless in H&E stains but pink with the Masson's trichrome. *Scale bars* **a**, **b**, **e** 500 μm; **c** 200 μm; **d**, **f–h** 50 μm

rostro-caudal axes (see below). This cross of bundles was named optic chasm by Cajal (1917). The bundles consist of numerous thin axons accompanied of glial cells and blood capillaries.

The ciliary proximal part of the retina is a simple epithelium formed of cuboidal–prismatic cells with the nucleus in basal location, large amounts of black pigment in the middle and an eosinophilic apical cytoplasm. This epithelial layer is continuous with that of supporting cells of the retina. The abrupt change from the neural retina to the ciliary epithelium reminds the ora serrata of vertebrates. More distally, this epithelial layer transforms toward the lens forming a numerous series of radial folds covered of characteristic epithelial cells and a vasculo-connective axis (ciliary papillae and ciliary ring). The shape and size of the papillary epithelial cells vary from small cells proximally to tall cell with large nucleus and highly basophilic cytoplasm sometimes with melanic granules that give rise to a thin process that extends in parallel with those of neighbor cells toward the lens. The accumulation of these long and thin cytoplasmic processes (crystalline processes) gives rise to the layers of the spherical lens, which is formed of two unequal halves, a small external and a large internal separated by a septum. Two series of papillary folds are responsible of these portions. A muscular ring joins the scleral cartilage to the ciliary ring, its contraction allowing eye accommodation by displacing the lens perpendicularly to the eye axis (Schaeffel et al. 1999).

Externally to the ciliary papillae, the pigment epithelium continues and covers the inner surface of the iris. In octopus, cuttlefish and squid, the iris is much thickened toward the pupil and contains a number of large iridophores filled of reflecting platelets (reflecting tissue, silver layer) in a central location. These platelets are unstained in H&E sections but appear brightly red-stained with the Masson's trichrome method. Iridocyte platelets contain condensed proteins of the reflectin family (Crookes et al. 2004; Andouche et al. 2013; DeMartini et al. 2015).

For the organization of statocysts, olfactory organs and other sensory structures, readers are referred to Young (1971), Wells (1978), Budelmann et al. (1997) and Polese et al. (2015).

4.13 The Nervous System (Figs. 4.23, 4.24, 4.25 and 4.26)

4.13.1 Brain

The nervous system of coleoid cephalopods (squid, cuttlefish and octopus) is very complex compared to other invertebrates, its level of complexity being comparable to those of fishes despite their very different designs. The cephalopod nervous system supports a number of complex behavioral traits with multiple dedicated systems for memory, learning and control of body movements, dynamic camouflage, reproductive behavior and visceral function (Young 1971, 1995; Wells 1978; Huffard 2013). The ganglionic nervous system of cephalopods has evolved from a more generalized mollusk organization as that observed in present-day gastropods. This nervous system is composed of cerebral ganglia joined by connectives and commissures with different pairs of ganglia: pallial, pedal, visceral and buccal. In coleoid cephalopods, the number of ganglia has increased by growth, condensation and subdivision of ancestral ganglia, forming a large mass ("brain") around the esophagus composed of numerous ganglia and lobes. This brain is partially encased by cartilage (cranial cartilage) and dense connective tissue. Here, only a brief description of selected ganglia, nerve cords and nerves stained with general methods will be provided. For further histological details, readers are directed to specialized monographs as that of Young (1971) on the nervous system of octopus.

In octopus, the different brain lobes (Fig. 4.23) exhibit a cortex of cell perikarya that surrounds an extensive neuropil and tract region. Large differences are noted among lobes in the number and size of perikarya, which is easily appreciable in sagittal sections of the brain. In some lobes, cords of cells enter the central neuropil, forming networks. The location, cell size and histological organization allow distinguishing lobes, although wide intermediate neuropil areas make difficult to trace boundaries between lobes. In the supraesophageal mass of the brain, the vertical lobes are most easily recognizable centers because the large amounts of small granule cells forming columns in the cortex and its superficial dorsal location. Rostral to it in superficial locations, the superior and inferior frontal lobes and the subfrontal lobe exhibit different cortical organization. Just rostral to the inferior frontal and subfrontal lobes, the superior buccal lobe exhibits a characteristic cortex with large neurons. Coarse labial nerves extend from this lobe rostrally. By comparison with these lobes, deeper regions of the supraesophageal mass appear as poorly delimited regions, including the subvertical lobe and several regions in the basal lobe system.

The optic lobes (Fig. 4.24) are easily recognizable in the three species by their lateral location with regard to the brain and relation with the eye, as ganglia that receive fibers of the optic nerves. The optic lobe is covered by a layered superficial region (cortex) that by analogy with deep layers of the vertebrate retina is named retina profunda, and a central region that shows a non-laminar organization with islands of neurons intermingled with extensive neuropil areas. The cortex is three-layered, with two dense bands of small neurons (granules) flanking an elaborated middle layer or plexiform layer. Optic nerve fibers end in this plexiform layer contacting with neurons of the granular layers. In both granular layers, some larger neurons can be distinguished among small cells, indicating a complex neuronal organization. Small axonal bundles cross these layers, giving them a columnar appearance. Below the inner granular layer, groups of neurons become arranged in radial columns

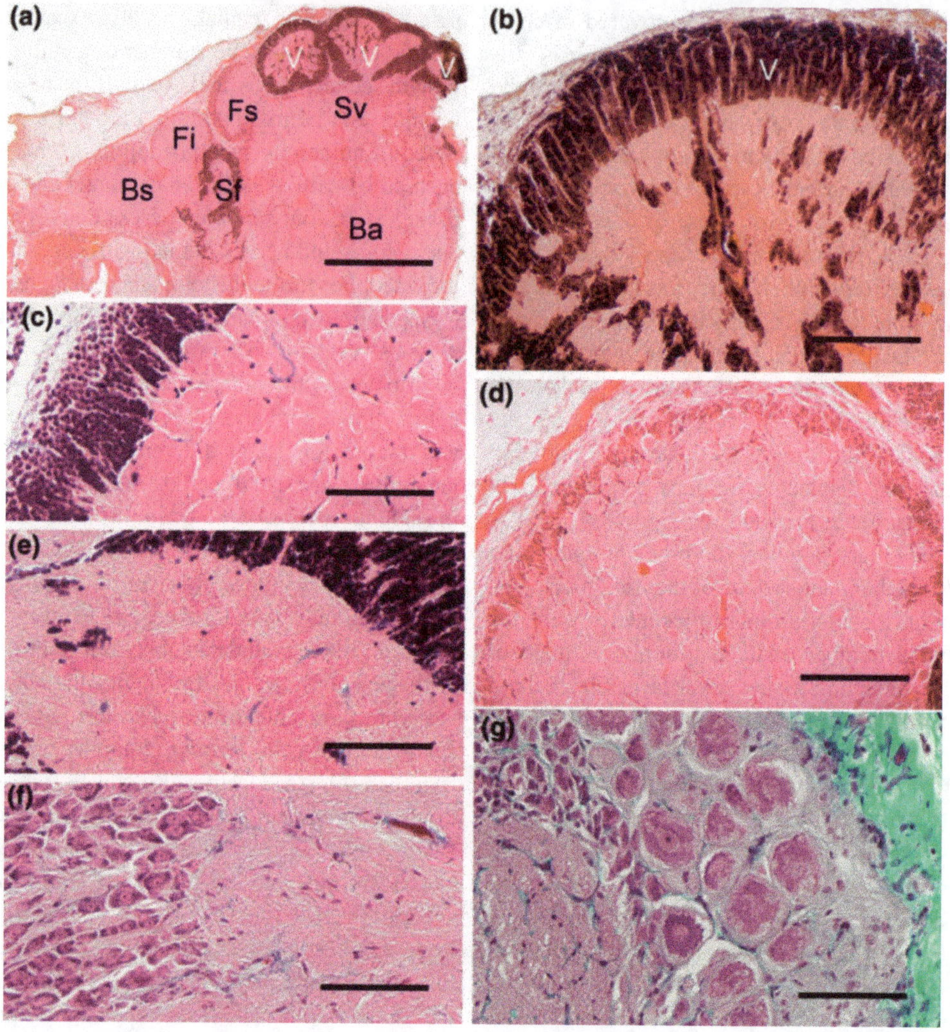

Fig. 4.23 **a** Photomicrograph of a parasagittal section of supraesophagic cerebral mass of octopus showing the different appearance of the main lobes. Rostral is at the left. Ba, Basal lobe; Bs, Superior buccal lobe; cb, cerebro-brachial connective; Fi, inferior frontal lobe; Fs, superior frontal lobe; Sf, Subfrontal lobe; V, vertical lobe. **b** Detail of the vertical lobe showing the cortex with small-celled columns extending cell cords to the central neuropil or medulla. **c** Detail of the frontal superior lobe showing the thick small-celled cortex and the central neuropil with glomerular appearance. **d** Detail of the inferior frontal lobe showing its glomerular neuropil. **e** Subfrontal lobe showing the small-celled cortex and a central region with numerous fiber bundles. **f** Detail of the buccal superior lobe showing large neurons in the cortex. **g** Detail of the magnocellular chromatophoric lobe of the pallioviscera complex showing big and small neuronal perikarya in the cortex. The connective layer covering the lobe is seen at right. **a–f** H&E stain; **f** Masson's trichrome. *Scale bars* **a** 1 mm; **b–g** 200 μm

separated by abundant neuropil. In more central regions of the lobe, the cords appear more heterogeneous forming a network and exhibiting large neurons. The optic lobes are among the most complex centers of the cephalopod central nervous system. The medial region of the optic lobes lacks the three-layered cortex and is joined with the basal complex of the supraesophagic mass via conspicuous optic tracts coursing in the optic peduncle, which includes small peduncle and olfactory lobes. In coleoids, the olfactory lobes receive sensory information of a peripheral chemosensory structure located in the skin behind the eye. Closely associated with the optic peduncle, there is a conspicuous optic gland that consists of endocrine cells and is innervated by a tract bearing fibers from peptidergic neurons of the posterior dorsal basal ganglion. These peptidergic neurons express the neuropeptides FMRFamide and/or GnRH, which appears to inhibit secretion (Di Cosmo and Di Cristo 1998). The secretion of gonadotropic mitogenic factor by this gland varies throughout the sexual cycle and is involved in the control of gametogenesis, being regulated by the axo-glandular innervation.

Most lobes of the subesophageal mass exhibit a simple histological organization with neuronal perikarya segregated to the cortex and a massive central region occupied by

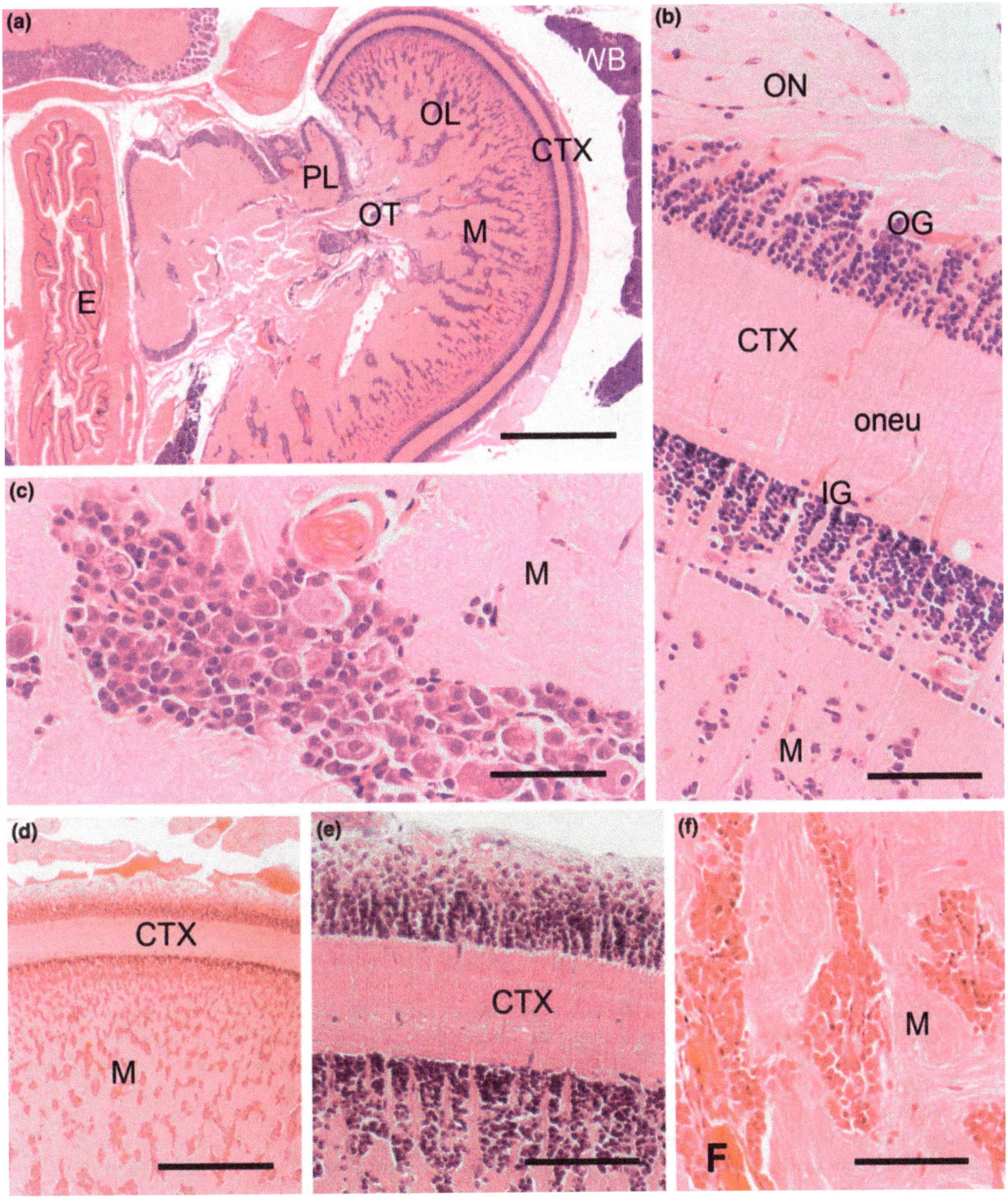

Fig. 4.24 Section of the cerebral mass of a squid showing the optic lobe (OL) and the optic tracts (OT) connecting with other lobes. Note the cortical laminas (CTX) embracing the core or medulla (M) of the lobe. Note also the esophagus (E) surrounded by cerebral masses and the white body (WB). PL, peduncular lobe. **b** Detail of the cortex of the squid optic lobe showing outer (OG) and inner (IG) granular layers and the thick outer neuropil (oneu). Note also the entrance of optic nerve (ON) bundles. **c** Detail of a cell cord of the medulla (M) with large and small neurons surrounded by neuropil. **d–f** Sections of the octopus optic lobe, showing similar organization as in squid, with small differences. Same abbreviations as used for squid. H&E stain. *Scale bars* **a** 1 mm; **d** 500 μm; **b**, **c**, **e**, **f** 200 μm

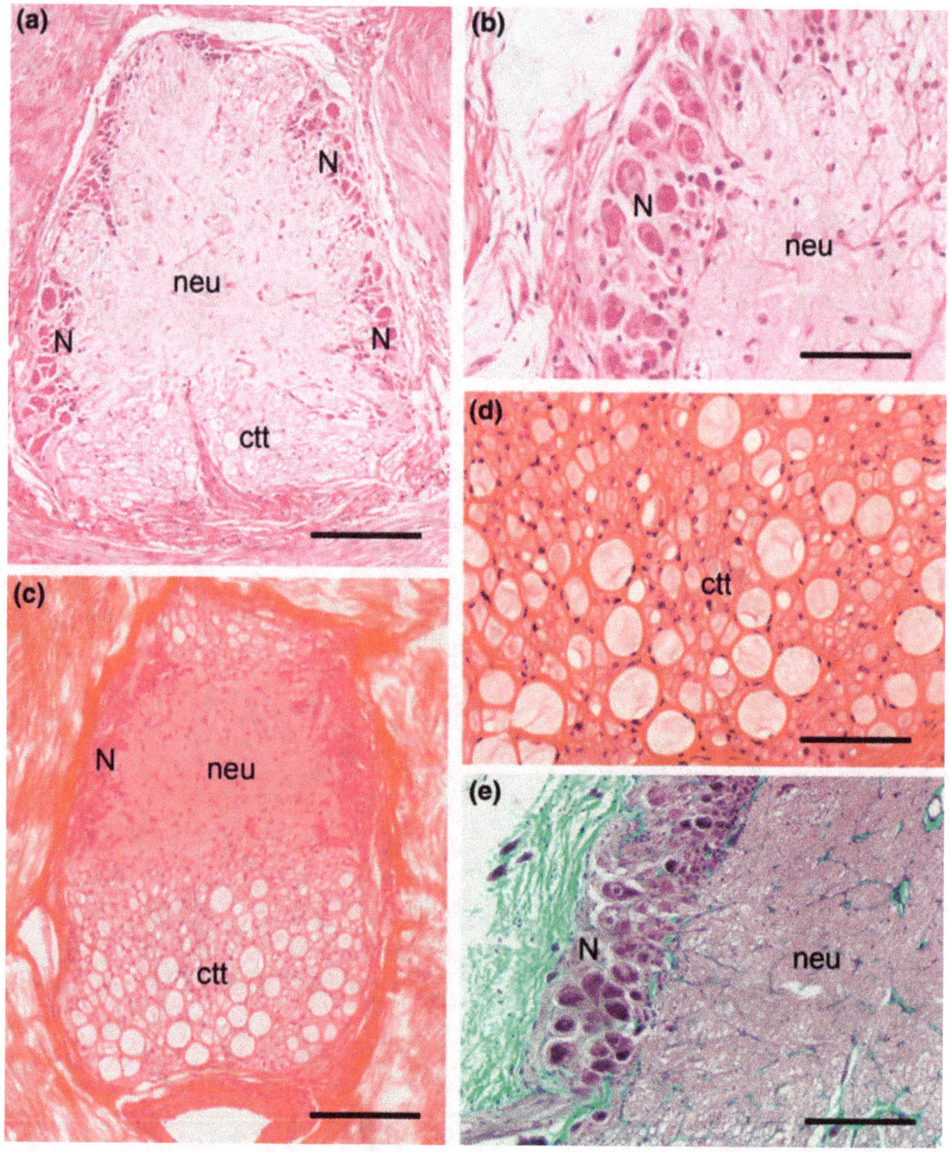

Fig. 4.25 Transverse section of the nerve cord of club (**a**, **b**) and tentacle (**c**, **d**) of a squid. **a**, **b** Panoramic view and detail showing the mantle of neuron perikarya that surround the central neuropil (neu). Glial and vascular processes are the better stained structures in the neuropil. Note the cerebral–tentacular tract (btt). **c**, **d** In the squid tentacle cord, the cerebro-tentacular tract is prominent exhibiting numerous coarse axons. With regard to the club, the cord neuropil is more scarce and the perikarya (N) small. **e** Section of octopus arm nerve cord showing the peripheral mantle of perikarya and the central neuropil. Masson's trichrome stains in green the vascular net entering the cord and the connective surrounding the cord. *Scale bars* **a**, **c** 200 μm; **b**, **d**, **e** 100 μm

neuropil with glial cells and capillaries. The size of neurons in the cortex varies from small to large or very large in the different ganglia. Some tracts of thickened fibers can be observed passing through the neuropil. These conspicuous tracts interconnect the different ganglia. Different nerves connect these ganglia with other structures. The subesophageal mass of cephalopods has evolved by fusion and specialization of several ganglia that are present in other mollusks. The anterior subesophageal mass of octopus gives rise to the eight thick arm nerves (ten in squid and cuttlefish), to large tracts joining the mass with the supraesophageal lobes (buccal, frontal) and to a large dorsal commissure. The arm nerves course toward the arms and to some distance of the brain acquire ganglionic cells and form the axial nerve cord that extends all along the center of the arms. The middle subesophageal mass receives the statocyst nerves. The subesophageal mass includes several conspicuous lobes dedicated to chromatophore control (chromatophoric lobes), as well as lobes dedicated to skin, vascular and body movements. The histological appearance of the chromatophoric lobes of octopus is unusual, with a very thick cortical layer with very numerous large neurons and a small core of cells and neuropil.

4.13.2 Ganglionic Nerve Cords of Arms and Tentacles (Fig. 4.25)

The control of the complex muscular system and coordination of arms and suckers, and the integration of sensory information, is provided by the brachial nerves and by additional arm ganglionic structures (Young 1971). The center of the arms and tentacles contains a ganglionic nerve cord that extends along the entire length and is continuous

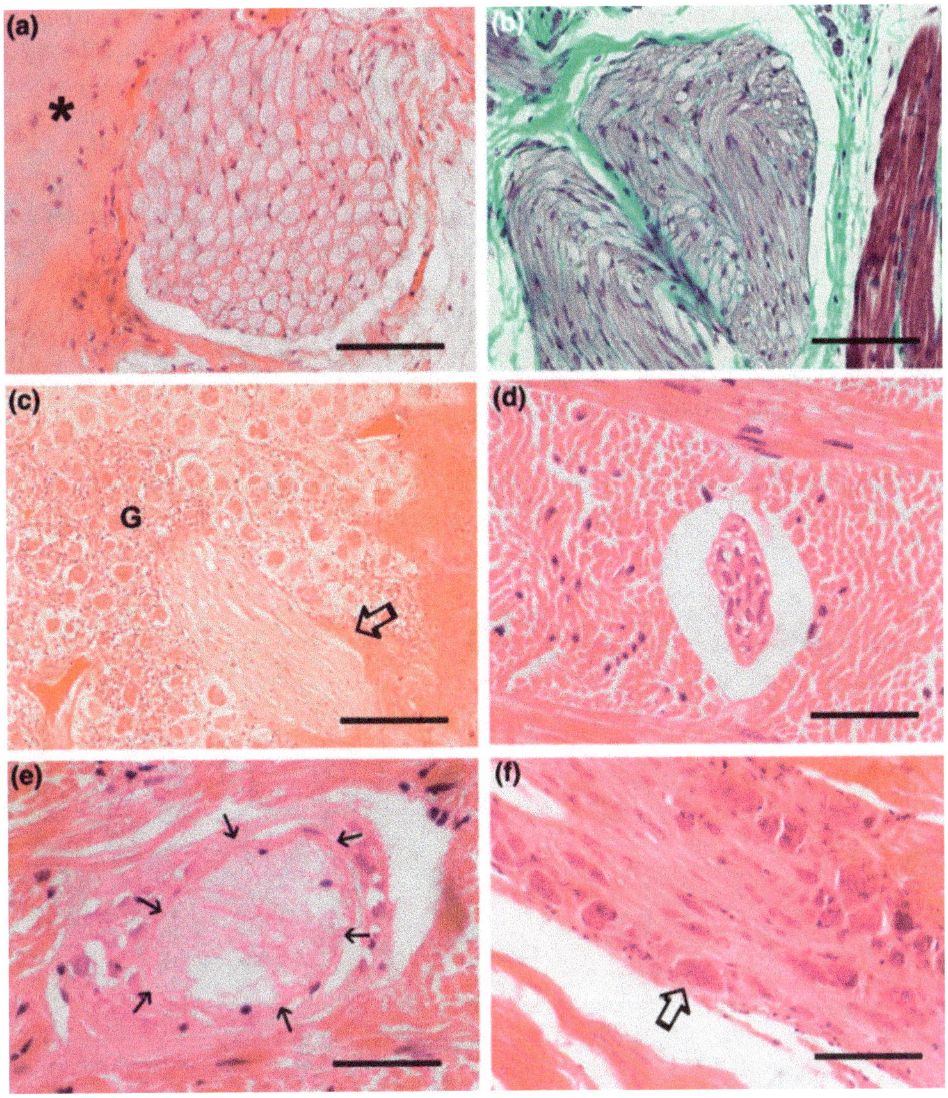

Fig. 4.26 Sections of nerves of octopus (**a**–**c**) and squid (**d**–**f**). **a**, **b** Transverse sections of nerves passing through the cranial skeleton showing the close arrangement and large diameter of non-myelinated fibers. Star, cartilage. **c**, Tangential section of the large-celled stellate ganglion (G) of octopus showing the exit of a stellar nerve (outlined arrow). **d**, **e** Mantle nerves of squid showing thin axons (**d**) and a giant axon (**e**), respectively. Thin arrows point to the profile of the giant axon. **f**, Branchial nerve cord with ganglion cells (outlined arrow). **a**, **c**–**f** H&E stain, **b** Masson's trichrome. *Scale bars* **a**, **b**, **d**–**f** 100 μm; **c** 200 μm

with the brachial nerve. The cord consists of a cortical region with perikarya mainly located at its lateral surfaces, a central region of neuropil and bundles of longitudinal fibers (cerebro-brachial tracts) on the oral and aboral sides. The cord innervates the complex musculature of the arms and suckers through numerous nerves, and also receives sensory fibers. The histological organization varies between arms and tentacles. In octopus arms, which bear two alternate lines of suckers, an alternate concentration of perikarya that innervate the suckers is noted along the cord (ganglionic cord). In squid tentacles, the shaft lacks suckers. In the nerve cord, almost a half of the oral side is occupied by thick fibers of the cerebro-brachial tract; those of the aboral side are smaller and scarcer. The lateral bands of neurons and central neuropil are located between tracts. Numerous glial cells are also observed. The cord is surrounded by connective tissue and accompanied of large blood vessels. In the tentacular club, the nerve cord is displaced toward the oral surface. The nerve cord organization is similar in cuttlefish tentacles.

4.13.3 Nerves, the Stellate Ganglion and the Giant Fiber System (Fig. 4.26)

Numerous nerves innervate the different parts of the cephalopod body. These consist of fibers of different diameters distinguishable from other tissues (muscle, connective) by its characteristic appearance. Some nerves consist of thick fibers, others of thin fibers and some of a mixture of thick and thin fibers. In the mantle of cuttlefish and squid, nerves containing a single giant nerve fiber are also recognizable.

The stellate ganglion is one of the larger peripheral ganglia of the coleoid nervous system. By its superficial location in the mantle, it is an accessible ganglion for experimentation. In octopus, it consists of a peripheral cortex with numerous large perikarya and a core neuropil that receives fibers from the palliovisceral lobe of the subesophageal mass through a coarse pallial nerve. The ganglion connects with the mantle through about 20 radial stellar nerves. This ganglion provides the motor fibers that innervate the mantle musculature. In cuttlefish and squid, the processes of some perikarya of this ganglion fuse to form the third-order giant fibers that innervate the mantle in these species. Most motor fibers arising in this ganglion, however, are not gigantic. In cuttlefish and squid, too, a pair of first-order gigantic neurons receiving statocyst fibers is situated in the magnocellular lobe of the subesophagic mass. These cells mediate the fast escape reflex in a way analogous to that of Mauthner neurons in many fishes. These first-order giant neurons contact second-order ganglion neurons located in the palliovisceral lobes that directly innervate some fast retractor muscles or contact the third-order giant axons in the stellate ganglion. Stellate nerves control respiratory movements of the mantle, jetting and the expansion of the mantle which causes water to be inhaled (Packard and Trueman 1974).

4.14 Reproductive System (Figs. 4.27, 4.28, 4.29, 4.30, 4.31, 4.32, 4.33, 4.34 and 4.35)

4.14.1 Females

The female reproductive system of coleoid cephalopods consists of an ovary and one (squid and cuttlefish) or two (octopus) oviducts with associated oviducal glands, which opens in the gonopore to the pallial cavity (Wells 1978).

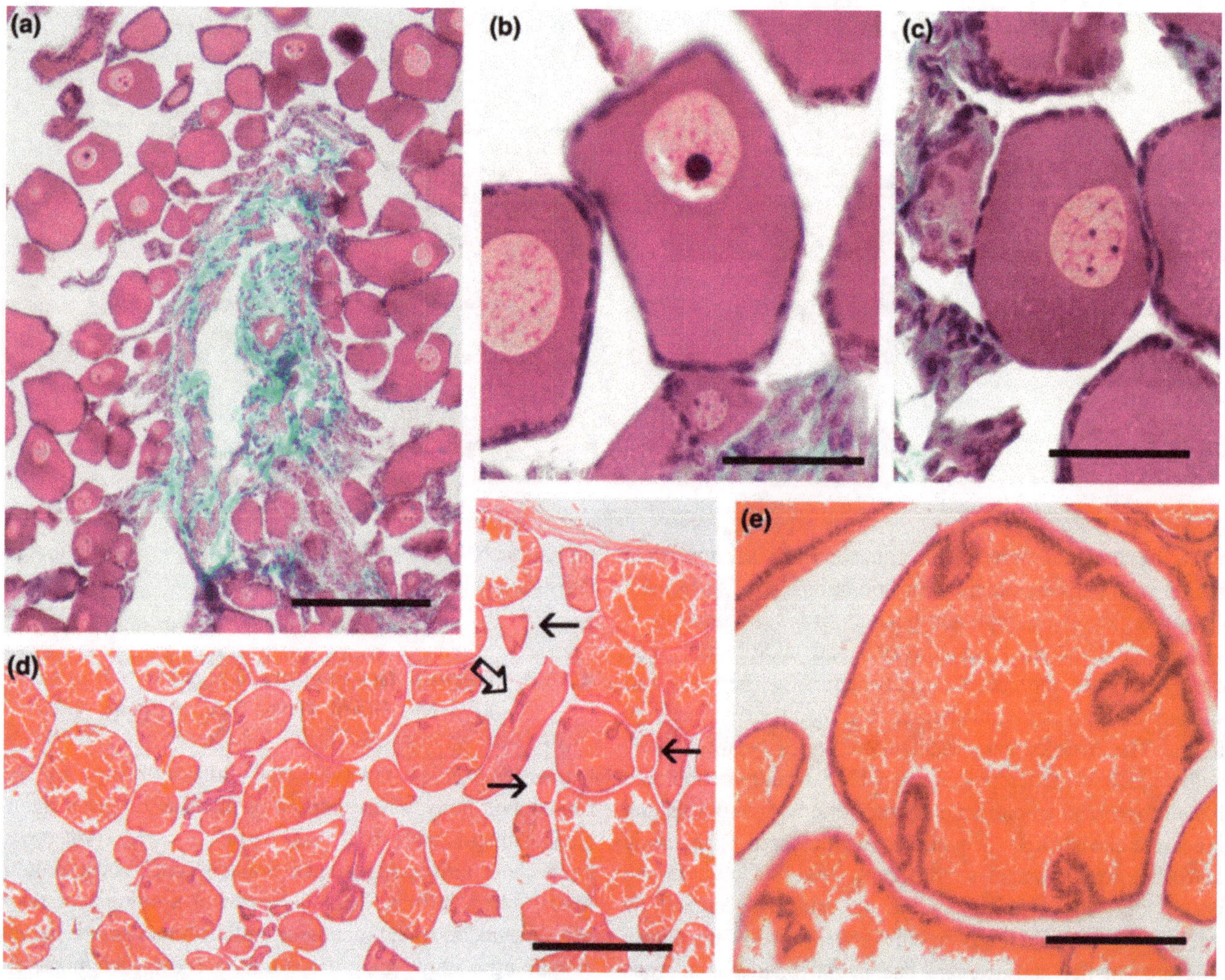

Fig. 4.27 Sections of ovaries of immature (**a–c**) and mature (**d**, **e**) female octopus. **a** Section of showing numerous oogonia and early oocytes attached to an ovarian cord. **b**, **c** Detail of an oogonia and oocytes in early folliculogenesis. Note in **b** a big nucleolus, and in **b** and **c** the meiotic chromosomes. **d** Section of a vitellogenic ovary showing abundant yolk inside oocytes and the follicular epithelium infolds forming elongated crests. Octopus follicles are elongated and pear-shaped, so that in sections of the long stalks show small diameter (arrows; most follicles are sectioned transversely). The outlined arrow points to an obliquely sectioned follicular stalk. **e** Detail of a vitellogenic follicle. **a–c** Masson's trichrome; **d**, **e** H&E stain. *Scale bars* **a** 200 μm; **b**, **c** 50 μm; **d** 800 μm; **e** 100 μm

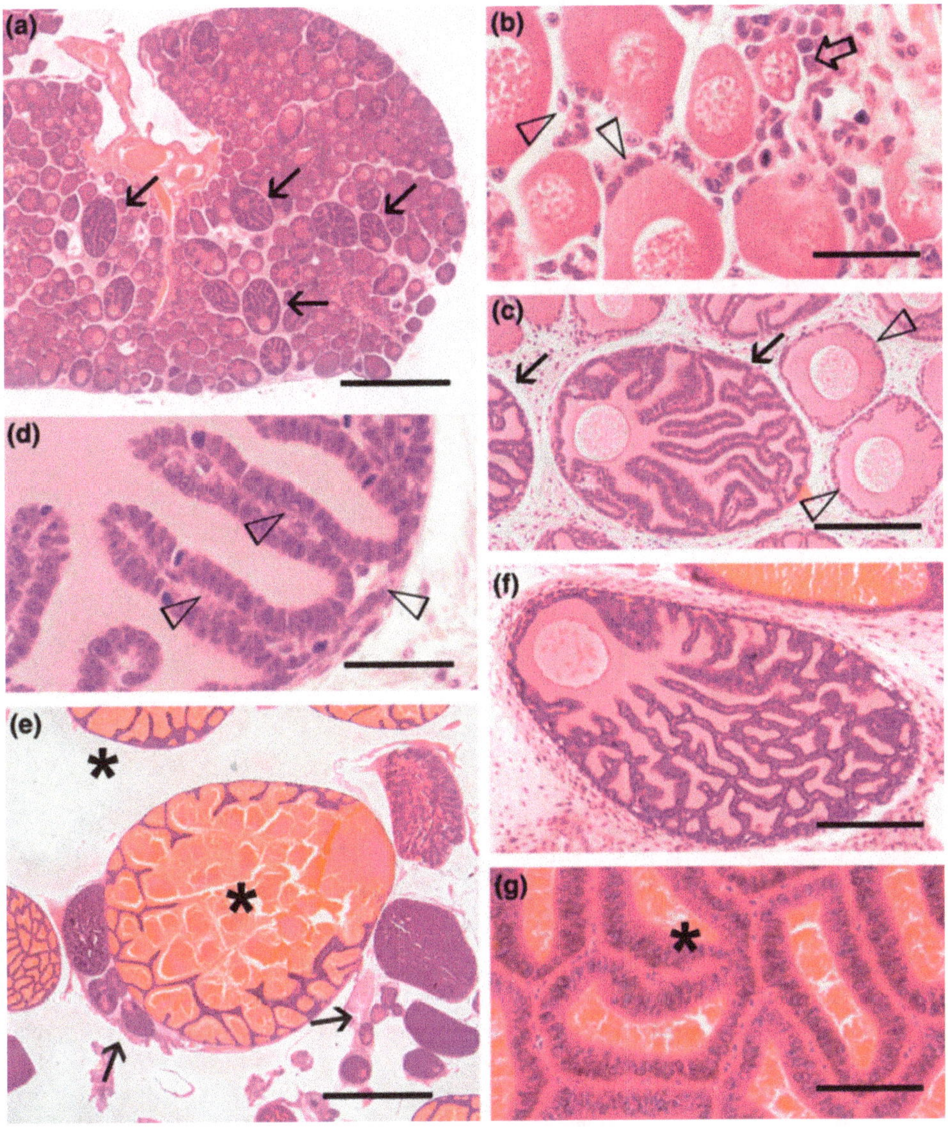

Fig. 4.28 Sections of ovaries of squid (**a–d**) and cuttlefish (**e–g**). **a** Panoramic view of an immature squid ovary showing some previtellogenic follicles (arrows) and a number of oocytes in early folliculogenesis. **b** Detail of a small oogonia (outlined arrow) and oocytes in early stages of folliculogenesis with a pole of follicular cells (arrowheads). Note that oocytes are in meiotic prophase (zygotene–pachytene) judging from the nuclear appearance. **c** Detail of previtellogenic follicles (thin arrows) and oocytes in folliculogenesis (arrowheads) of the same ovary. **d** Wall of a previtellogenic follicle showing deep infolds of the follicular epithelium accompanied of vasculo-connective tissue (arrowheads). Note frequent mitotic figures in the follicular epithelium. **e** Section of a mature cuttlefish ovary showing large vitellogenic follicles (stars) and smaller follicles in previtellogenic stages (arrows). Note the yellow-stained yolk inside the cytoplasm of large oocytes. **f** Previtellogenic follicle of cuttlefish showing the reticular appearance of follicular infolds. **e** Detail of the follicular infolds of a large vitellogenic follicle. H&E stain. *Scale bars* **a** 0.8 mm; **b**, **d**, **g** 50 μm; **c**, **f** 200 μm; **e** 1.2 mm

Spermatophore receptacles or spermathecae of octopus are part of the oviducal gland, whereas receptacles of cuttlefish and squid females are located in the head. In decapods, a pair of large nidamental glands and accessory nidamental glands opens directly in the pallial cavity near the gonopore. These accessory glands lack in octopus. Oviducal and nidamental glands form the egg case that is essential in the reproductive strategy of cephalopods (Boletzky 1986).

4.14.1.1 The Ovary of Octopus (Fig. 4.27)

The ovary has the appearance of a racemose gland with numerous ovarian follicles surrounded by the gonadial coelom. A comparison of the ovaria of immature and mature octopus illustrates the huge changes occurring in ovarian follicles (Di Cosmo et al. 2001). In sections of an octopus immature ovary sac, a large number of small developing follicles can be appreciated. These follicles are pear-shaped,

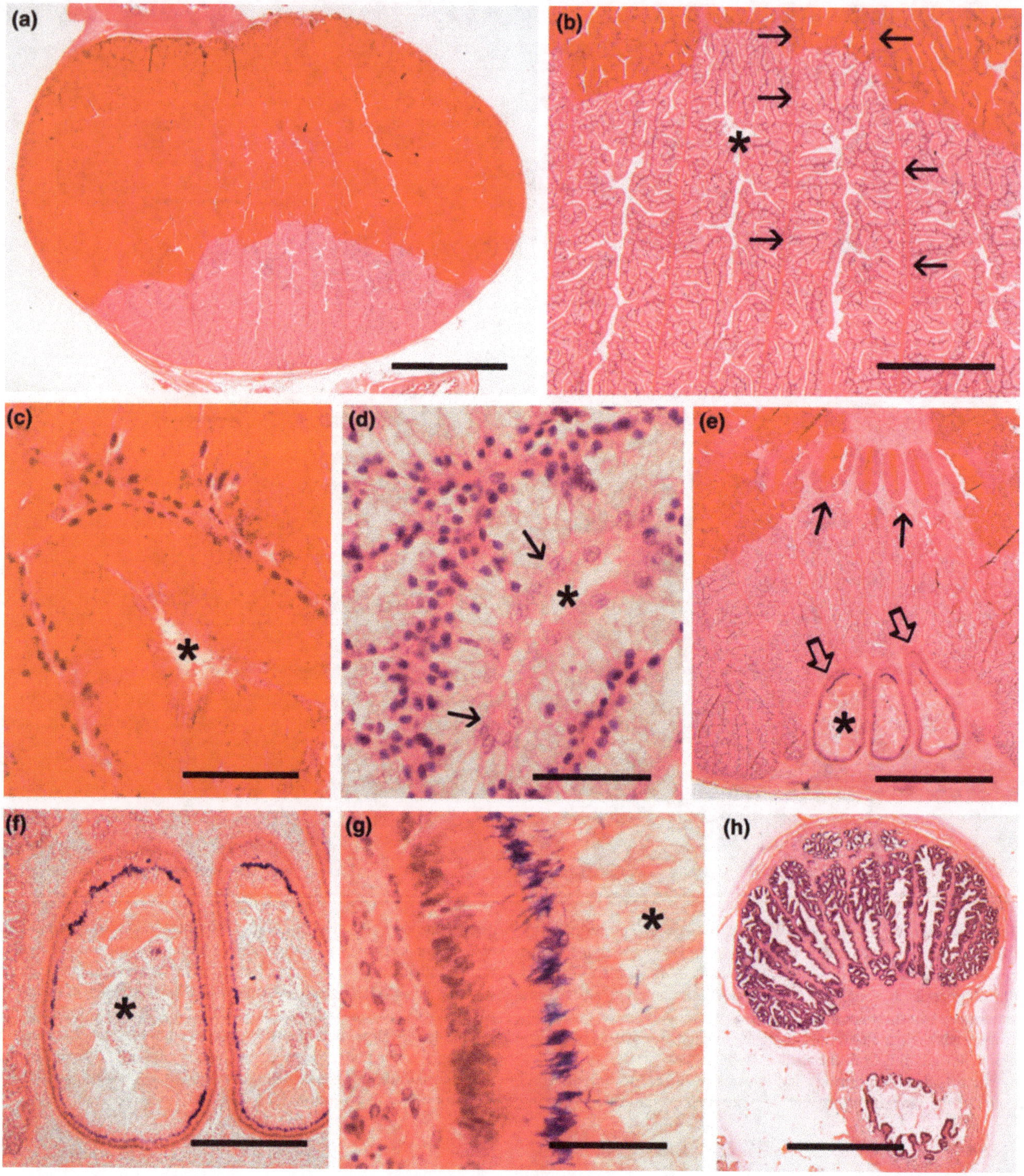

Fig. 4.29 **a**, **b** Longitudinal tangential section of the oviducal gland of a mature female octopus shows the organization in sectors consisting of glandular units of two types, proximal and distal with respect to the ovary. Distal units stain brightly red and the proximal units pale pink. Note the sharp limit between the units extending in each gland sector (arrowed) (**b**). Star, lumen of mucous region. **c** Detail of the distal glandular epithelium showing gland cells filled of red-stained secretory granules. Note the basal location of cell nuclei. Star, lumen. **d** Detail of proximal secretory units filled of pale mucous granules. Note pale nuclei of cells lining the lumen (arrows) and dense nuclei of gland cells. **e** Section passing more centrally showing secretory ducts of the distal portion (arrows) and sections of three spermathecae (outlined arrows). **f** Spermathecae with sperm released from spermatophores waiting for egg fertilization. **g** Detail of the spermatheca tall epithelium with attached sperm heads and long sperm tails directed to the lumen (bundles of tails are appreciable in **f**). **h** Tangential section of the oviducal gland and oviduct (ov) of an immature female octopus showing sectors of branching tubules that are broadly separated by connective stroma. Star, lumen. H&E stain. *Scale bars* **a**, **e** 1.2 mm; **b** 400 μm; **f** 500 μm; **c**, **d**, **g** 50 μm; **h** 1 mm

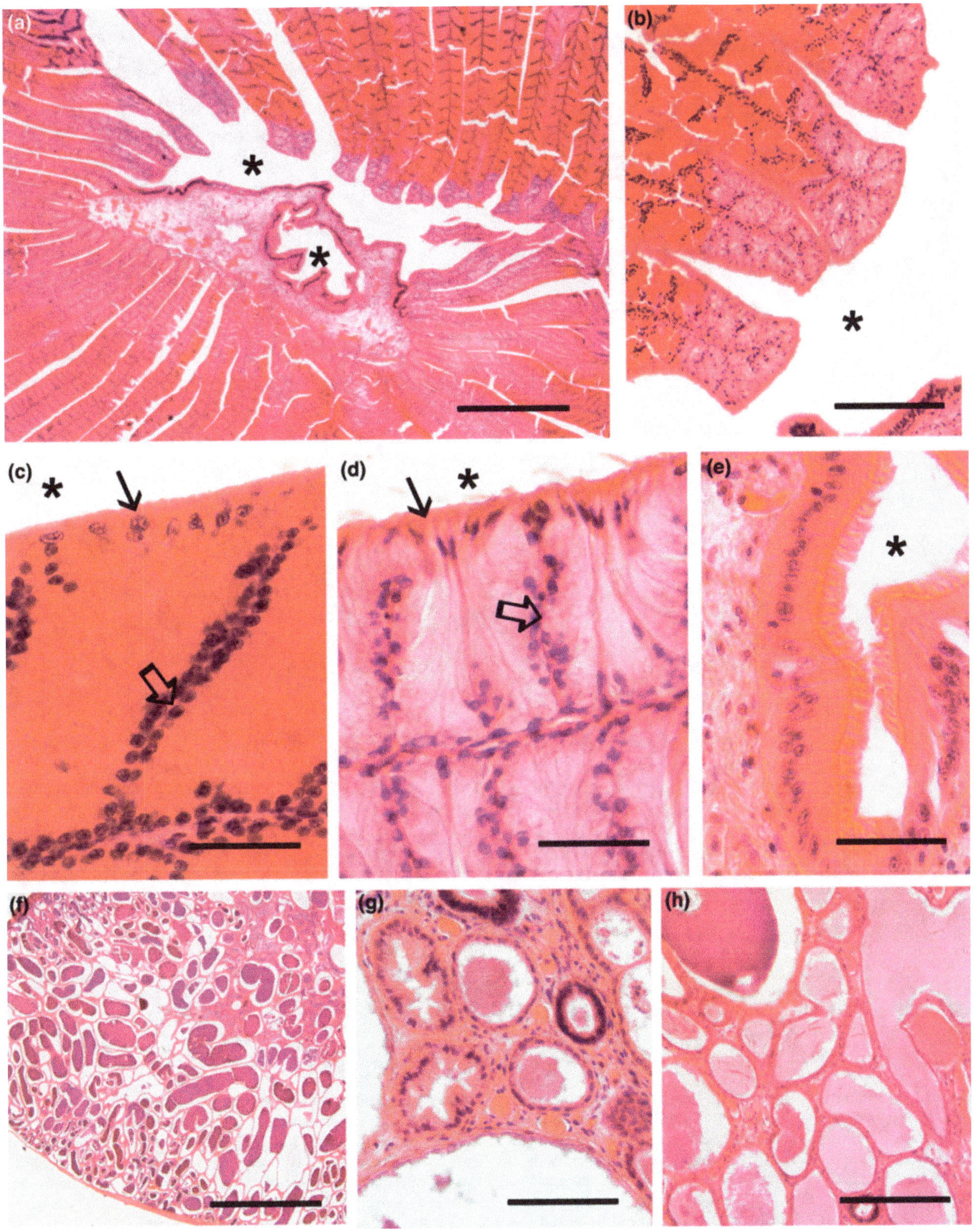

Fig. 4.30 **a** Section of the nidamental gland of a mature female cuttlefish showing leafs of glandular tissue around a central region showing the gland duct. **b** Detail of the inner region of leafs showing two different glandular regions. **c** Detail of the basal region of the leaf showing closely apposed parallel bands of tall glandular cells with cytoplasm filled of red-stained granules and a dense basal nucleus. Note apical non-glandular cells (arrow). **d** Detail of the apical region of the leaf showing parallel bands of tall mucous cells with basal nuclei and apical supporting cells (arrow). The outlined arrows in **c**, **d** point to the thin connective layers separating glandular bands excepting apically. **e** Section of the nidamental gland duct showing the tall ciliated epithelium. Stars in **a–e** indicate the glandular and duct lumen. **f–h**, Panoramic view and details of the accessory nidamental gland of a mature female cuttlefish showing numerous glandular tubules filled of secretion. H&E stain. *Scale bars* **a**, **f** 500 µm; **b**, **h** 200 µm; **c–e** 50 µm; **g** 100 µm

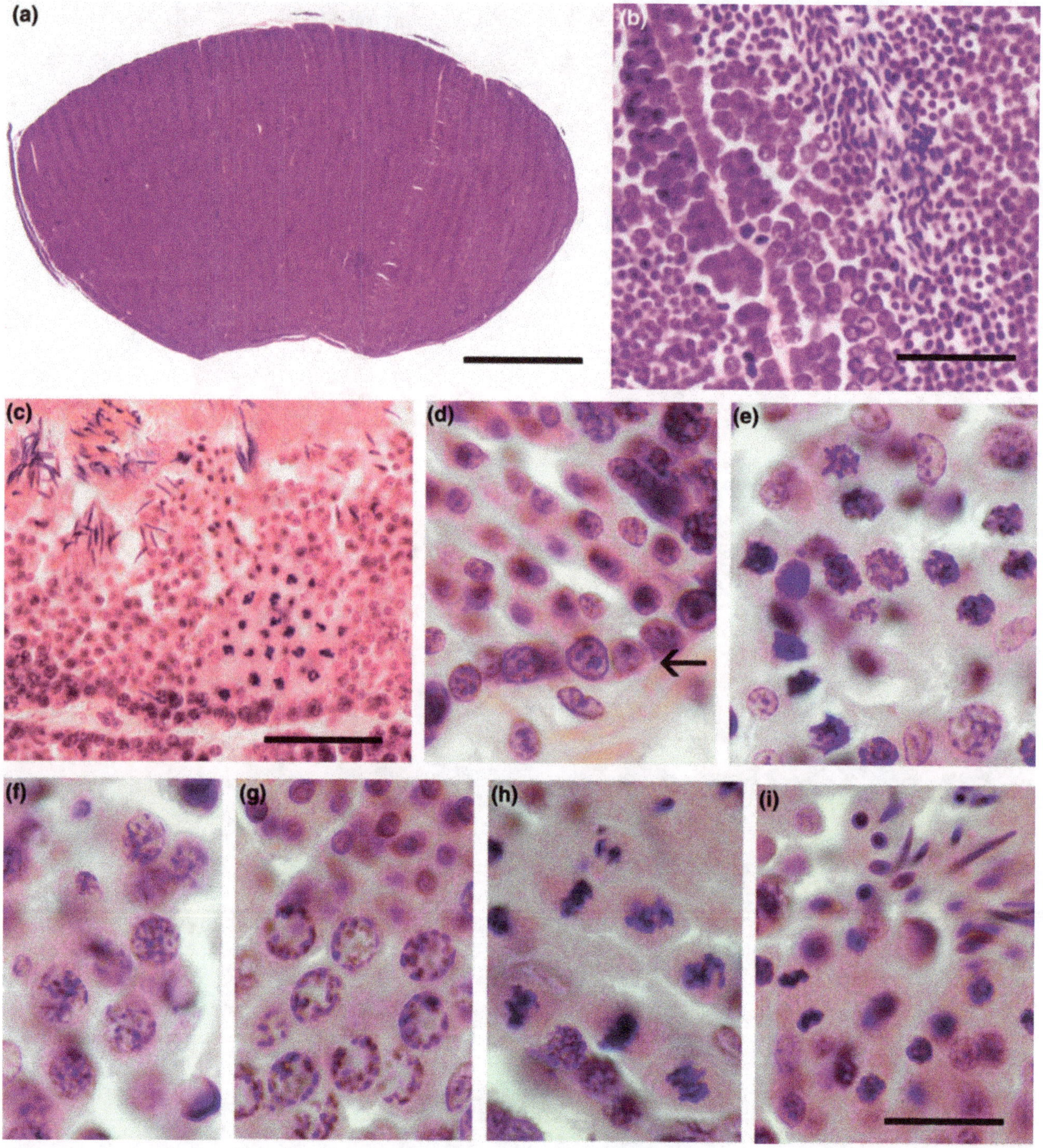

Fig. 4.31 **a** Section of the testis of an immature squid showing the compact organization of testicular cords. **b** Detail of adjacent testicular cords (tubules) showing a zonal organization with spermatogonia in the outer layers, followed of cysts of spermatocytes and spermatids in maturation. **c** Section of the wall of a testicular tubule of a mature octopus showing cysts of germ cells in different maturation stages, including mature spermatozoa. **d–i** Details of spermatogenic cells in different stages of maturation. **d** Layer of spermatogonia (arrow) in the tubule border. **b** Cluster of spermatocytes in leptotene (prophase **I** of meiosis). **f** Cluster of spermatocytes **I** in zygotene. **f** Cluster of spermatocytes in pachytene (bottom) and early spermatids (top). **h** Cluster of spermatocytes in metaphase **I**. **i** Spermatocytes in telophase **I** (bottom), and spermatids with elongating nuclei (top). H&E stain. *Scale bars* **a** 1 mm; **b** 40 µm; **c** 50 µm; **i** 16 µm, this bar also applies to **d–h**

with a long stalk continuous by its proximal end with the septal ingrowths of the ovary wall and protrude in the ovarian cavity. The octopus oocytes are flask-shaped with a thin part entering the stalk and a thicker distal region. The oocyte is covered by an inner follicular epithelium surrounded by a flattened ovarian epithelium with thin blood vessels that enter in the stalk between these layers. The nucleus of immature oocytes is rounded and exhibits a large nucleolus and a granular appearance. In mature octopus, the ovary contains very large yolk-filled oocytes, which are covered by a thick follicular epithelium that shows some longitudinal infoldings. The number of follicular cells covering each oocyte is enormous. These follicular cells synthesize among others the main protein of yolk, vitellogenin and other substances as lipids that form this egg reserve material. With high magnification, a number of yolk platelets are appreciable in the otherwise homogeneous yolky region. Nuclei are very infrequently observed in sections of these big oocytes.

4.14.1.2 The Ovary of Squid and Cuttlefish (Fig. 4.28)

The pictured sections of squid ovary were from an immature female. In this ovary, a large number of immature, previtellogenic oocytes of several sizes, are observed. Smaller oocytes only present very flattened follicular cells and may appear to contact other oocytes, whereas in larger oocytes a thicker follicular epithelium was clearly appreciable. Only a few oocytes show infolds of their surface accompanied of a pleated sheet of follicular cells. In larger follicles, numerous mitotic figures are appreciable in the follicular epithelium. The nucleus of oocytes shows chromatin with granular appearance but not a conspicuous nucleolus.

Sections of ovaries of mature female cuttlefish show ovarian follicles in different stages of development, the most advanced being in vitellogenic stages. The presence of follicles in different stages of development indicates that cuttlefish females may breed at different times. Small previtellogenic oocytes are surrounded by a layer of follicular cells whose height increases with development. In more advanced vitellogenic follicles, the follicular epithelium becomes pleated accommodating in the infolds of the oocyte surface, having a meandering appearance. These infolds are anastomosed forming a complex network. The follicular cells are short and are mostly occupied by a round condensed nucleus. In some sections, the large and round oocyte nucleus can be appreciated with uncondensed chromatin showing an appearance similar to that of lampbrush chromosomes (uncondensed bivalents), and the cytoplasm becomes slightly basophilic. In large vitellogenic follicles, the follicular cells are tall and intensely basophilic, with a granular nucleus that occupies the middle of the cell. The entire follicle is surrounded by connective tissue (follicular theca), and connective tissue and blood vessels enter in the axis of infoldings of the follicular epithelium. This is unlike octopus, where the covers of follicles are inconspicuous. The oocyte is filled of eosinophilic yolk that by places appears formed of rounded platelets. The follicle diameter increased considerably from early vitellogenic stages. Atretic follicles can also be observed in the ovary.

4.14.1.3 The Oviduct

The oviduct of female cuttlefish is a duct with folded inner surface that consists of a high ciliated epithelium that lies on a thick connective-vascular tissue. The thin and tall epithelial cells show basal nuclei. Muscular layers surround externally the connective tissue.

4.14.1.4 The Oviducal Gland and Seminal Receptacle of Female Octopus (Fig. 4.29)

The oviducal gland of mature female octopus is a compact ovoid-shaped gland that exhibits two different sectors, an outer sector consisting of highly eosinophilic gland cells and an inner one with light gland cells, with a clear limit between. These sectors produce cement (a mucoprotein) and mucopolysaccharides that act as a polymerizer of the cement, to form an egg string for its fixation to appropriate substrates. The gland appears organized in compact lobes separated by thin connective septa that extend through both sectors, and it is covered with a thin connective-muscular capsule. The lobes consist of branched glandular epithelial tubules with thick walls and small lumen that are separated by very thin septa, giving the gland a quite compact appearance. The tubules branch from the central region of the lobe, where the lumen of the tubules is larger. The tubules of the eosinophilic sector consist of two types of cell, glandular and supporting, the glandular cells showing the abundant cytoplasm filled of round secretory granules that are highly eosinophilic, whereas the small and condensed nucleus is located basally close to the septa. The supporting cells have larger nuclei located apically and basal processes coursing among glandular cells, but they are masked by the large amount of secretory granules. The non-eosinophilic sector is also formed of closely apposed thick branched epithelial tubules with small lumen. In this sector, the supporting cells show clearly their apical nuclei and the basal processes because the light glandular cells do not mask them. The light gland cells exhibit condensed nuclei in the basal region. No continuity between eosinophilic and light tubules was observed in the sections examined. In the central region of the eosinophilic lobes, some short tubules showed regions without gland cells covered by ciliated epithelial cells, forming a transition toward the gland ducts that are covered by a tall ciliated epithelium with undulated surface. In sections showing the ducts, they appear filled of a mass of eosinophilic granules including condensed nuclei, suggesting that secretion of this gland sector is of holocrine type.

The seminal receptacle of female octopus consists of the spermathecae, which are closely associated with the oviducal gland. They are elongated sacs of smooth surface covered of a columnar epithelium with nuclei located basally. In mated females, the epithelium is associated with large numbers of sperm cells attached through their head, whereas the long sperm tails fill the sac cavity accompanied of numerous eosinophilic globules. Sperm waits there until oviposition.

Unlike in mature females, the oviducal glands of immature octopus show a very different appearance, with wide ducts of pleated and branched walls, forming numerous alveolar structures. These ducts exhibit a radial arrangement around the oviduct, and each duct and its lobules are separated from those adjacent by abundant connective tissues. The ducts are covered of a tall ciliated epithelium, and the walls do not show the appearance of glandular epithelium.

4.14.1.5 Nidamental Glands (Fig. 4.30)

The nidamental gland of cuttlefish is a large gland of massive appearance formed of a number of laminas extending from the periphery toward the center. The lamina is formed of two closely apposed thick layers of glandular–epithelial tissue separated by a thin vasculo-connective axial region with an unusual appearance. The glandular cells are organized in parallel bands partially separated by processes of ciliated epithelial cells. In these bands, the gland cell nuclei are displaced toward the limit of the axial sheet or to the limit between adjacent bands, whereas the abundant cytoplasm with secretory granules is located toward the centro-apical region. This organization produces a characteristic pattern of parallel bands when sections are tangential to the lamina surface. The elongated glandular units may be anastomosed at some points. The covering cells are small cells with nuclei located mostly apically in the epithelium and long basal processes coursing mostly among gland cells toward the basis of the epithelium or to the lines between adjacent secretory bands. These cells are ciliated. Toward the tip of the lamina, the epithelium becomes progressively thinner, most glandular cells disappear and the epithelium changes to a thin highly ciliated epithelium similar to that covering the gland duct. Areas of ciliated epithelium can also be observed toward the base of laminas. The outer surface of the gland is formed of connective-vascular layers.

The accessory gland of cuttlefish is a large glandular structure filled of numerous wide tubular and alveolar structures surrounded with layers of connective and vascular tissue. Tubular parts of small diameter are covered with a simple cuboidal epithelium and have reduced lumen, whereas the dilated tubules and alveoli are covered by a flattened epithelium. Abundant amorphous secretory material can be appreciated inside of alveoli and tubules. Among tubules and alveoli run thin sheets of connective-vascular tissue with numerous blood vessels.

In immature female squid, the elongated nidamental gland shows a large number of closely parallel laminas formed of two apposed cuboid epithelia with a thin connective-vascular lamina between them. At the border of laminas, each layer of

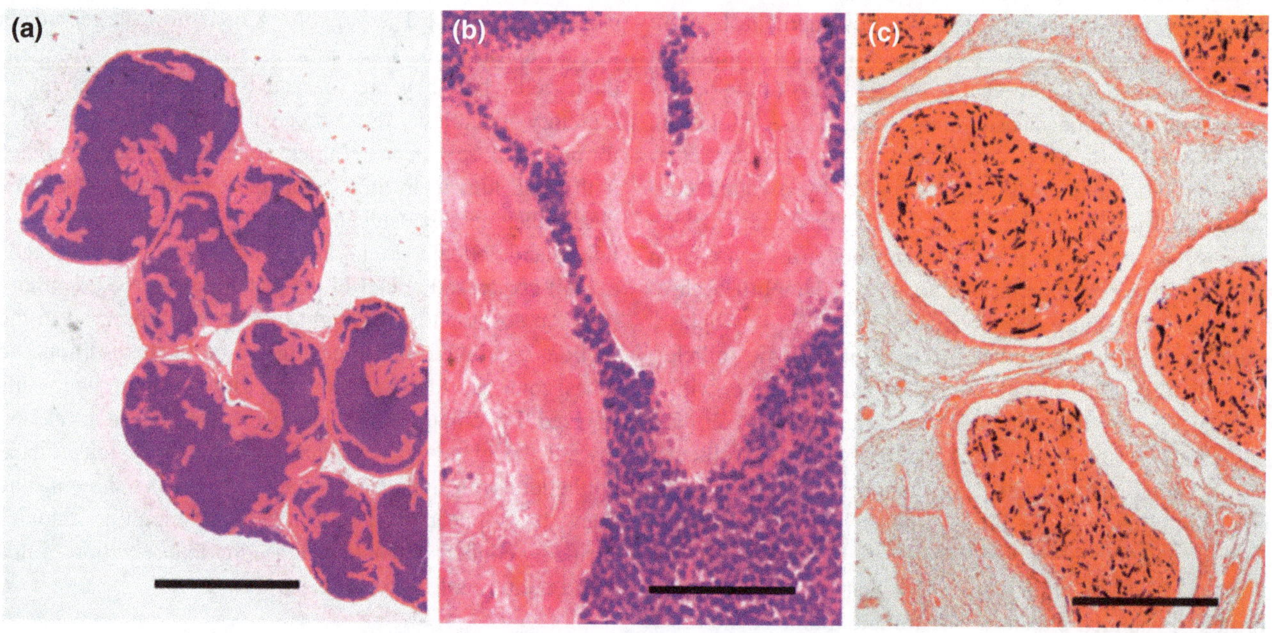

Fig. 4.32 Sections of the ependyme (coiled male duct) of cuttlefish (**a**, **b**) and octopus (**c**). Note large amounts of spermatozoa and in **b**, the thick epithelium covering the trabeculas that are characteristic of cuttlefish and squid. H&E stain. *Scale bars* **a** 1 mm; **b** 50 μm; **c** 500 μm

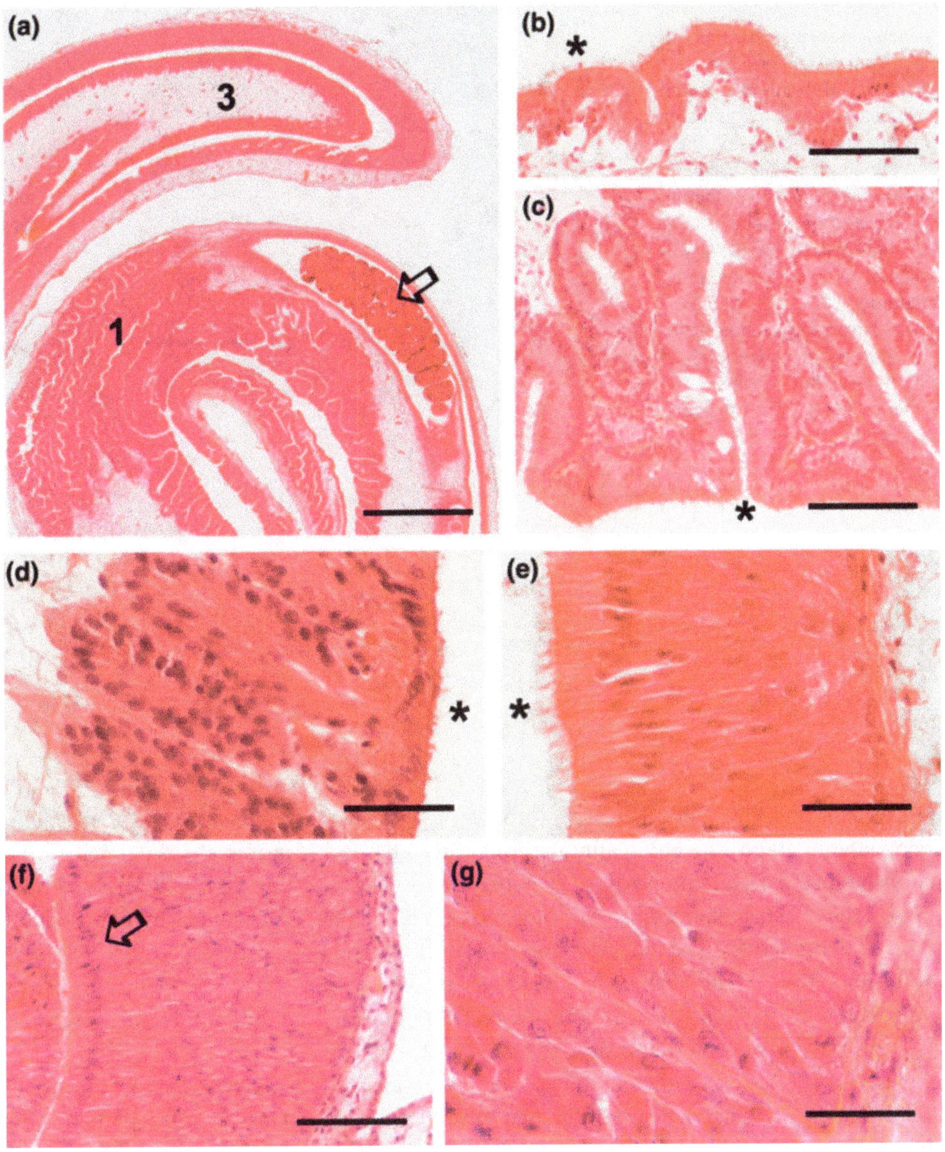

Fig. 4.33 **a** Section of the spermatophoric gland of a mature male octopus showing different parts, including a convoluted glandular region (1; Section 1), a thick-walled secretory part (3; Section 3) and a part of the proximal vas deferens with a sperm rope inside (outlined arrow) abutting Section 1. **b** Detail of the ciliated epithelium of the vas deferens. Star, lumen. **c** Detail of the convoluted glandular epithelium in Section 1. **d**, **e** Detail of glandular epithelia of Section 3 covering the convex wall (**d**) and the thicker outer region (**e**). Note the different appearance of basal regions, with solid invaginations in **d** and smooth in **e**. The apical epithelial cells are ciliated, as better shown in **e**. Stars, duct lumen. **f** Section of the thick glandular epithelium of the spermatophoric gland of a cuttlefish, with an appearance similar to that octopus. The outlined arrow points to superficial epithelial (supporting) cells. **g** Detail of basal columns of gland cells that form most of the epithelium. H&E stain. *Scale bars* **a** 1 mm; **d**, **e** 50 μm; **b**, **c**, **f** 100 μm; **g** 30 μm

epithelium is continuous with that of the adjacent lamina. The epithelium shows frequent apical mitosis and lacks any glandular appearance at this immature stage.

4.14.1.6 Male Reproductive Organs (Figs. 4.31, 4.32, 4.33, 4.34 and 4.35)

The male reproductive system of coleoid cephalopods consists of a single testis and the gonoduct, which comprises the proximal deferent canal (male duct, spermiduct), blind-end seminal vesicles (spermatophoric glands) and associated accessory gland, the distal deferent canal and a dilatation that, in mature animals, contains spermatophores, the Needham's sac. It opens into the pallial cavity through the gonopore (Mann et al. 1970; Wells 1978).

The Testis (Fig. 4.31)

In immature males of cuttlefish, the testis is massive and formed of closely apposed testicular cords or tubules. The cords show a large number of germinal cells in different phases of maturation. In a mature male octopus, the massive testis consists of a number of thick-walled testicular tubules with maturing spermatozoa inside the lumen. The tubules are separated by a thin connective-vascular space. The walls of tubules show a sequence of stages of spermatogenesis from gonial stages outside to spermiogenesis near the lumen. Cysts of cells are easily recognized because they show the same appearance. The outermost cell layer is formed of spermatogonia attached to a connective membrane that at some places look like an epithelium. Mitosis is occasionally

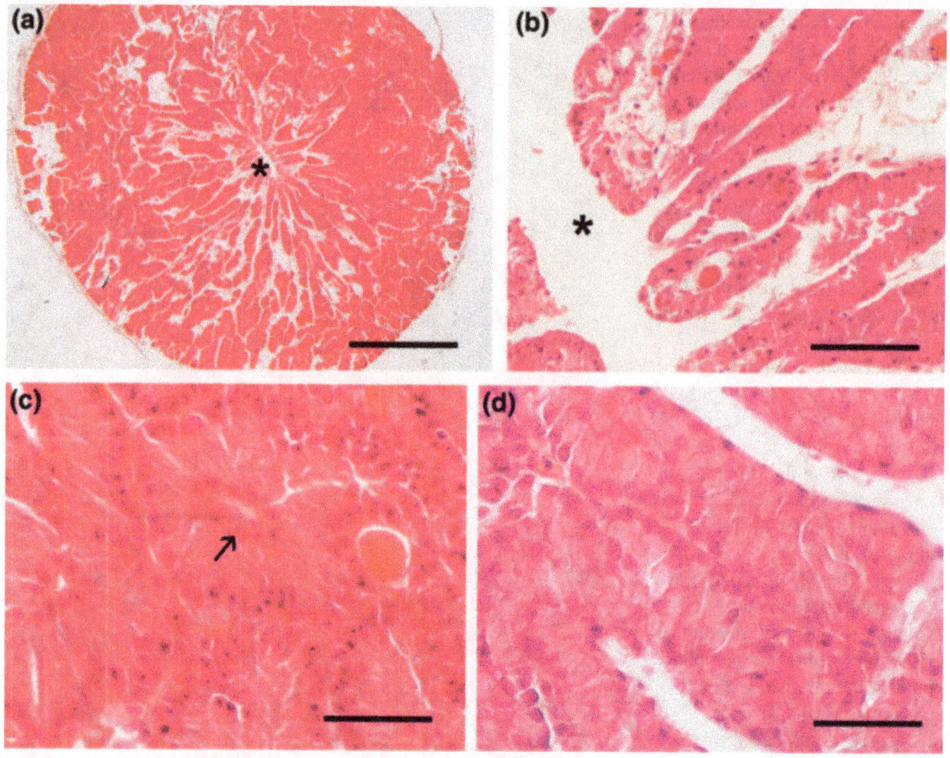

Fig. 4.34 **a** Transverse section of the accessory spermatophoric gland (spermatophoric gland system II, prostrate) of a mature male octopus showing numerous glandular tubules abutting the central duct. **b** Detail of the junction of tubules with the duct (star). **c** Section of tubules showing the secretory cells with nuclei in the outer region and supporting cells close to the lumen (arrow). **d** Section of the accessory spermatophoric gland of cuttlefish showing the glandular tissue. H&E stain. *Scale bars* **a** 800 µm; **b** 100 µm; **c**, **d** 50 µm

observed in this layer. In other areas, groups of secondary spermatogonia with fine chromatin are prophasic cells. Primary spermatocytes are numerous occupying next locations. These cells are characterized by their large size (they are the largest cells in the testis) and characteristic chromatin inside the nucleus that reveals that cells of each group are in the same phase of the long first meiotic prophase (leptotene, zygotene, pachytene and diplotene). Some cysts also appear in metaphase I showing paired chromosomes with a lozenge shape. This is the longest phase of the first meiotic division, and the anaphase I and telophase I are rarely observed. Most cells over the region of primary spermatocytes are small spermatids with small round nuclei, because spermatocytes II and second meiotic division are short-lived stages. Cysts of spermatids changing its nuclear shape (elongating) in various stages of transformation to spermatozoa can also be observed close to the lumen. Clumps of spermatozoa with long filamentous nucleus and tangles of long sperm flagella occupy the lumen of the tube.

Proximal Vas Deferens and Ependymus (Fig. 4.32)

In male cuttlefish, the ependymus appears as a tortuous dilated tube filled of spermatozoa, which in sections appears to consist of a pale cubic or flattened epithelium over a thin vasculo-connective lamina. In cuttlefish, the tube exhibits sparse meandering infolds of the epithelium, which is unlike the octopus. The large amounts of spermatozoa preclude a clear observation of the apical surface of these epithelial cells.

The spermatozoa leaving the octopus testis pass into the proximal vas deferens (Mann et al. 1970). In mature octopus, this highly convoluted duct consists of a ciliated epithelium surrounded by connective tissue. The duct is dilated by the presence of large masses (rope) of spermatozoa and has a rather smooth inner surface with opposite indentations. Numerous blood vessels enter the axis of the tubular complex.

Spermatophoric Gland I (Seminal Vesicle) (Fig. 4.33)

This complex part of the spermiduct follows the proximal vas deferens containing a beaded rope of spermatozoa in Fig. 4.33a. It is a convoluted structure in which three sectors can be distinguished from proximal to distal (Mann et al. 1970). A proximal region is characterized by the labyrinth formed by its finely pleated walls. Its inner walls consist of a high ciliated epithelium showing two layers of nuclei, those of ciliated cells in the apical region, and those of the numerous glandular cells in the basal region of the epithelium. The epithelium is finely pleated and a thin basal vasculo-connective layer separates its different folds. The third sector shows a C-shaped lumen because a side of the tube wall protrudes toward it. In this third region, the ciliated glandular epithelium is very thick and shows a striking appearance. Differences are noted between the thicker epithelium covering the outer, concave lumen surface and the thinner convex inner surface. In the outer lumen surface, a large number of nuclei are distributed through most of the epithelium thickness. Several rows of dense spindle-shaped

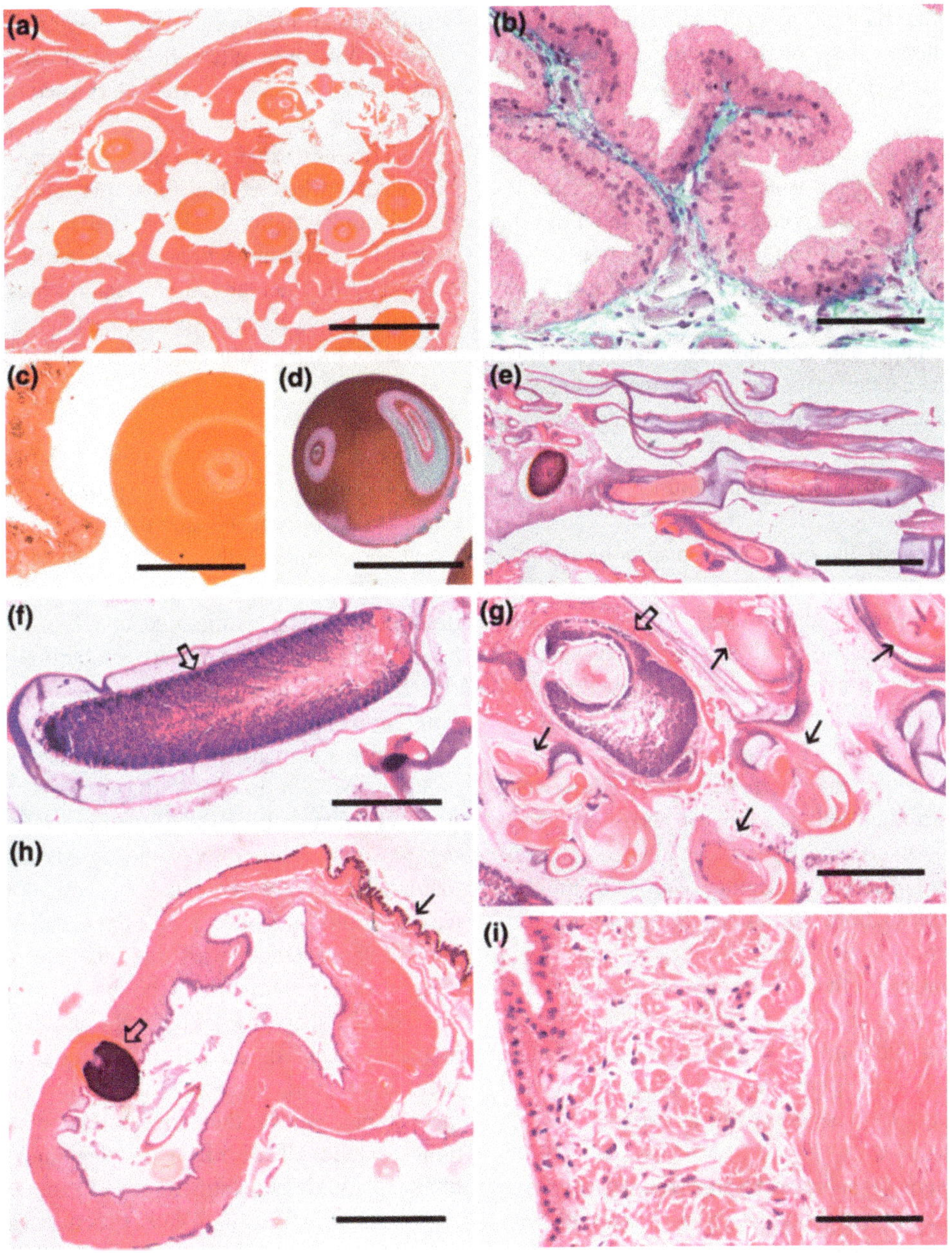

Fig. 4.35 **a** Transverse section showing a part of the octopus Needham's (spermatophoric) sac with spermatophores among extensive wall folds. **b** Detail of the simple thick epithelium covering the branched folds and the connective-vascular axes. **c, d** Sections of the "female oriented" ejection apparatus of octopus spermatophores showing the secretion spiral in **d**. Note the layered organization of the ejaculatory apparatus. **e** Section of cuttlefish elongated spermatophores in Needham's sac showing different regions. **f** Section passing trout the cuttlefish spermatophore "male-oriented" pole containing the coiled rope of spermatozoa. **g** Sections of spermatophores passing through the transition between the rope and the ejaculatory apparatus (outlined arrow) and through different levels of this apparatus (thin arrows). Note the complex spermatophore organization. **h** Transverse section of the terminal organ (penis) of a squid showing a spermatophore (outlined arrow) lodged in one of the longitudinal grooves of the wall. Note skin papillae (thin arrow). **i** Detail of the covering epithelium and the longitudinal and circular muscle layers. **a**, **c**, **e–i** H&E stain; **b**, **d** Masson's trichrome. *Scale bars* **a** 500 μm; **b** I, 50 μm; **c**, **d**, **f**, **g**, 100 μm; **e**, **h** 200 μm

nuclei are located apically, corresponding to nuclei of ciliated epithelial cells and apical mucous cells. Other glandular cells with larger and less-condensed nuclei are distributed along most of the thickness. Deep glandular cells appear grouped forming vertical columns corresponding with the lobes of the basal border of the epithelium. The distribution of glandular cells in the convex surface of this sector is clearly lobular, with basal lobes extending in the loose connective submucosa. Deep glandular cells show an eosinophilic cytoplasm but do not show secretory granules. In tangential sections through the apical part of the epithelium, a mosaic of necks of glandular cells of two types is appreciable. In some parts of the thick epithelium, there are large cells with large nuclei often showing a conspicuous nucleolus. These cells probably correspond to intraepithelial sensory neurons. In the region containing these cells, small intraepithelial nerve bundles are also seen coursing horizontally near the base of the epithelium. Below the epithelium, there is a layer of loose connective tissue that links the major turns of the glandular conduct.

In mature male cuttlefish, the thick epithelium of the spermatophoric sector 3 appears quite similar to that of octopus. The lobed appearance of the basal glandular region is more pronounced than in octopus, and thin connective laminas ascend among lobes till the subapical region.

Spermatophoric Gland II *(*Accessory Gland, Prostrate*)* (Fig. 4.34)

This is a massive gland that in octopus consists of a highly branched system of thick-walled convoluted glandular tubules that radiate from a central canal. The gland is surrounded by a thin connective capsule, whereas thin laminas of vasculo-connective tissue extend from it inside the gland and branch separating glandular tubules. Blood vessels are numerous. The tubules consist of two types of cell. Most of the thickness of the epithelium is formed of glandular cells with basal nuclei. Other cells are ciliated and show apical nuclei located near the central lumen. The ciliated nature of these cells is better observed in sagittal sections of tubules, since in transverse sections the lumen is narrow or very narrow. At the junction of proximal tubules with the gland duct, the glandular epithelium diminishes its thickness and transforms in a ciliated cuboidal epithelium.

In mature male cuttlefish, the massive accessory gland consists of tubules with glandular and ciliated epithelial cells that are similar to those described in octopus.

Distal Vas Deferens (Transition to the Needham's Sac)

In octopus, this part of the gonoduct consists of a tube with the lumen invaded by long epithelial laminas accompanied of a vasculo-connective axis. Secondary laminas are numerous along the longest primary laminas. The epithelium is formed of cuboidal cells with numerous apical cilia, showing a homogeneous appearance.

Needham's (Spermatophoric) Sac, Spermatophores and Penis (Fig. 4.35)

The Needham's pouch or sac of mature male octopus is a wide sac of pleated inner walls covered in most parts of a thick glandular epithelium that contains the mature spermatophores waiting for breeding. The epithelium consists of tall ciliated cells with round nuclei. Nuclei of these cells are dense and locate at the basal pole of glandular cells, whereas a granular secretion occupies most of the apical cytoplasm. At the transition of this glandular epithelium to non-glandular regions, the tall glandular cells disappear, whereas covering cells form then all the epithelium. The glandular zone lies over a rich vasculo-connective layer. The folds of the inner wall of the sac in the glandular zone consist of long primary and short secondary folds sometimes bifurcated, whereas the folds are short and simple in non-glandular regions. The folded region surrounds spermatophores that in sections appear as long rods or circles depending on the plane of the section. Surrounding the sac, there is a loose connective wall containing numerous blood vessels, but apparently lacking muscular tissue.

Spermatophores

Spermatophores of octopus and cuttlefish are very long slender structures bearing large packets of spermatozoa that consist of two moieties, one that bears the rope of spermatozoa at one end and the other, the ejaculatory apparatus, in the other. The spermatophores of cuttlefish were first described in the seventieth century by Swammerdam, who represented five different parts including the long anterior flagellum, the coiled ejaculatory apparatus, a vitreous portion, a white substance and a posterior "perlucida" part. Since spermatophores are very large structures (about 2–3 cm long in octopus), histological sections provide details of parts but make difficult to understand the whole organization. Here, only some details of cuttlefish spermatophores will be presented. In sections through the posterior region, the coiled rope of spermatozoa shows a thin laminar appearance with thin laminas of eosinophilic material separating turns. The heads of spermatozoa are oriented obliquely toward the walls and the mass of tails and including materials toward the center and anteriorly. This spermatangium is surrounded by a thick slightly basophilic inner tunica and a thin eosinophilic outer tunica. These tunics extend till the tip of the flagellum surrounding the other spermatophore structures. The anterior limit of the spermatangium is a flask-like structure called the cement body of complex shape that after a constriction continues in a coiled layered structure that stains differentially. It disappears in the flagellum. For further data on spermatophores and the spermatophore reaction, see Mann et al. (1970), Marian and Domaneschi (2012) and Marian (2012).

Terminal Organ or Penis

From the spermatophoric sac, octopus spermatophores enter singly in the terminal spermatophoric duct consisting of the diverticulum and terminal organ or "penis" (Mann et al., 1970). In sections, the duct appears covered with a thick epithelium that consists of ciliated and mucous glandular cells. In the lumen, the single spermatophore is appreciable. The epithelium shows small undulations and invaginations. The epithelial duct is surrounded by connective tissue containing a large number of blood vessels.

4.15 Concluding Remarks

The chapter presents a basic histological and functional study of the various tissues of fascinating cephalopods. For those readers studying aspects of the cephalopod biology, it intends to be a convenient guide on the basic knowledge on the histological organization of their various functional systems. For readers unfamiliar with cephalopods, it may uncover them the strange organization of tissues and systems in these successful soft-bodied carnivorous mollusks, which show both some surprising convergences and most often large divergences with the body organization of vertebrates, including man.

Acknowledgements We thank José Manuel Antonio Durán (IIM-CSIC) for his technical assistance in necropsies and tissue processing for histological analysis.

References

Andouche A, Bassaglia Y, Baratte S, Bonnaud L (2013) Reflectin genes and development of iridophore patterns in *Sepia officinalis* embryos (Mollusca, Cephalopoda). Dev Dyn 242:560–571. https://doi.org/10.1002/dvdy.23938

Beuerlein K, Schipp R (1998) Cytomorphological aspects on the response of the branchial heart complex of *Sepia officinalis* L. (Cephalopoda) to xenobiotics and bacterial infection. Tissue Cell 30:662–671

Beuerlein K, Schimmelpfennig R, Westermann B, Ruth P, Schipp R (1998) Cytobiological studies on hemocyanin metabolism in the branchial heart complex of the common cuttlefish *Sepia officinalis* (Cephalopoda, Dibranchiata). Cell Tissue Res 292:587–595

Boletzky SV (1986) Encapsulation of cephalopod embryos—a search for functional correlations. Am Malacol Bull 4:217–227. http://biostor.org/reference/143198

Boucaud-Camou E, Boucher-Rodoni R (1983) Feeding and digestion in cephalopods. In Saleuddin ESM, Wilbur KM (eds) The Mollusca, vol 5, part 2. Academic Press, New York

Budelmann BU, Schipp R, Boletzky S (1997) Cephalopoda. In: Harrison FW, Humes AG (eds) Microscopic Anatomy of Invertebrates, vol 6A, Mollusca II. Whiley-Liss, New York, pp 119–414

Cajal SR (1917) Contribución al conocimiento de la retina y centros ópticos de los cefalópodos. Trab Lab Invest Biol Univ Madrid 15:1–82

Castellanos-Martínez S, Prado-Álvarez M, Lobo-da-Cunha A, Azevedo C, Gestal C (2014) Morphologic, cytometric and functional characterization of the common octopus (*Octopus vulgaris*) hemocytes. Dev Comp Immunol 44:50–58. https://doi.org/10.1016/j.dci.2013.11.013

Checa AG, Cartwright JH, Sánchez-Almazo I, Andrade JP, Ruiz-Raya F (2015) The cuttlefish *Sepia officinalis* (Sepiidae, Cephalopoda) constructs cuttlebone from a liquid-crystal precursor. Sci Rep 5:11513. https://doi.org/10.1038/srep11513

Chun C (1914) The Cephalopoda. 1975 English translation freely available in https://archive.org/details/cephalopoda00chun

Cole AG, Hall BK (2009) Cartilage differentiation in cephalopod molluscs. Zoology (Jena) 112:2–15. https://doi.org/10.1016/j.zool.2008.01.003

Costa PM, Rodrigo AP, Costa MH (2014) Microstructural and histochemical advances on the digestive gland of the common cuttlefish. Zoomorphology 133:59–69

Crookes WJ, Ding LL, Huang QL, Kimbell JR, Horwitz J, McFall-Ngai MJ (2004) Reflectins: the unusual proteins of squid reflective tissues. Science 303(5655):235–238

Cuvier G (1817) Mémoires pour servir á l'histoire et a l'anatomie des mollusques. Chez Deterville, Paris. Freely available at https://archive.org/details/mmoirespourser00cuvi

DeMartini DG, Izumi M, Weaver AT, Pandolfi E, Morse DE (2015) Structures, organization, and function of reflectin proteins in dynamically tunable reflective cells. J Biol Chem 290:15238–15249. https://doi.org/10.1074/jbc.M115.638254

Derby CC (2014) Cephalopod ink: production, chemistry, functions and applications. Mar Drugs 12:2700–2730. https://doi.org/10.3390/md12052700

Di Cosmo A, Di Cristo C (1998) Neuropeptidergic control of the optic gland of *Octopus vulgaris*: FMRF-amide and GnRH immunoreactivity. J Comp Neurol 398:1–12

Di Cosmo A, Di Cristo C, Paolucci M (2001) Sex steroid hormone fluctuations and morphological changes of the reproductive system of the female of *Octopus vulgaris* throughout the annual cycle. J Exp Zool 289:33–47

Dilly PN, Nixon M (1976) The cells that secrete the beaks in octopods and squids (Mollusca, Cephalopoda). Cell Tissue Res 167:229–241

Ding D, Guerette PA, Hoon S, Kong KW, Cornvik T, Nilsson M, Kumar A, Lescar J, Miserez A (2014) Biomimetic production of silk-like recombinant squid sucker ring teeth proteins. Biomacromol 15(9):3278–3289. https://doi.org/10.1021/bm500670r

Girod P (1881) Recherches sur la poche du noir des Céphalopodes des côtes de France. Typographie A. Hennuyer, Paris. https://archive.org/search.php?query=recherchessurlap00giro

Guerette PA, Hoon S, Ding D, Amini S, Masic A, Ravi V, Venkatesh B, Weaver JC, Miserez A (2014) Nanoconfined β-sheets mechanically reinforce the supra-biomolecular network of robust squid sucker ring teeth. ACS Nano 8:7170–7179

Guérin M (1908) Contribution à l'étude des systèmes cutané, musculaire et nerveux de l'appareil tentaculaire des Céphalopodes. Arch Zool Exp Gen 8:1–178. https://archive.org/details/contributionl00gu

Hanlon R (2007) Cephalopod dynamic camouflage. Curr Biol 17(11):R400–R404

Hensen V (1865) Über das Auge einiger Cephalopoden. Wilhelm Engelmann, Leipzig

Hiew SH, Guerette PA, Zvarec OJ, Phillips M, Zhou F, Su H, Pervushin K, Orner BP, Miserez A (2016) Modular peptides from the thermoplastic squid sucker ring teeth form amyloid-like cross-β supramolecular networks. Acta Biomater 46:41–54. https://doi.org/10.1016/j.actbio.2016.09.040

Huffard CL (2013) Cephalopod neurobiology: an introduction for biologists working in other model systems. Invert Neurosci 13:11–18. https://doi.org/10.1007/s10158-013-0147-z

Isgrove A (1909) *Eledone*. Williams & Norgate: London. Freely available in https://archive.org/stream/eledone00isgr#page/n5/mode/2up

Johnsen S, Kier WM (1993) Intramuscular crossed connective tissue fibres: skeletal support in the lateral fins of squid and cuttlefish (Mollusca: Cephalopoda). J Zool Lond 231:311–338

Kier WM (1985) The musculature of squid arms and tentacles: ultrastructural evidence of functional differences. J Morphol 185:223–239

Kier WM (2016) The musculature of coleoid cephalopod arms and tentacles. Front Cell Dev Biol 4:10. https://doi.org/10.3389/fcell.2016.00010

Kier WM, Curtin NA (2002) Fast muscle in squid (*Loligo pealei*): contractile properties of a specialized muscle fibre type. J Exp Biol 205:1907–1916. http://jeb.biologists.org/content/205/13/1907

Kier WM, Smith KK (1985) Tongues, tentacles and trunks: the biomechanics of movement in muscular-hydrostats. Zool J Linn Soc 83:307–324

Kier WM, Stella MP (2007) The arrangement and function of octopus arm musculature and connective tissue. J Morphol 268:831–843

Kurth JA, Thompson JT, Kier WM (2014) Connective tissue in squid mantle is arranged to accommodate strain gradients. Biol Bull 227:1–6

Le Pabic C, Goux D, Guillamin M, Safi G, Lebel JM, Koueta N, Serpentini A (2014) Hemocyte morphology and phagocytic activity in the common cuttlefish (*Sepia officinalis*). Fish Shellfish Immunol 40:362–373. https://doi.org/10.1016/j.fsi.2014.07.020

Lee DG, Park MW, Kim BH, Kim H, Jeon MA, Lee JS (2014) Microanatomy and ultrastructure of outer mantle epidermis of the cuttlefish, *Sepia esculenta* (Cephalopoda: Sepiidae). Micron 58:38–46. https://doi.org/10.1016/j.micron.2013.11.004

Mann T, Martin AW, Thiersch JB (1970) Male reproductive tract, spermatophores and spermatophoric reaction in the giant octopus of the North Pacific, *Octopus dofleini martini*. Proc R Soc Lond B 175:31–61. https://doi.org/10.1098/rspb.1970.0010

Marian JEAR (2012) Spermatophoric reaction reappraised: novel insights into the functioning of the loliginid spermatophore based on *Doryteuthis plei* (Mollusca: Cephalopoda). J Morphol 273:248–278. https://doi.org/10.1002/jmor.11020

Marian JEAR, Domaneschi O (2012) Unraveling the structure of squids' spermatophores: a combined approach based on *Doryteuthis plei* (Blainville, 1823) (Cephalopoda: Loliginidae). Acta Zool Stockholm 93:281–307

Matus AI (1971) Fine structure of the posterior salivary gland of *Eledone cirrosa* and *Octopus vulgaris*. Z Zellforsch Mikrosk Anat 122:111–121

Messenger JB, Young JZ (1999) The radular apparatus of cephalopods. Phil Trans R Soc Lond B 354:161–182

Meyer WTh (1913) Tintenfishche mit besondere Berücksichtigung von *Sepia* und Octopus. Verlag von Dr. Werner Kinkhardt, Leipzig. Freely available in https://archive.org/details/tintenfischemitb00meye

Mommsen TP, Ballantyne J, Macdonald D, Gosline J, Hochachka PW (1981) Analogues of red and white muscle in squid mantle. Proc Natl Acad Sci USA 78:3274–3278

Osorio D (2014) Cephalopod behaviour: skin flicks. Curr Biol 24(15): R684–R685. https://doi.org/10.1016/j.cub.2014.06.066

Owen R (1855) Lectures on the comparative anatomy and physiology of the invertebrate animals: delivered at the Royal College of Surgeons. Longman, London. Freely available in https://archive.org/details/lecturesoncompar1855owen

Packard A (1995) Organization of cephalopod chromatophore systems: a neuromuscular image generator. In: Abbott NJ, Williamson R, Maddock L (eds) Cephalopod neurobiology: neuroscience studies in squid, octopus and cuttlefish. Oxford UP, London, pp 331–367

Packard A, Trueman ER (1974) Muscular activity of the mantle of *Sepia* and *Loligo* (Cephalopoda) during respiratory movements and jetting, and its physiological interpretation. J Exp Biol 61:411–419

Palumbo A (2003) Melanogenesis in the ink gland of *Sepia officinalis*. Pigment Cell Res 16:517–522

Polese G, Bertapelle C, Di Cosmo A (2015) Role of olfaction in *Octopus vulgaris* reproduction. Gen Comp Endocrinol 210:55–62. https://doi.org/10.1016/j.ygcen.2014.10.006

Rosenbluth J, Szent-Györgyi AG, Thompson JT (2010) The ultrastructure and contractile properties of a fast-acting, obliquely striated, myosin-regulated muscle: the funnel retractor of squids. J Exp Biol 213:2430–2443

Ruder T, Sunagar K, Undheim EA, Ali SA, Wai TC, Low DH, Jackson TN, King GF, Antunes A, Fry BG (2013) Molecular phylogeny and evolution of the proteins encoded by coleoid (cuttlefish, octopus, and squid) posterior venom glands. J Mol Evol 76:192–204. https://doi.org/10.1007/s00239-013-9552-5

Schaeffel F, Murphy CJ, Howland HC (1999) Accommodation in the cuttlefish (*Sepia officinalis*). J Exp Biol 202:3127–3134

Schipp R, Schäfer A (1969) Vergleichende elektronenmikroskopische Untersuchungen an den zentralen Herzorganen von Cephalopoden (*Sepia officinalis*). Z Zellforsch 101:367–379

Swammerdam J (1737) Biblia Naturae. Leyden. Freely available in https://archive.org/details/BybeldernatuureISwam

Tan Y, Hoon S, Guerette PA, Wei W, Ghadban A, Hao C, Miserez A, Waite JH (2015) Infiltration of chitin by protein coacervates defines the squid beak mechanical gradient. Nat Chem Biol 11:488–495. https://doi.org/10.1038/nchembio.1833

Tramacere F, Beccai L, Kuba M, Gozzi A, Bifone A et al (2013) The morphology and adhesion mechanism of *Octopus vulgaris* suckers. PLoS ONE 8(6):e65074. https://doi.org/10.1371/journal.pone.006507

Tramacere F, Kovalev A, Kleinteich T, Gorb SN, Mazzolai B (2014) Structure and mechanical properties of *Octopus vulgaris* suckers. J R Soc Interface 11:20130816. https://doi.org/10.1098/rsif.2013.0816

Troncone L, De Lisa E, Bertapelle C, Porcellini A, Laccetti P, Polese G, Di Cosmo A (2015) Morphofunctional characterization and antibacterial activity of haemocytes from *Octopus vulgaris*. J Nat Hist 49:1457–1475. https://doi.org/10.1080/00222933.2013.826830

Uyeno TA, Kier WM (2005) Functional morphology of the cephalopod buccal mass: a novel joint type. J Morphol 264:211–222

Wells MJ (1978) Octopus. Physiology and behaviour of an advanced invertebrate. Chapman and Hall, London

Wells MJ, Wells J (1982) Ventilatory currents in the mantle of cephalopods. J Exp Biol 99:315–330

Williams LW (1909) The anatomy of the common squid *Loligo pealii* Lesueur. Brill, Leiden. Freely available in https://archive.org/details/anatomyofcommons00will

Young JZ (1965) The nervous pathways for poisoning, eating and learning in octopus. J Exp Biol 43:581–593

Young JZ (1971) The anatomy of the nervous system of *Octopus vulgaris*. Clarendon Press, Oxford

Young JZ (1995) Multiple matrices in the memory system of Octopus. In: Abbott NJ, Williamson R. Maddock L (eds) Cephalopod neurobiology: neuroscience studies in squid, octopus and cuttlefish. Oxford UP, London, pp 431–443

Young RE, Vecchione M (2002) Evolution of the gills in the Octopodiformes. Bull Mar Sci 71:1003–1017

5 Tissues of Paralarvae and Juvenile Cephalopods

Raquel Fernández-Gago, Pilar Molist, and Ramón Anadón

Abstract

Cephalopods have a different development to other molluscs and hatch as modified miniature adults called larvae, juveniles or, in some octopuses, paralarvae. The terminology used to describe young cephalopods is varied. In *Octopus vulgaris* and other members of Octopoda and Teuthida (squids), hatchlings are called paralarvae. They are planktonic stages that swim actively and prey on live planktonic organisms while undergoing morphological changes mainly due to the fast growth of the arms relative to the mantle. *Sepia officinalis* and other members of the Sepioidea are called hatchlings until they are a week old. All of the specimens studied in this chapter are newly hatched. For a better understanding of the correct terminology, we will refer to the cuttlefish and squid specimens as juveniles and to the *O. vulgaris* specimens as paralarvae. In this chapter, we provide a detailed view of the anatomy of premature hatchlings of the squid (*Loligo vulgaris*) and the cuttlefish (*S. officinalis*) and of paralarvae of *O. vulgaris.* We organize this into sections of the functional "systems" (e.g. respiratory system, excretory system).

Keywords

Histology • Anatomy • Squid • Cuttlefish • Octopus • Normal structure

5.1 Introduction

Cephalopods have a different development to other molluscs and hatch as modified miniature adults called larvae, juveniles or, in some octopuses, paralarvae (Young and Harman 1988). The terminology used to describe young cephalopods is varied. In *Octopus vulgaris*, the hatchlings are called paralarvae. They are squid-like, swim actively and prey on live planktonic animals while undergoing strong morphological changes mainly due to the fast growth of the arms relative to the mantle (Iglesias et al. 2007). Hanlon and Messenger (1988) named the early *Sepia officinalis* stages hatchlings until they are a week old. All of the specimens studied in the following chapter are newly hatched. For a better understanding of the correct terminology, we will refer to the cuttlefish and squid specimens as juveniles and to the *O. vulgaris* specimens as paralarvae. In this chapter, a detailed view of the anatomy of premature hatchlings of squid (*Loligo vulgaris)* and cuttlefish (*S. officinalis)* and of paralarvae of octopus (*O. vulgaris)* is presented by "systems" (e.g. respiratory system, excretory system), following a functional approach.

5.2 Skin and the Body Wall (Fig. 5.1)

The skin consists of epidermis and dermis. The epidermis of hatchling octopodiformes, *O. vulgaris*, and decapodiformes, *L. vulgaris* and *S. officinalis*, show differences in morphology. In octopus paralarvae, the epidermis of the head and arms is

R. Fernández-Gago (✉)
Department of Ecology and Animal Biology, University of Vigo, Lagoas-Marcosende, Vigo, Spain
e-mail: raquelfernandezgago@gmail.com

P. Molist
Department of Functional Biology and Health Sciences, University of Vigo, Lagoas-Marcosende, Vigo, Spain
e-mail: pmolist@uvigo.es

R. Anadón
Department of Functional Biology, University of Santiago de Compostela, Campus Vida, Santiago de Compostela, Spain
e-mail: ramon.anadon@usc.es

C. Gestal et al. (eds.), *Handbook of Pathogens and Diseases in Cephalopods*,
https://doi.org/10.1007/978-3-030-11330-8_5

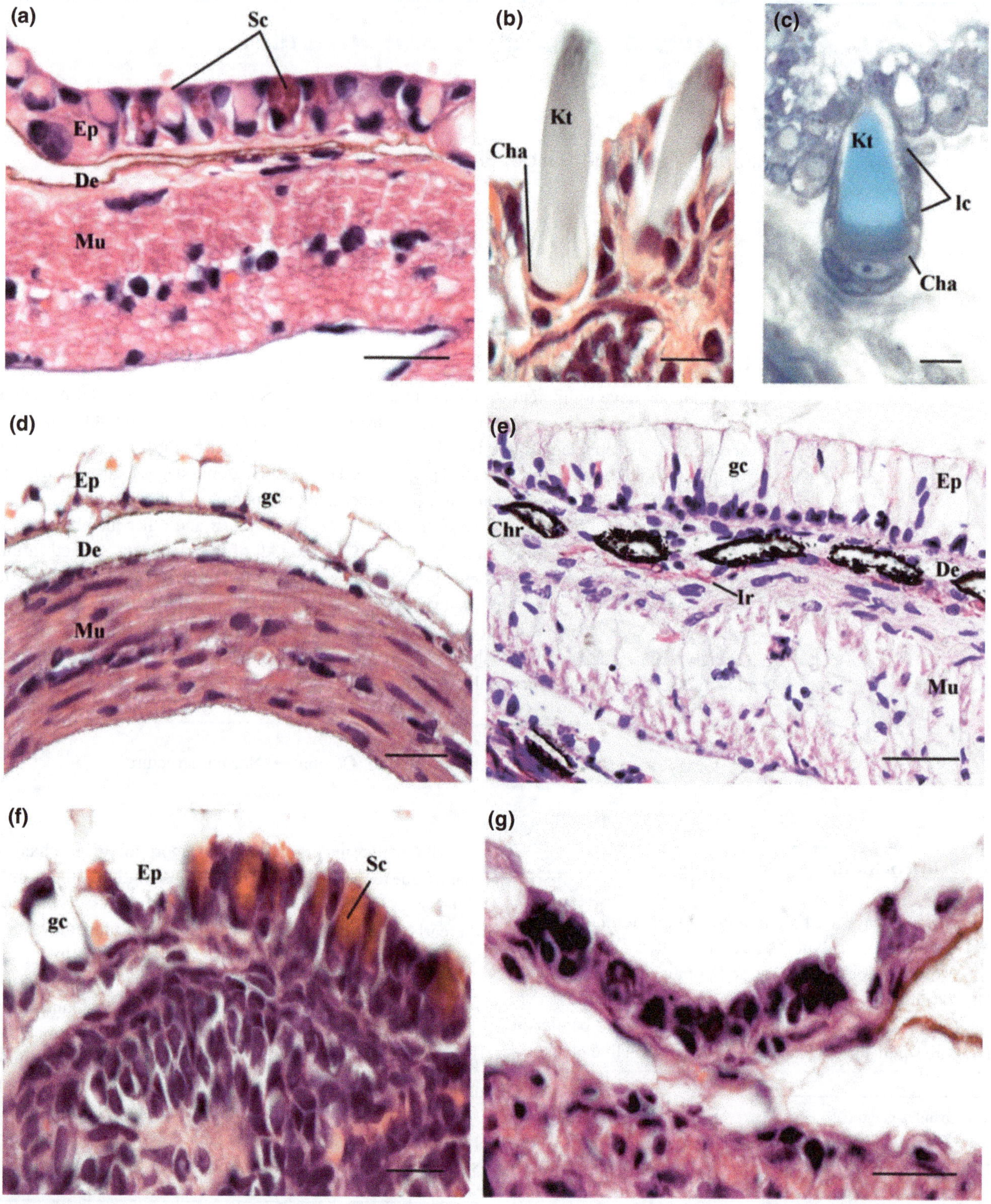

Fig. 5.1 Longitudinal section of the skin of octopus mantle (**a**). Kölliker organ detail (**b**, **c**). Transversal section of the skin of squid mantle (**d**). Longitudinal section of the skin of cuttlefish mantle (**e**). Sections of the skin of squid arm (**f**). Detail of epidermal line epithelium (**g**). Cha, chaetoblast; Chr, chromatophoric organs; Ed, dermis; Ep, epidermis; gc, goblet cell; Kt, Kölliker organ tufts; lc, lateral cell; Mu, musculature; Ir, iridophores (reflecting cells); and Sc, secretory cell. **a–b**, **d–g** H&E stain and **c** Richardson blue. Scale bars: **a**, **f**, **g** 20 µm; **b–c** 10 µm; **d** 30 µm; and **e** 50 µm

formed by a simple columnar epithelium (Fig. 5.1a). This epithelium is lower than in the mantle. Bi-stratified regions of this epithelium can be seen in some areas. Among the epithelial columnar cells, there are two types of secretory cells (Fig. 5.1a) and a characteristic cell of hatchling cephalopods, the Kölliker organs (Fig. 5.1b, c). Boletzky (1973) and Brocco et al. (1974) electron microscopy studies show that these organs are mainly composed of the epidermis and a dermal muscular layer. The epidermis consists of numerous follicles with specialized epidermal cells (Fig. 5.1c) producing an extracellular fascicle of cannular rodlets (Kölliker's tufts; Fig. 3.1b, c) (Boletzky 1973). The follicle is centred in a specialized basal cell called cystoblast or chaetoblast (Brocco et al. 1974) (Fig. 5.1b, c) that is surrounded by several follicular cells or wall cells (Boletzky 1973) (Fig. 5.1c). The chaetoblast has a large nucleus and apical microvilli that penetrate the base of each rodlet (Brocco et al. 1974). The lateral follicular cells (Fig. 5.1c) are similar to chaetoblasts except for the lack of microvilli. The muscular apparatus consists of a group of striated muscle fibres allowing evagination and spreading of the bundles.

These organs are widely distributed over the surface of paralarvae until 30–35 days post-hatching (Boletzky 1973), although they are more abundant in the mantle than in the head, syphon and arms (Brocco et al. 1974). Kölliker's organs disappear after the first few months of post-embryonic life, so it is assumed they have a function associated with planktonic life. There have been several theories regarding its function: Naef (1923) proposed that these structures help passive planktonic transport in the water column and are a basis for the formation of more complex structures in juveniles and adults, Portmann (1933), Boletzky (1973) and Mangold et al. (1971) hypothesized that these organs help the embryo survival out of the chorion, and Villanueva (1995) suggested that light reflection by tufts of Kölliker's organs could help in the camouflage of the planktonic paralarvae.

In early juvenile squid and cuttlefish, the epidermis (Fig. 5.1d, e) is generally composed of large goblet cells with an ovoid basal nucleus, but in the arms and surrounding eyes, this epithelium is something modified. In the internal region of the arms, the epidermis presents gland cells with eosinophilic secretory granules (Fig. 5.1f). In some regions of the post-embryonic specimens, it is possible to see the lines of epidermal cells that have a rectilinear arrangement (Sundermann 1983). These lines are seen in the arms' external region epithelium and around the eyes. These epidermal lines consist of ciliated and accessory cells (Fig. 5.1g). Accessory cells are slender and elongated with dense cytoplasm and a microvillous apical border. This type of cell has a small and dark nucleus. The ciliated cells are very voluminous and have a central nucleus.

The dermis is a narrow layer below the epidermis, formed by a network of connective tissue with collagen fibres, fibroblasts and various amounts of extracellular matrix. In this layer, there are small chromatophores with the same appearance as in adults. The presence of iridophores, leucophores, photophores and reflecting cells was not observed in octopus and squid hatchling specimens. However, in the cuttlefish dermis, there are abundant chromatophores and iridophores or reflecting cells (Fig. 5.1e).

5.3 Musculature (Fig. 5.2)

The muscular mantle wall in octopus consists of three sets of muscular layers orientated in longitudinal, circular and radial directions (Fig. 5.2a). In decapods (Fig. 5.2b, c), the

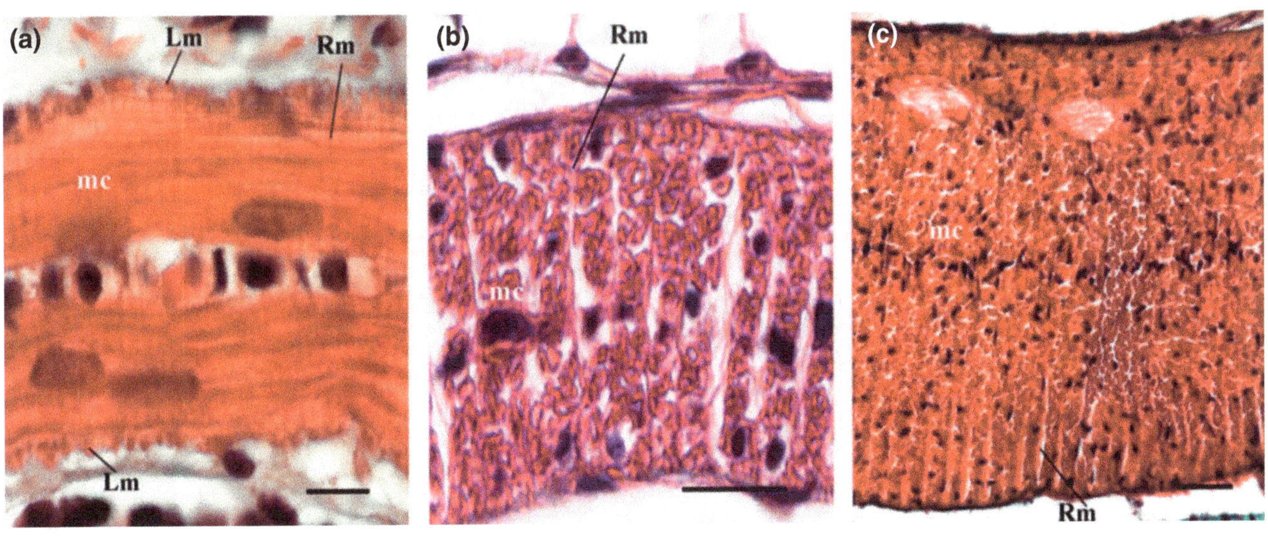

Fig. 5.2 Arrangement of muscle fibres in the muscular layer of the mantle. Transversal sections of octopus (**a**). Longitudinal sections of squid (**b**) and horizontal section of cuttlefish (**c**) mc, circular muscular layer; Lm, longitudinal muscular layer; Rm, radial muscular layer and radial muscle fibres. **a–c** Masson's trichome stain. Scale bars: **a** 10 μm; **b** 20 μm; and **c** 50 μm

situation is strikingly different, with two layers in circular and radial orientations (Budelmann et al. 1997). As similarly observed in adults, muscle fibres are arranged in different directions although this arrangement is less significant in hatchling cephalopods. Specifically, the longitudinal and radial musculature is less developed than in adults (Fig. 5.2).

5.4 Shell (Fig. 5.3)

The internal cephalopod shells can be classified into chitinous pen or gladius and calcified (cuttlebone).

5.4.1 *Chitinous Pen* (*L. vulgaris*)

The squid exoskeleton is a chitinous pen constituted mostly of β-chitin (Hunt and El Sherief 1990; Yun et al. 2013), which is in the dorsal part of the mantle. The loliginid pens are broad and are almost as long as the mantle (Budelmann et al. 1997). The squid pens contain a central axis or rachis, lateral expansions (vane) and the terminal conus. The shell sac in *L. vulgaris* consists of an invaginated monolayer of ectodermal cells with two distinct zones: primary or ventral and secondary or dorsal zones (Hopkins and Boletzky 1994; Fig. 5.3a). The main function of this structure is maintaining rigidity about the longitudinal axis of the animal during swimming.

In larval squid, the shell sac extends along the dorsal midline of the mantle. This sac is a membranous envelope that surrounds the gladius, whose epithelium presents dorsal and ventral differentiation (Fig. 5.3a, b). In the shell sac, the dorsal epithelium is characterized by flat cells with an elongated nucleus, while the ventral epithelium consists of cubic cells with a dark cytoplasm (Fig. 5.3b). The shell sac ultrastructure in hatchling *L. vulgaris* has been described by Hopkins and Boletzky (1994). These authors identified five kinds of cells: basal cells at the margin in the dorsal and ventral regions low cells of two distinct morphologies in the dorsal zone and tall cells of two distinct morphologies in the ventral zone. In adults, Bizikov (1987) observed three shell layers: the inner layer or hypostracum, the ostracum or medium shell layer and the periostracum or outer shell layer. In larvae, the shell is formed by an eosinophilic homogenous material without any layer.

5.4.2 *Calcified Shell* (*S. officinalis*)

The sepia cuttlebone is a flat, elongated shell with an oval form (Budelmann et al. 1997). Its dorsal surface is heavily calcified, while the ventral surface has a smooth anterior part and a striped posterior part (siphuncular zone). Each siphuncular stripe is the posterior edge of an interseptal space or shell chamber (Budelmann et al. 1997).

The cuttlebone develops early in embryogenesis (Fioroni 1990). In hatchling cuttlefish, eight to nine complete shell chambers are present (Boletzky 1983). The septa are more spaced than in adults. The lamellar structure provides an indicator of growth because it lays down at fairly regular intervals (Boletzky and Wiedmann 1978).

5.5 The Digestive System (Figs. 5.4, 5.5, 5.6, 5.7, 5.8 and 5.9)

The digestive system of larval and paralarval cephalopods is composed of the alimentary canal and digestive glands (anterior and posterior salivary glands, and digestive gland).

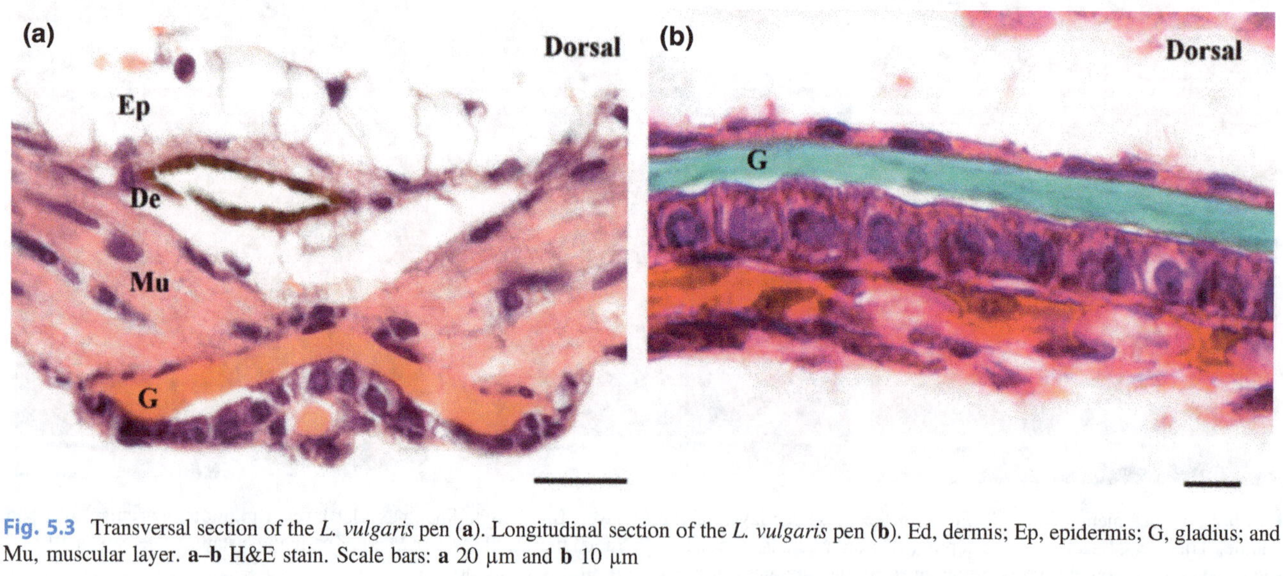

Fig. 5.3 Transversal section of the *L. vulgaris* pen (**a**). Longitudinal section of the *L. vulgaris* pen (**b**). Ed, dermis; Ep, epidermis; G, gladius; and Mu, muscular layer. **a**–**b** H&E stain. Scale bars: **a** 20 μm and **b** 10 μm

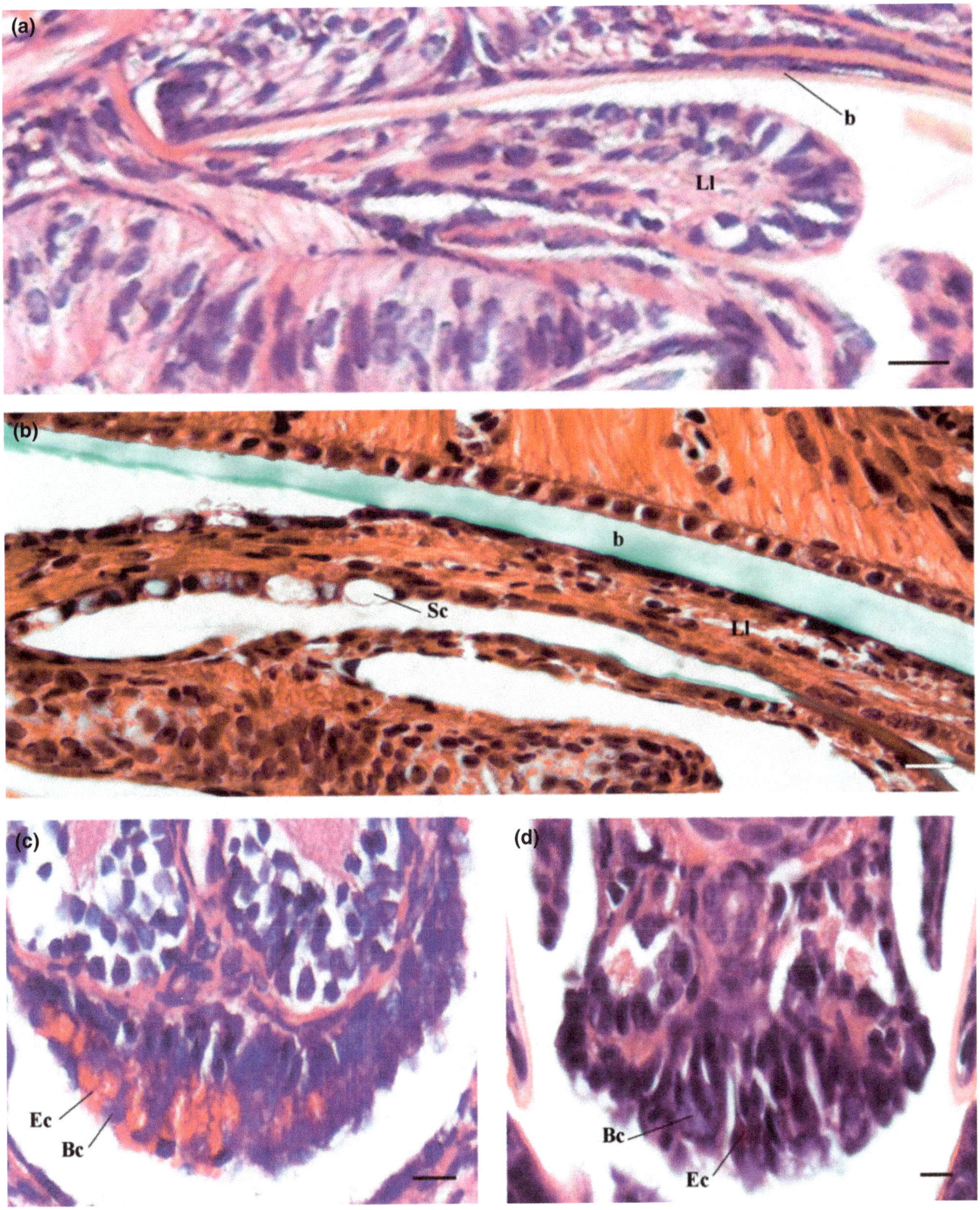

Fig. 5.4 Longitudinal section of *O. vulgaris* lateral lobe (**a**). Horizontal section of *S. officinalis* lateral lobe (**b**). Detail of *O. vulgaris* submandibular gland (**c**). Detail of *L. vulgaris* submandibular gland (**d**). B, beak; Bc, basophilic cell; Ec, eosinophilic cell; Ll, lateral lobe; and Sc, secretory cell. **a**, **c**, **d** H&E stain and **b** Masson's trichome stain. Scale bars: **a**, **c** 10 μm and **b**, **d** 20 μm

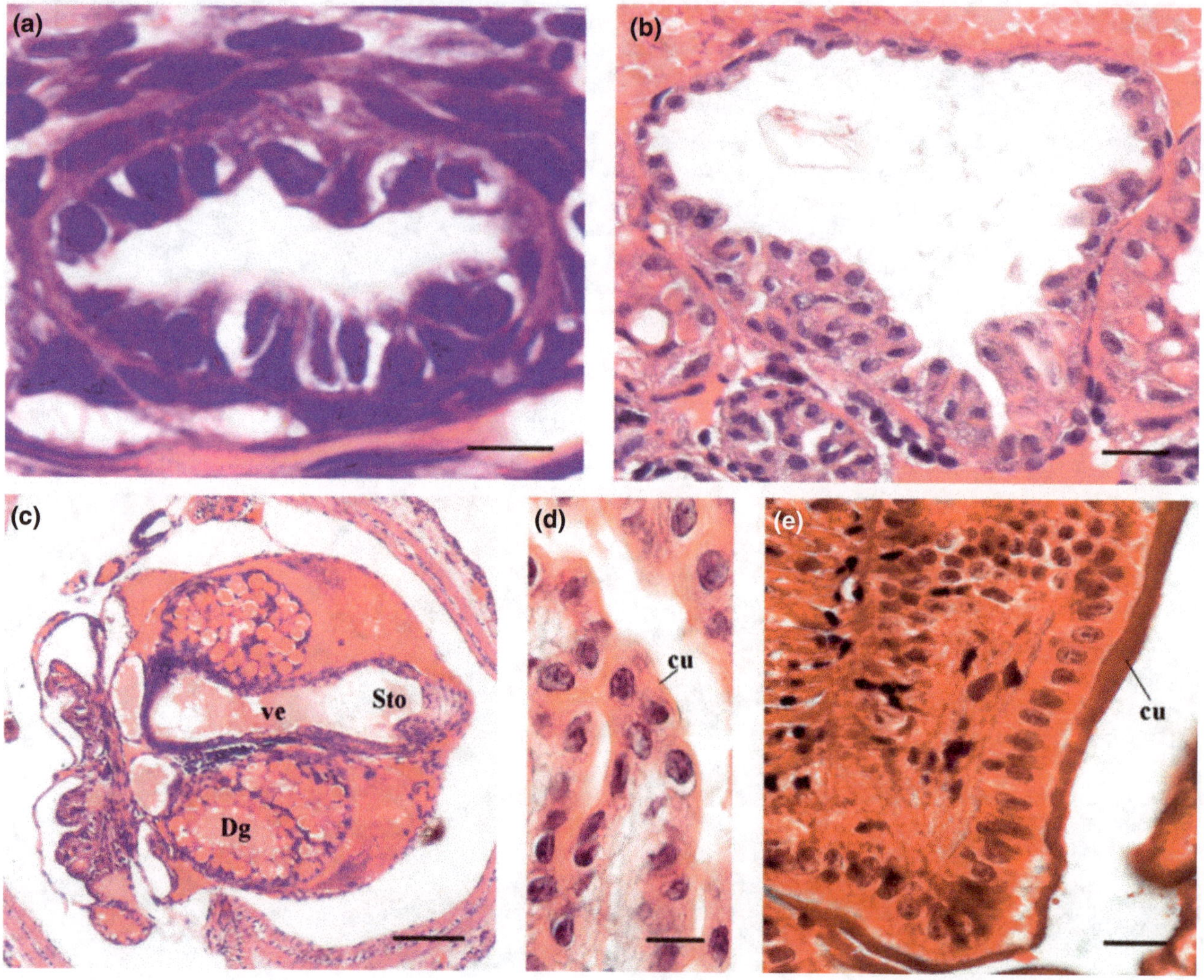

Fig. 5.5 Transversal section of *L. vulgaris* oesophagus (**a**). Transversal section of *O. vulgaris* crop (**b**). Transversal section of *O. vulgaris* stomach and vestibule (**c**). Detail of *O. vulgaris* stomach epithelium (**d**). Detail of *S. officinalis* stomach epithelium (**e**). Cu, cuticle; Dg, digestive gland; eW, external wall; Sto, stomach; and ve, vestibule. **a–d** H&E stain and **e** Masson's trichome stain. Scale bars: **a**, **d** 10 μm; **b** 20 μm; and **c** 100 μm

Different regions are distinguishable in the canal: buccal mass, oesophagus, stomach, caecum and intestine. Functionally, the digestive system is a complex system that plays an important role in the absorption of essential nutrients (Fernández-Gago et al. 2017).

The digestive system of octopus paralarvae and of squid and cuttlefish larvae is a U-shaped tube, as in the adults and juveniles of the species. The descending U-branch is in dorsal position and consists of the buccal bulb and oesophagus. A crop is also found in octopus (Fernández-Gago et al. 2017). The stomach and the caecum are located in the curve of the U-shaped tube. The ascending U-branch, which is ventral, is formed by the intestine and the anus. Between the ascending and the descending branches of the U, the digestive gland and the posterior salivary glands are visible. All regions of the digestive system are already formed one day post-hatching. Although the histology of the digestive tube varies along its length, the following layers can be observed from inside out: the mucosa, the submucosa, the muscular layer and the serosa.

Similarly to adults, the buccal mass is formed by different structures that contribute to the feeding process, namely: mandibles, radula, salivary papilla, submandibular gland and the secretory ducts of the posterior and anterior salivary glands. The overall anatomy of the different parts of the buccal bulb is very similar to adults, although with some histological

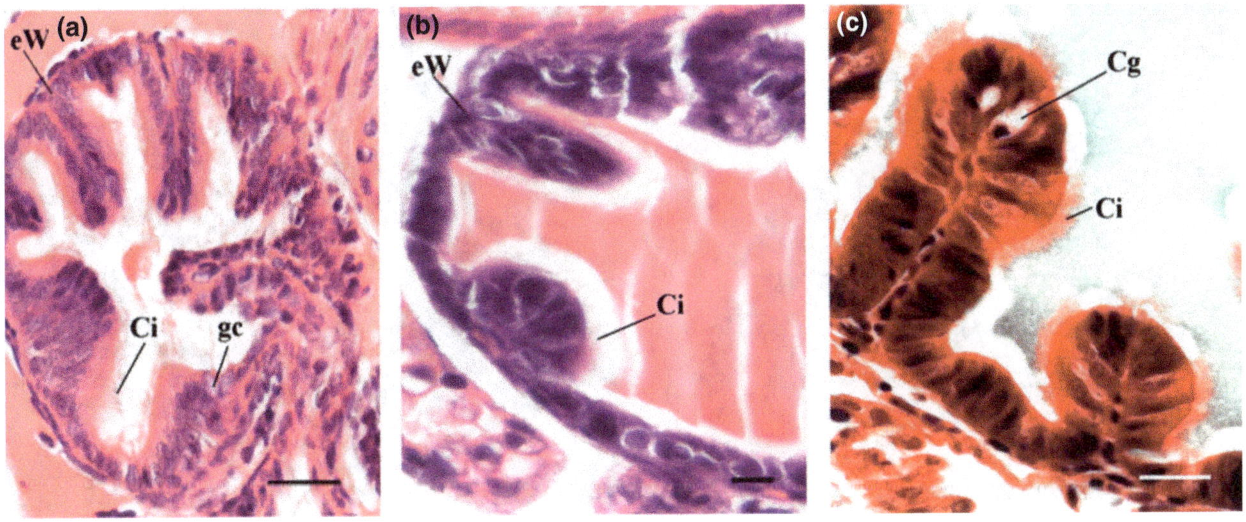

Fig. 5.6 Transversal sections of *O. vulgaris* caecum (**a**). Detail of *L. vulgaris* caecum epithelium (**b**). Detail of *S. officinalis* caecum epithelium (**c**). Cg, caecal gland; Ci, cilia; eW, external wall; and gc, goblet cell. **a–b** H&E stain and **c** Masson's trichome stain. Scale bars: **a**, **c** 25 μm and **b** 10 μm

differences. The buccal lateral lobes, which form the food passage, are underdeveloped in larvae and paralarvae.

The food passage is lined by a simple cubic epithelium with cubical cells instead of the typical prismatic cells of adults (Fig. 5.4a, b). The glandular epithelia associated with the posterior part of the lateral lobes and jaws are absent at these stages. The submandibular gland consists of a simple glandular epithelium formed by two types of secretory cells: granular and mucous. In octopus paralarvae, the zonal arrangement of these two types of cell is characteristic. The granular cells are located in the middle of the epithelium, while mucous cells are in the lateral regions of the gland (Fig. 5.4c). However, in squid, both types of cell appear mixed (Fig. 5.4d).

The oesophagus is a muscular tube formed by a mucosa with folds or villi of different sizes. Unlike in adults, it is lined by a low simple epithelium with a thin cuticle. Moreover, in the hatchling squid, the oesophagus does not have folds in its mucosa (Fig. 5.5a). The crop of octopus paralarvae is a tubular structure with a distended lumen. In the crop, the mucosa forms small villi or longitudinal folds that differ from the adult in the fact that they are not branched (Fig. 5.5b).

In hatchling cephalopods, the stomach is a sac-like organ with a simple folded mucosal epithelium (Fig. 5.5c). In octopus and squid, the stomach epithelium is formed by cubic cells with a large and central nucleus (Fig. 5.5d), but in cuttlefish, the stomach epithelium is formed by cylindrical cells (Fig. 5.5e). The three species have the apical region of the cells covered by a thin non-stratified cuticle.

The caecum of cuttlefish and octopus hatchlings, as in adults, shows a histological differentiation between the external and internal walls. The external wall contains only primary folds of the mucosa that consist of a pseudostratified epithelium, whereas in the internal wall the unfolded mucosa is formed by a simple epithelium (Fig. 5.6a). The caecum of juvenile squid presents the differentiated regions of the ciliated organ and the caecal sac. The ciliated organ has the same differentiation between the internal and external walls (Fig. 5.6b), but these are missing in the caecal sac (Bidder 1950). No secretory cells have been found in the ciliated organ of the squid, unlike in the adults. The only gland cells present in the caecum of paralarvae are located at the entrance or exit of this organ to the vestibule (Fig. 5.6a), lacking secretory cells in the internal and external walls, as well as the caecal glands typical of adults. However, in hatchling cuttlefish, the caecum has secretory cells and the caecal glands in the apical region of the folds (Fig. 5.6c).

The octopus and squid intestines are a tubular organ that presents structural differences at the level of the mucosa. In the ventral region of the mucosa, there are two broad longitudinal folds that resemble the adult typhlosoles (Fig. 5.7a, b), but they are comparatively less developed. These folds present a thick ciliated pseudostratified epithelium

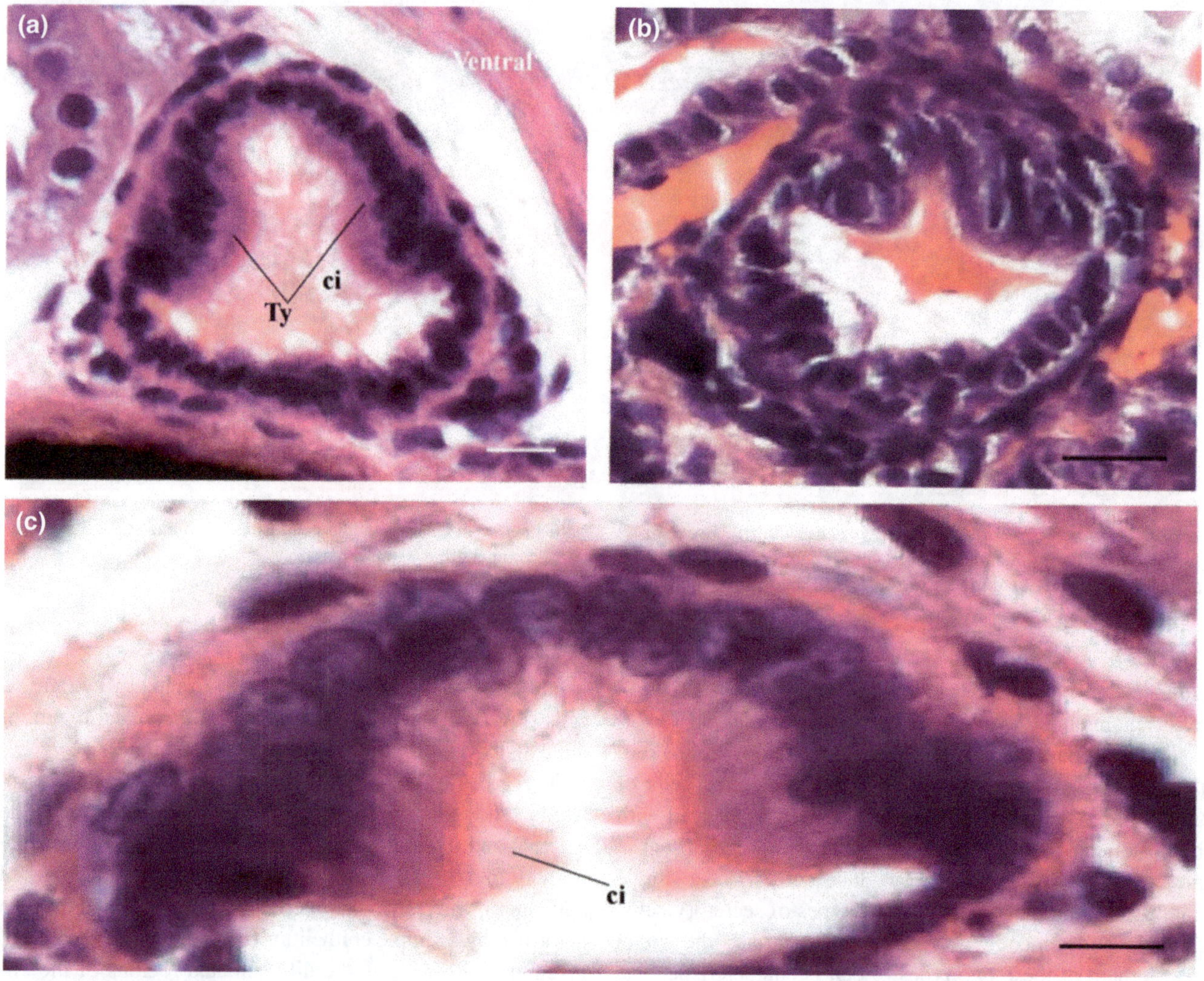

Fig. 5.7 Transversal section of the intestine of *Octopus vulgaris* paralarvae (**a**). Transversal section of the intestine of squid (**b**). Detail of the typhlosole epithelium (**c**). ci, cilia and Ty, typhlosole. **a–c** H&E stain. Scale bars: **a** 10 μm; **b** 20 μm; and **c** 5 μm

(Fig. 5.7c). The two folds are only present in the region of the intestine close to the vestibule, whereas, in the remainder tube, there are no folds or villi in the mucosa, which consists of a simple squamous epithelium. In the dorsal region, a thickening of this wall was observed (Fig. 5.7a, b). No secretory cells are present in the intestinal mucosa.

5.5.1 Annex Glands

Unlike the adults, the anterior salivary glands of the squid and octopus hatchlings are simple and have no ramifications (Fig. 5.8a, b). These glands show, in octopus, two types of glandular cells with granular secretion, eosinophils and basophils as well as a type of gland cell with mucous secretion. The epithelium lining this gland shows a greater proportion of eosinophilic gland cells than the other two types (Fig. 5.8b). Due to the absence of secretory cells, the anterior salivary gland in squid does not yet have a secretory function, which may be due to its premature state (Fig. 5.8a).

The posterior salivary glands (Fig. 5.8c, d) of the hatchlings have a morphological structure similar to those in adults. The secretory units of these glands show two types of gland cells: (i) cells with granular eosinophilic secretion and (ii) cells with mucous basophilic secretion. However, in the case of *O. vulgaris* paralarvae the yellow granular cells, typical in adults, are not present.

The single digestive gland of newly hatched octopus paralarvae has tubules with a simpler structure than those in

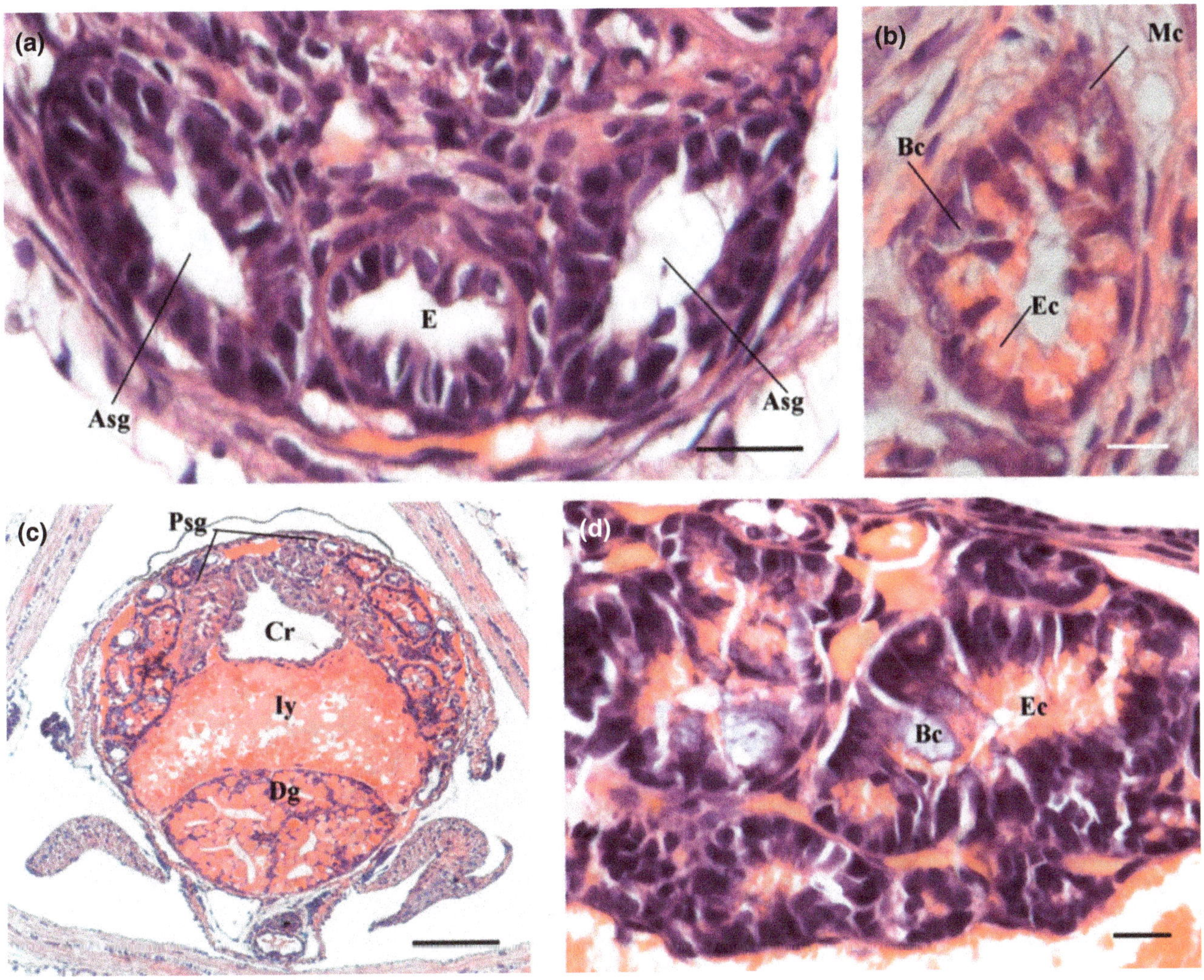

Fig. 5.8 Transversal section of the anterior salivary glands of a squid larva (**a**). Detail of the anterior salivary gland of an octopus paralarva (**b**). Transversal section of octopus showing the posterior salivary glands (**c**). Detail of the posterior salivary gland of a squid larva (**d**). Asg, anterior salivary gland; Bc, basophilic cell; Cr, crop; Dg, digestive gland; E, oesophagus; Ec, eosinophilic cell; Iy, internal yolk; and Psg, posterior salivary gland. **a–d** H&E stain. Scale bars: **a** 50 μm; **b** 10 μm; **c** 100 μm; and **d** 20 μm

adults (Fig. 5.9a). These tubules are characterized as having a lumen and a poorly defined cellular organization, showing only a basement membrane and two types of cell: immature digestive cells and storage cells (Fig. 5.9b). The latter cells show an appearance similar to mature digestive cells of adults, but its cytoplasm appears expanded due to abundant yolk plaques and inclusions of different sizes. Lemaire et al. (1977) described storage cells and cells that have boules in the basal region and a microvilli border in the apical region. In squid, the two digestive glands appear at both sides of the internal yolk. They are tubular and lack yolk plaques (Fig. 5.9c). However, this absence seems indicate that they are premature hatchlings (early juvenile) than a distinctive feature of this stage of development. The digestive gland of cuttlefish has a similar structure to that in octopus (Fig. 5.9d). The internal yolk of squids and octopuses is composed of a cluster of yolk platelets of different sizes (Fig. 5.9a, c) with the sizes decreasing from the centre to the periphery. This internal yolk is separated from the digestive gland by a thin membrane. While the paralarvae internal yolk is formed by a single elongated mass running parallel to the digestive gland, the juvenile squid internal yolk consists

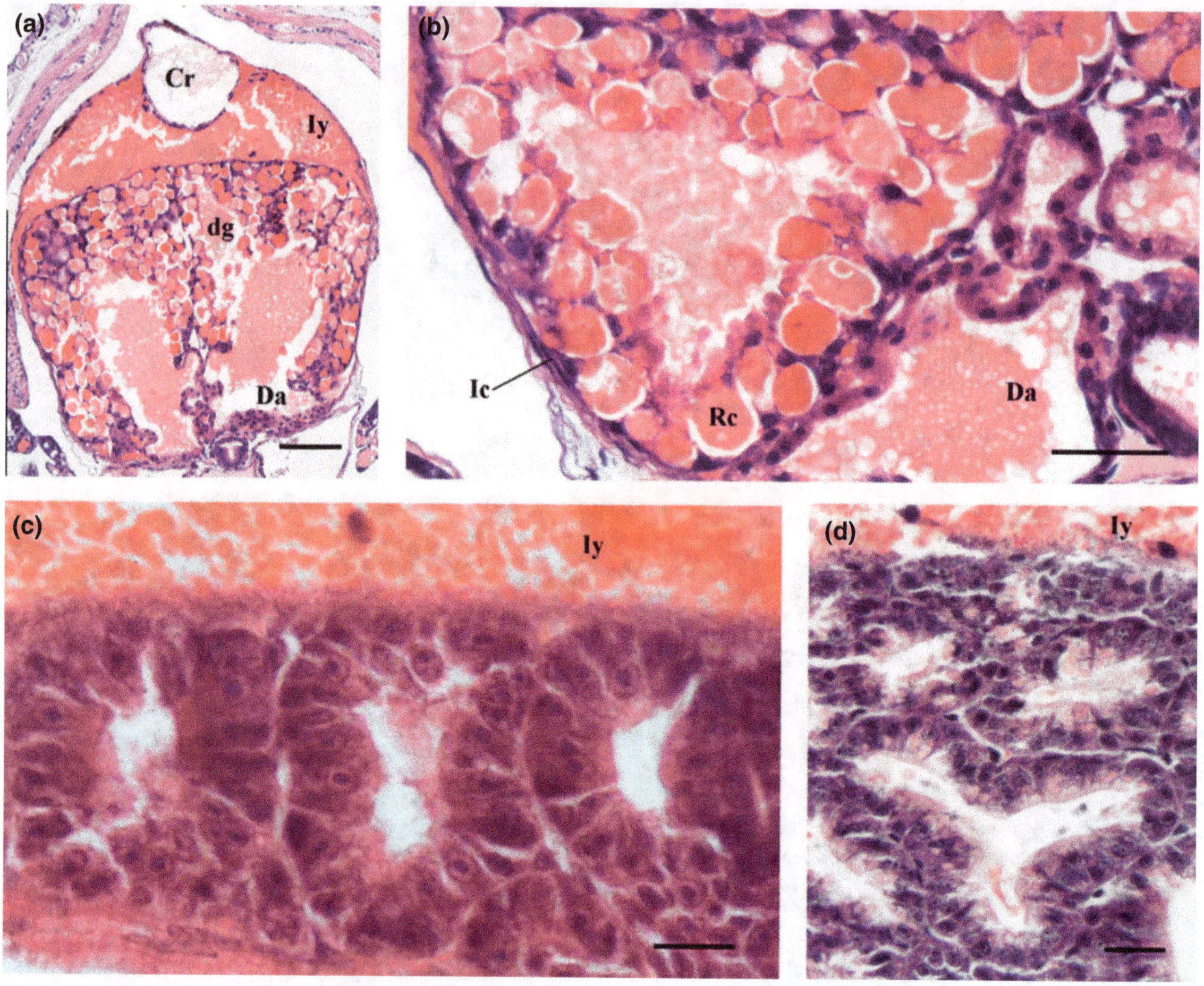

Fig. 5.9 Transversal section of the digestive gland of paralarval octopus (**a**). Detail of octopus main digestive gland and digestive gland appendages (**b**). Longitudinal section of *L. vulgaris* digestive gland (**c**). Longitudinal section of the digestive gland of larval cuttlefish (**d**). Cr, crop; Da, digestive appendages; dg, digestive gland; lc, basal cell or immature cell; ly, internal yolk; and Rc, reserve cell. **a–d** H&E stain. Scale bars: **a** 100 μm; **b** 50 μm; **c** 20 μm; and **d** 25 μm

of anterior and posterior masses located at the back of the mantle.

5.6 Circulatory System (Fig. 5.10)

5.6.1 Branchial Glands

In adults, the branchial glands are a dense paired structure. These glands extend the whole length of the gills. The branchial gland is contained in a capsule consisting of a columnar cell epithelium (Dilly and Messenger 1972). It presents a uniform appearance with numerous acini groups of cells. These acini are formed by some characteristic basophilic cells with a large nucleus near the base of the cell. In hatchling cephalopods, the branchial glands are present (Fig. 5.10a). Similarly to adults, these are dense structures formed by basophilic cells with a central round large nucleus (Fig. 5.10b). However, the well-developed cord structure present in adults is not seen in hatchlings. These glands have a similar structure in squid and octopus.

5.6.2 *White Body* (Hematopoietic Organ)

The hematopoietic organ or white body is a multilobular gland behind the eyeball in cephalopod adults. In octopods

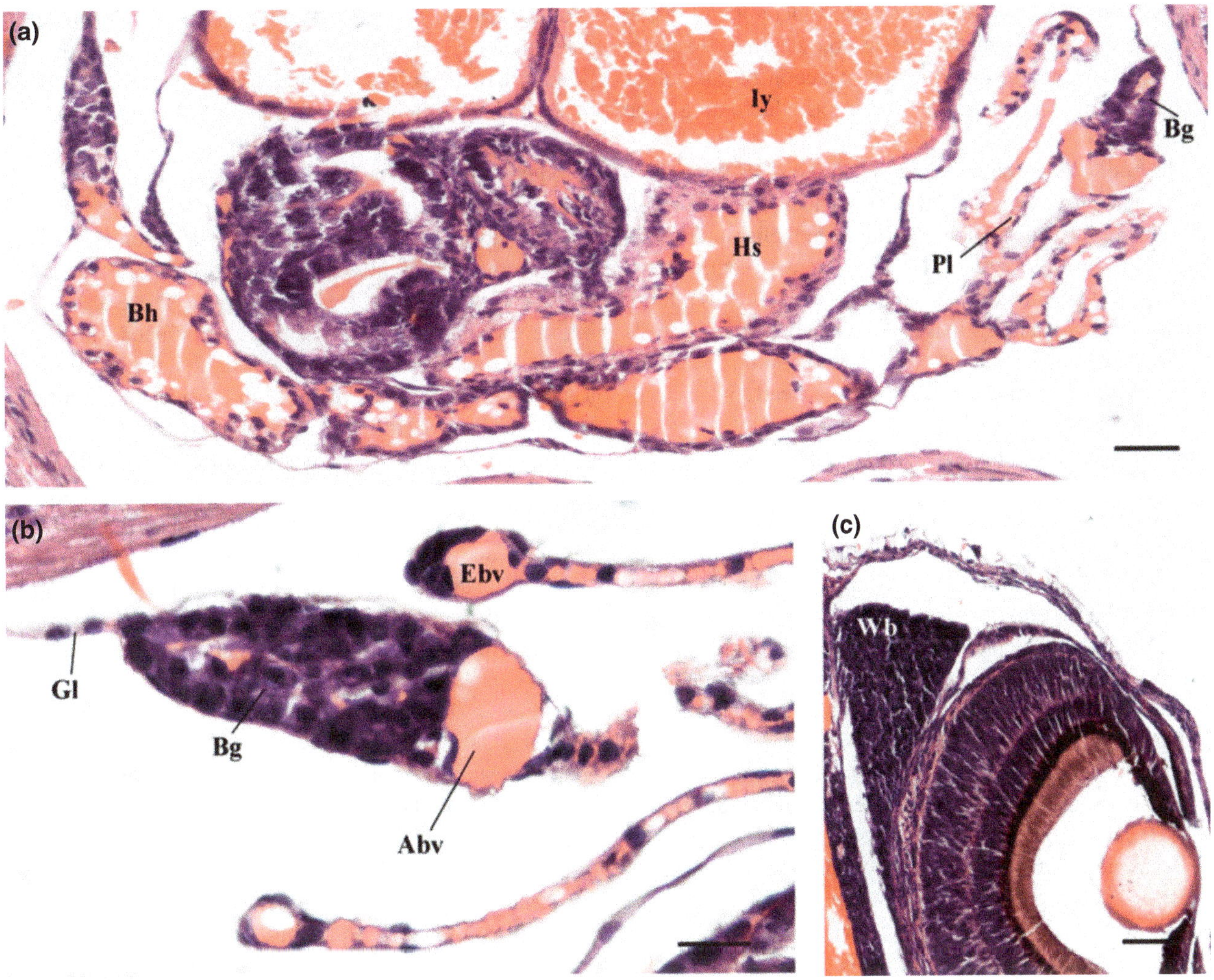

Fig. 5.10 Transversal section of *L. vulgaris* circulatory and respiratory systems (**a**). Detail of *L. vulgaris* branchial gland (**b**). Transversal section of the *L. vulgaris* head showing the eye and the associated white body (**c**). Abv, afferent blood vessel; Bg, branchial gland; Bh, branchial heart; Ebv, efferent blood vessel; Gl, gill ligament; Hs, systemic heart; Iy, internal yolk; Pl, primary lamella; and Wb, white body. **a–c** H&E stain. Scale bars: **a–c** 50 µm and **b** 100 µm

and decapods, this gland is well vascularized and has relatively few collagen fibres (Johnson 1987). Similarly to adults, the white body of the hatchling cephalopods is located between the eye and the optic lobe and is made up of a tight group of small blood cells (Fig. 5.10c).

5.6.3 Systemic and Branchial Hearts

The cephalopods have a completely closed circulatory system which is well developed with an extended artery and vein net. The system is like the circulatory system of vertebrates (Schipp 1987). Among the Cephalopoda, the Coleoidea have two auricles, branchial hearts, and a single ventricle, systemic heart. The vessel system is formed of arteries and veins which are linked by a capillary network and a peripheral sinus and lacunae where a gas exchange occurs.

The systemic heart is a powerful muscle with a lumen which is divided by a muscular heart septum into two equally large chambers (Kling and Schipp 1987). The main moving force of blood circulation is produced by the heart and is supported by other contractile organs (Kling and Schipp 1987). Therefore, the function of this is to be the central motor of the high-pressure circulatory system. The branchial hearts are deep red to yellow-brown colour with a much branched narrow lumen (Schipp and Schäfer 1969).

This organ also has other different functions: to assist filtration for the formation of primary urine, to store important substances, to aid in the excretion of catabolites and in the immune defence mechanism (Fielder and Schipp 1987).

The wall of the ventricle and the auricles has three main layers: epicardium, myocardium and endocardium. The epicardium is formed by flat extended epithelial cells with microvilli. The myocardium has a different structure in the systemic and branchial hearts (Budelmann et al. 1997). It is a spongy layer containing muscle fibres and polygonal cells rich in the cytoplasm and containing an ovoid nucleus. This layer is more developed in the systemic heart and is composed of many muscle layers. However, in the branchial heart, this layer is only formed by one or two layers of densely innervated muscle fibres (Budelmann et al. 1997). As it is observed in adults, the myocardium is formed by cardiomyocytes similar to the vertebrate cardiomyocytes (Schipp and Schäfer 1969). The third layer is an incomplete endothelium towards the lumen, but sometimes it is not developed at all (Fielder and Schipp 1987). This layer is formed by a continuous basal lamina with flattened endothelial cells and myocytes (Kling and Schipp 1987; Budelmann et al. 1997).

The post-hatching cephalopod ventricles and auricles have a large lumen. These organs have poorly developed walls. Paralarvae and juveniles have a strong musculature in the systemic heart similar to adults. The branchial heart in hatchling cephalopods has a large lumen, unlike in adults. In the organ wall, it is possible to see the typical cells of this organ with a dense black vacuole (Fig. 5.10a).

5.7 The Respiratory System (Figs. 5.10 and 5.11)

The dibranchiate cephalopods (coleoids) have a pair of gills protruding from an expandable mantle cavity where the flow of respiratory water passes through their folds. This water flow is produced by the powerful contractions of a highly elastic mantle muscle system (Budelmann et al. 1997). A pair of branchial hearts generate part of the circulatory pressure and pump the blood via the afferent branchial vessel (branchial artery) that lies in the gill ligament, to the gill lamellae where it is oxygenated. It is passed to the systematic heart by active pulsations of the efferent branchial vein (Schipp et al. 1979). The cephalopod gills serve for respiratory and excretory functions (Schipp et al. 1979).

The gills are composed by lamellae, which are organized symmetrically in Sepia and asymmetrically in octopods (Budelmann et al. 1997). In *O. vulgaris*, each gill has a central cavity, with the primary lamellae on each side. The primary lamella is folded along its long axis so that a series of secondary lamellae are formed, alternating on the two sides of the primary ones (Wells and Wells 1982). The secondary lamellae are branched and form tertiary lamellae. The main afferent vessel runs along the dorsal margin of the gill and down the inner surface of each primary lamella. From here, it branches along the crest of the secondary lamella. Cuttlefish gills are less complex. These are divided into a series of compartments by membranous partitions. One such runs vertically along the length of the gill, dividing it into two. The afferent vessel from the branchial heart runs along the groove formed at the bottom of the gill. The corresponding efferent vessel is external (Thompsett 1939). The secondary and tertiary lamellae are crossed by the arteries and veins of the second and third orders. Between the veins and arteries of the third order, the blood runs in "lacunae". This is the region of gas exchange (Schipp et al. 1979; Wells and Wells 1982).

In the hatchlings of octopus and squid, the gills are scarcely branched, in contrast to the deeply branched gills of the cuttlefish (Fig. 5.11). Paralarvae and juveniles only have a primary lamella (Fig. 5.11a), which in its distal portion ends in a bulbous protrusion, where a blood sinus is found (Fig. 5.10b). Similarly to adults, it is possible to observe the gill gland as well as the afferent vessels from the branchial heart (Fig. 5.10b). The epithelium of the lamellae varies from cubic to squamous in different gill areas of octopus, while this epithelium is squamous in squid (Fig. 5.11a, c). In juvenile cuttlefish, the gill shows differences in height and inner structure of the concave and convex epithelial surfaces of secondary folds (Fig. 5.11b). The height of the epithelium of the concave side is nearly twice that of the outer side epithelium and appears more vacuolated (Schipp et al. 1979). The inner epithelium (concave side) is formed by tall cells exhibiting some vesicles and a large vacuole (Fig. 5.11d). The outer (convex) epithelium is a simple squamous epithelium with a well-developed microvillous apical border (Budelmann et al. 1997).

5.8 The Excretory System (Fig. 5.12)

In cephalopod excretion, the organs involved are the renal complex, with the renal and digestive appendages, and the branchial heart complex, with their appendages or pericardial glands and the brachial heart (Furuya et al. 2004). The digestive gland and the white body also collaborate in this function (Boucher-Rodoni and Mangold 1988).

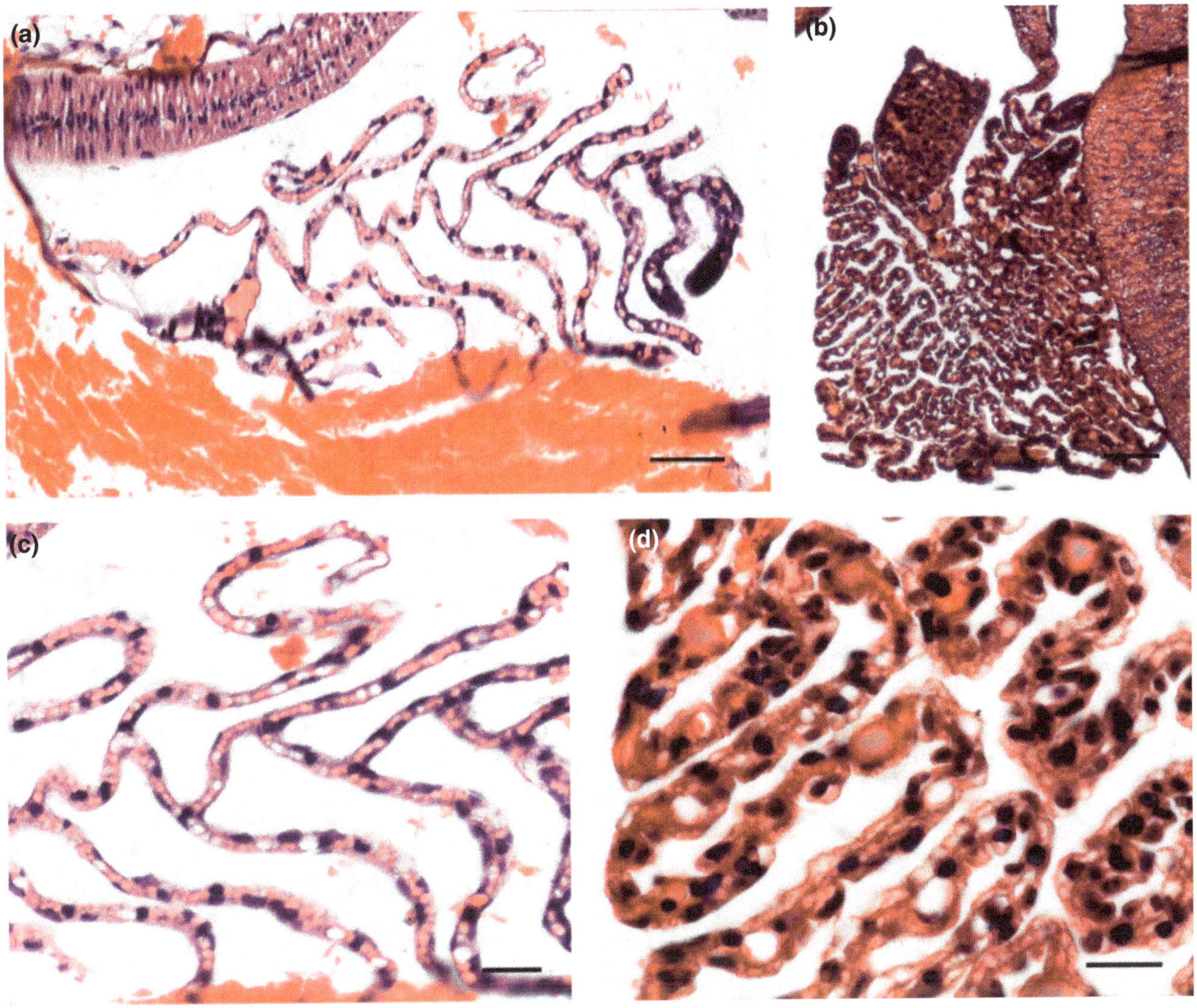

Fig. 5.11 Longitudinal section of the *Loligo vulgaris* gill (**a**). Horizontal section of *S. officinalis* gill (**b**). Detail of the *L. vulgaris gill* epithelium (**c**). Detail of the *S. officinalis* gill epithelium (**d**). **a**, **c** H&E stain and **b**, **d** Masson's trichrome stain. Scale bars: **a** 50 μm; **b** 100 μm; and **c–d** 25 μm

5.8.1 Renal Appendages

In adult octopods, the renal appendages are protrusions in the coelom cavity with grooves and folds that cover the vena cava and its branches. These appendages consist of a single-layered columnar epithelium with apical microvilli. The renal appendages of decapods have the same structure that has been observed in octopus, with deep grooves and folds (Furuya et al. 2004) coated by a columnar epithelium with microvilli. However, these cells are characterized as the presence of numerous mitochondria in the apical region and in the area of the basal labyrinth, as well as by many large dense lysosomes with high acid phosphatase activity (Budelmann et al. 1997). Below the epithelium lies a blood "lacuna" with an incomplete layer of endothelial cells (only a few fibroblasts and collagenous fibres), but also an extensive network of fine oblique striated muscle cells is observed. This network of muscle fibres is responsible for the rhythmic contractions of the renal appendages, which support the flow of the haemolymph and urine (Budelmann et al. 1997).

Furuya et al. (2004) established that the renal appendages differ between juveniles and adults of different species, the latter always exhibiting a more complex surface of renal appendages than in juveniles. In octopus paralarvae, the

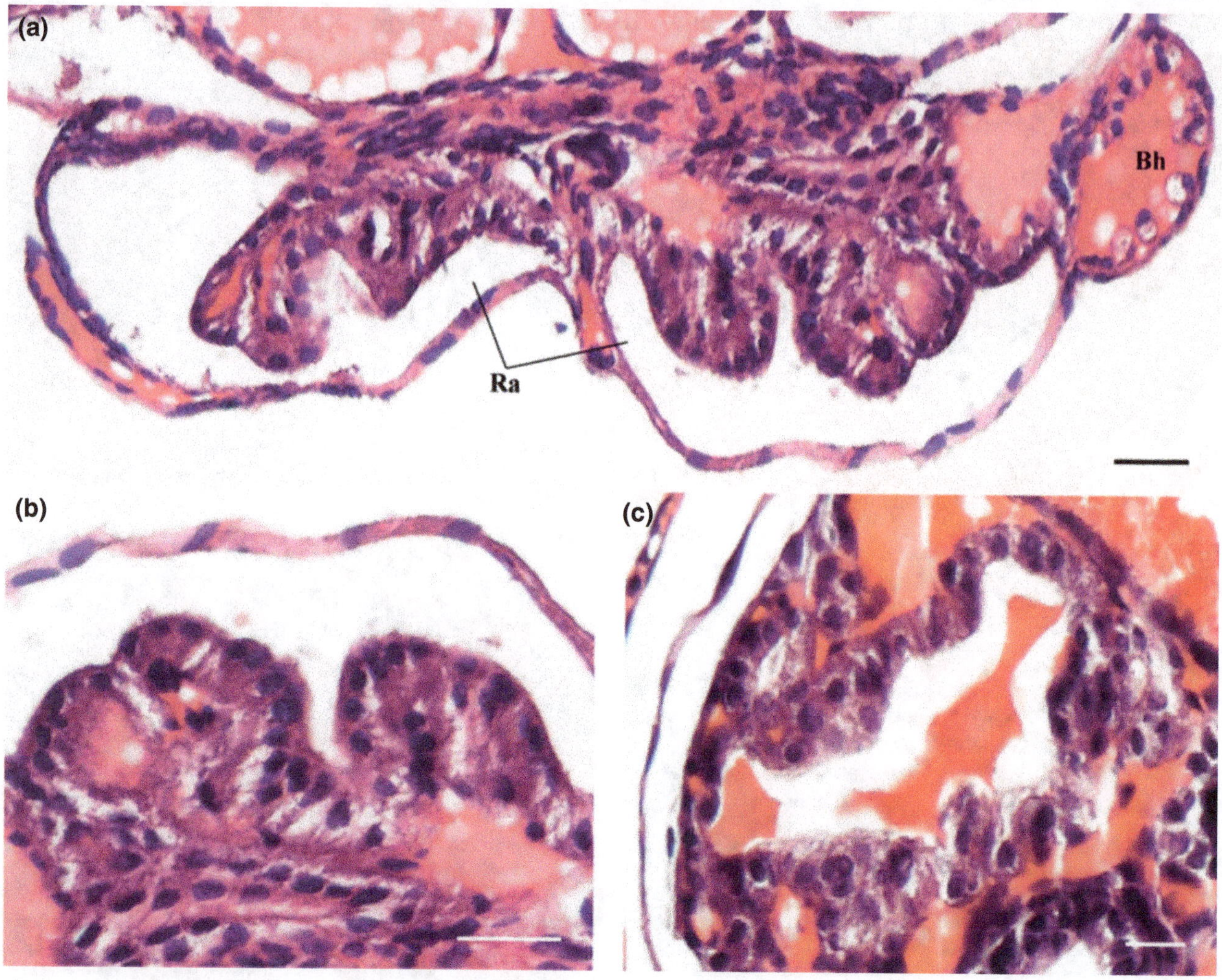

Fig. 5.12 Transversal section of renal appendages of an *O. vulgaris* paralarva protruding in the renal coelom (**a**). Detail of the epithelium of renal appendages (**b**). *L. vulgaris* digestive appendages, transversal view (**c**). Bh, branchial heart and Ra, renal appendages. H&E stain. Scale bars: **a–b** 25 μm and **c** 10 μm

renal appendage consists of a single-layered columnar epithelium covering the vena cava and its branches (Fig. 5.12a, b). In comparison with the adult, it is a simple saccular structure without groove and folds. The renal appendages of squid show the same organizational structure as in octopus paralarvae, but these are more developed than in adult octopus.

5.8.2 Digestive Appendages

In squid, the digestive appendages consist of two different epithelia. The outer epithelium consists of a single-layered columnar epithelium with microvilli. It is connected to the terminal epithelia of the renal appendages. In the centre, two pancreatic epithelial sheets (the outer renal and the inner pancreatic epithelium) lie in parallel, separated by a capillary system and a small amount of connective tissue (Budelmann et al. 1997). The juvenile pancreatic appendages are less folded and show a simple cubic epithelium (Fig. 5.12c).

5.8.3 Branchial Heart Appendages or Pericardial Glands

The cephalopod pericardial gland is a structure connected with the branchial heart that projects into the coelom. In cuttlefish, these appendages are conical and have grooves and folds. Apparently, these structures are not developed in post-hatching stages (Derby 2014).

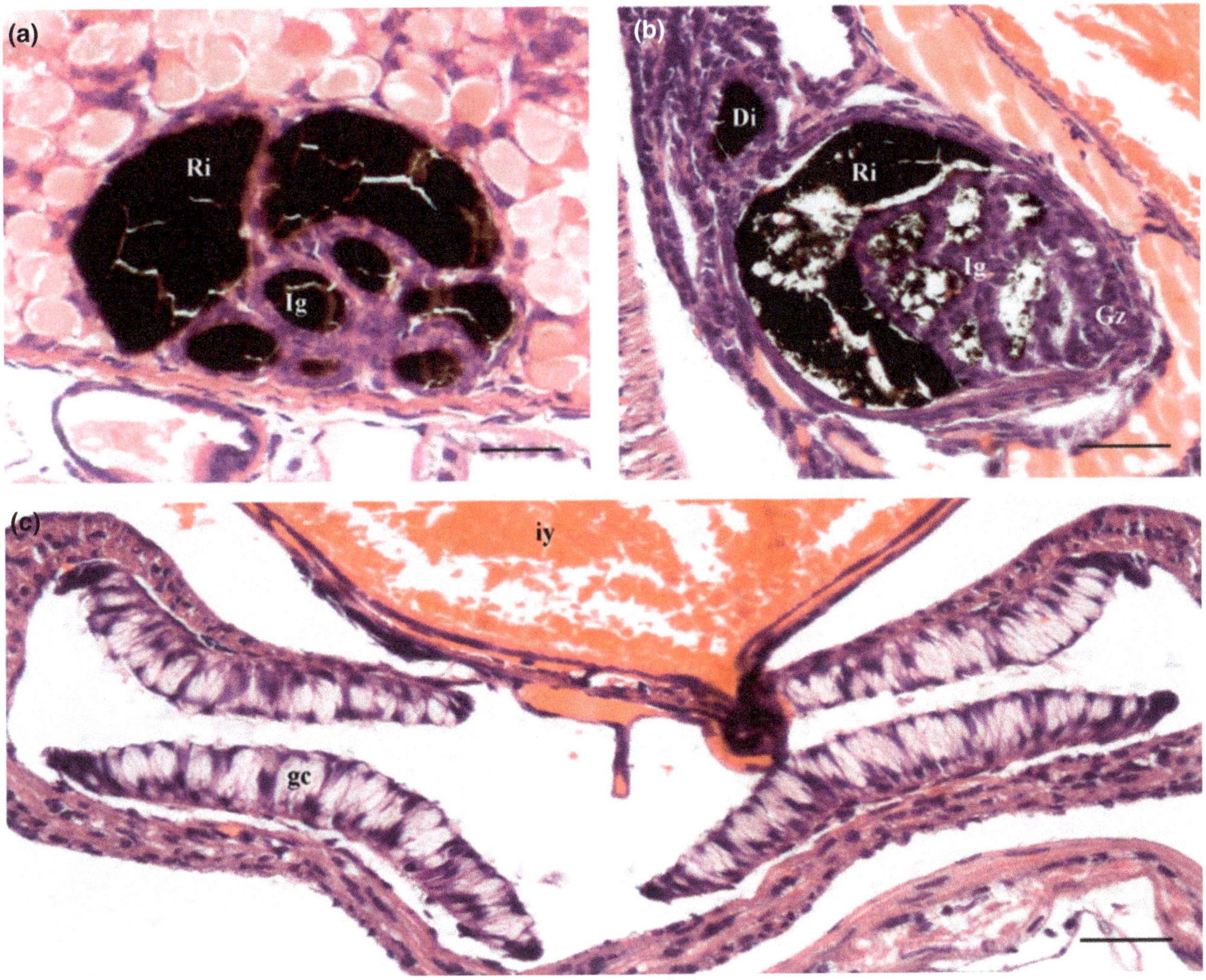

Fig. 5.13 Transversal section of *O. vulgaris* showing the ink sac (**a**). Longitudinal section of the *L. vulgaris* ink sac (**b**). *L. vulgaris* funnel organ, transversal view (**c**). Gc, goblet cell; Gz, basal germinal zone; Di, ink sac duct; Ig, ink gland; iy, internal yolk; and Ri, ink sac or reservoir. **a–c** H&E stain. Scale bars: **a** 25 µm and **b–c** 50 µm

5.8.4 Ink Gland Complex (Fig. 5.13)

The Coleoidea species have ink sacs and produce ink, but some coleoids have lost their ink sac. For example, this is true in the case of the octopod species in the Cirrata suborder (Budelmann et al. 1997). The ink gland complex consists of three parts: the ink gland, the ink reservoir and the ink sac duct (Budelmann et al. 1997). The ink is produced by the secretions of two glands, the ink gland (in the ink sac) and the funnel gland (Derby 2014). The combined secretion of these two glands, produced in different quantities, leads to ink different forms (Derby 2014).

5.8.5 Ink Sac

This gland is exocrine and produces the ink. The epithelium of the gland complex inner wall is formed by a columnar glandular epithelium, whereas the outer wall is formed by iridophores (Mangold et al. 1989). The ink gland is divided by lamellae that are composed of muscle and collagenous fibres. The gland centre has a tubuloalveolar structure with a cubical epithelium (Budelmann et al. 1997). In hatchling cephalopods, it is possible to see the ink gland complex and its structures (gland sac and duct). The gland presents a cubic epithelium, while the ink sac wall is formed by a squamous epithelium (Fig. 5.13a, b).

5.8.6 Funnel Organ

The funnel organ is the second gland contributing to the ink secretion (Derby 2014). This is a mucous gland on the funnel inner surface (Budelmann et al. 1997). In adult squids, this gland is formed by columnar goblet cells with a dark cytoplasm and a nucleus in the basal region (Laurie 1888). This organ has morphological differences between different species. This organ is usually W-shaped in octopuses, but in Sepioidea it consists of a dorsal inverted V-shaped and paired lateral pads (Voss 1963).

This organ is present in hatchling squid, cuttlefish and octopus. In juvenile squids (Fig. 5.13c), this organ has the same morphology as observed by Voss (1963) for Sepioidea. This gland has a glandular epithelium composed of columnar goblet cells with clear cytoplasm and a basal nucleus.

5.9 Central Nervous System or Brain (Fig. 5.14)

Cephalopods have the most complex brain of all invertebrates (Young 1977, 1979). The central nervous system can

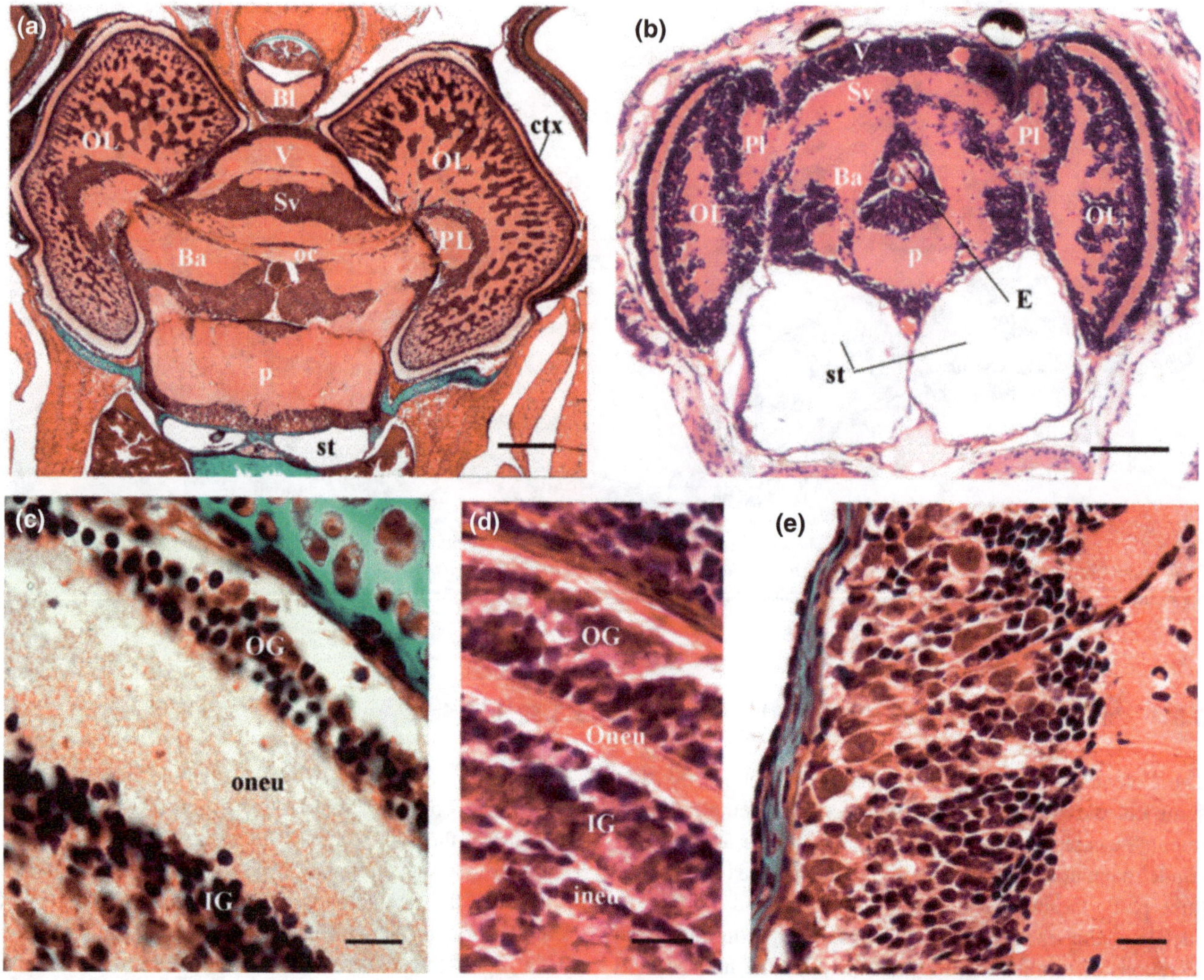

Fig. 5.14 Horizontal section of the *S. officinalis* brain at the level of the optic commissure (**a**). Horizontal section of the *O. vulgaris* brain (**b**). Detail of *S. officinalis* optic lobes (**c**). Detail of *L. vulgaris* optic lobes (**d**). Detail of the outer layer of the *S. officinalis* pedal lobe (**e**). Ba, basal lobe; ctx, cortical laminas; E, oesophagus; IG, inner granular; ineu, inner neuropil; oc, optic commissure; OG, outer granular; OL, optic lobes; oneu, outer neuropil; p, pedal lobes; PL, peduncular lobe; st, statocyst; Sv, subvertical lobe; and V, vertical lobe. **a**, **c–e** Masson's trichrome stain and **b** H&E stain. Scale bars: **a** 300 μm; **b** 100 μm; and **c–d** 20 μm

morphologically be divided into sub- and supra-oesophageal areas, partitioned by the oesophagus. On each side of the peri-oesophageal lobes are the large optic lobes which comprise an outer cortex and a central medulla. The brain areas are divided into many lobes (Young 1977, 1979); in the Coleoidea, brain has been characterized by twenty-five major lobes (Young 1971). The central mass lobes have a pattern of central neuropil (nerve fibres) and a surrounding cortex (cell bodies). The brain lobe proportions change between hatchling, juveniles and adult stages of life (Frösch 1971). These changes have been correlated with morphological developments and changes in behaviour and habitat (Messenger 1973; Nixon and Mangold 1996; Shigeno et al. 2001). The modes of brain development vary between species (Yamazaki et al. 2002). The tactile memory centres grow faster than the swimming centres in benthic species. However, the optic lobes increase with growth in pelagic species (Yamazaki et al. 2002). Basically, the eyes and nervous system of a variety of hatchling cephalopod species follow the same pattern; they vary interspecifically in size, proportion and complexity (Wild et al. 2015).

The optic lobes of hatchling squid, cuttlefish and octopus are similar in relative size and tissue organization to those of adults (Fig. 5.14a, b). The outer cortex is formed by three layers: two of them contain small neurons that are densely packed (outer and inner granular layers), and in the middle, there is a layer of optic nerve fibres (outer neuropil or plexiform layer) (Fig. 5.14c). Below the inner granular

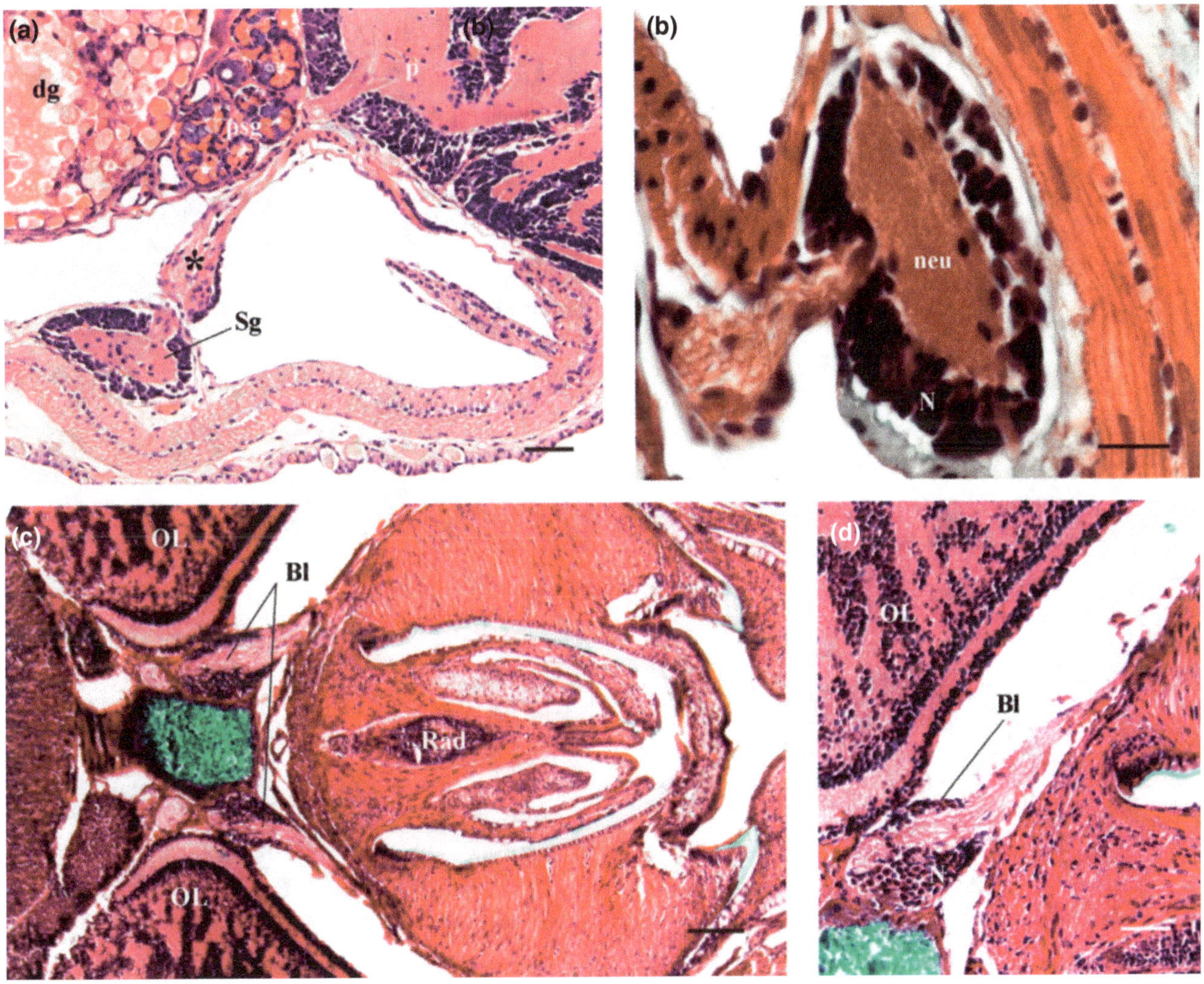

Fig. 5.15 Horizontal section of *O. vulgaris* connection (*) between the pedal lobe and stellate ganglion (**a**). Detail of *O. vulgaris* stellate ganglion (**b**). Horizontal section of *S. officinalis* buccal ganglion (**c**). Detail of *S. officinalis* buccal ganglion (**d**). Bl, buccal lobe; dg, digestive gland; N, neurons; neu, neuropil; OL, optic lobes; p, pedal lobes; psg, posterior salivary gland; Rad, radula sac; and Sg, stellate ganglion. **a** H&E stain and **b–d** Masson's trichrome stain. Scale bars: **a**, **c** 100 µm; **b** 20 µm; and **d** 50 µm

layer, the neurons are arranged in columns separated by neuropil which are more abundant in the medulla (Fig. 5.14a, b). However, in the hatchlings of *L. vulgaris* a thin second plexiform layer (inner) is seen just below the inner granular layer (Fig. 5.14d) (Wild et al. 2015). From each optical lobe, an optic tract crosses the brain forming the optic commissure (Fig. 5.14a). The optic commissure is well developed and can be divided into dorsal (Fig. 5.14a) and ventral optic commissures (Wild et al. 2015). The peduncle commissure lies tightly adjacent to the dorsal optic commissure (Wild et al. 2015).

The cerebral ganglia in hatchling cephalopods are less developed, lacking the complex organization observed in the adults. Nevertheless, the general architecture of the brain formed by suboesophageal and supra-oesophageal lobes has been observed (Fig. 5.14a, b). Moreover, ganglia which are connected with the cerebral ganglia via connectives and commissures are also observed along the body.

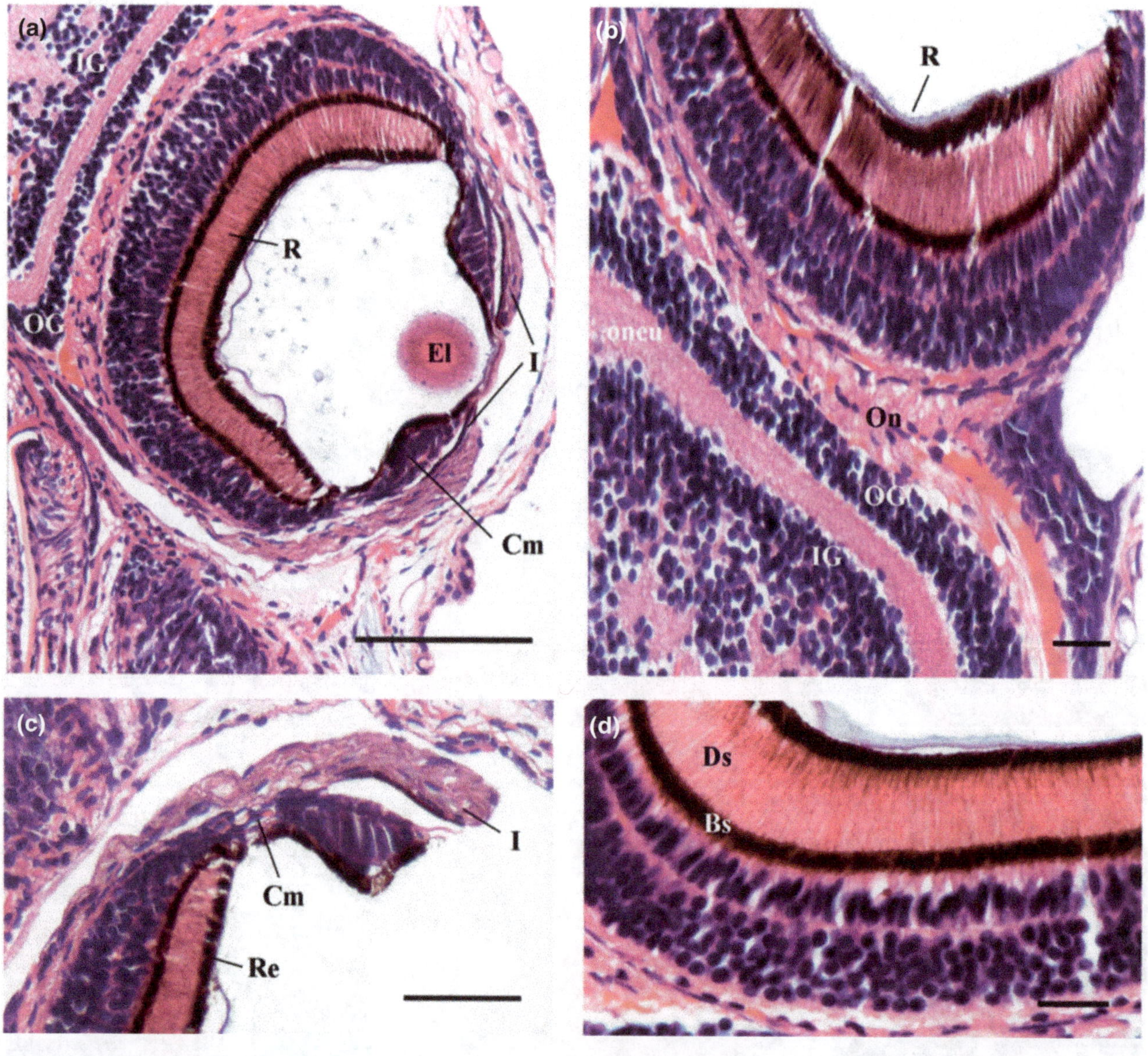

Fig. 5.16 Longitudinal section of the *O. vulgaris* head showing an eye (**a**). Longitudinal section of the *O. vulgaris* optic nerves and optic lobe (**b**). Detail of *O. vulgaris* ciliary body and iris (**c**). Detail of the *O. vulgaris* retina (**d**). Bs, basal region of distal segments of the visual cell filled with pigment granules; Cm, ciliary body; Ds, distal region of photoreceptor segments bearing rhabdomeres and pigment granules; El, eye lens; I, iris; IG, inner granular cells; OG, outer granular cells; oneu, outer neuropil; and R, retina. **a–e** H&E stain. Scale bars: **a** 100 μm; **b** 25 μm; **c** 50 μm; **d** 10 μm

Concerning the suboesophageal mass, the hatchlings show a developed pedal lobe (Fig. 5.14a, b). A brachial lobe entailing short brachiopedal connectives is described in hatchling cuttlefish (Wild et al. 2015). The supra-oesophageal mass is more complex, and it is composed laterally by the basal and peduncular lobes and anteriorly by the vertical and subvertical lobes (Fig. 5.14a, b). Moreover, in the most anterior part posteriorly to the buccal mass, a buccal lobe can also be observed (Fig. 5.14a). The arrangement of these lobes is simpler than those in adults. The vertical lobe, in adults, has a very characteristic shape with five lobules. Most of the lobes in the hatchlings are formed by a central extended neuropil surrounding by densely packed groups of neurons. The size of the neurons varies from small to large (Fig. 5.14c). Group of fibres forming nerves connect these lobes with small ganglia located along the body. In the hatchling cuttlefish and octopus, it is possible to see the neuropil of the stellate ganglia receiving fibres from the pedal lobe through a coarse pallial nerve (Fig. 5.15a, b). Moreover, the muscular organ (bolsters) of the buccal mass receive innervation from the buccal lobe (5.15c, d). The connection of the buccal lobe in adults has been described by Young (1971), "the superior buccal lobes send nerves directly to the posterior salivary glands and, via inferior buccal ganglia (which are connected to the superior buccal lobes by inter-buccal connectives) to the anterior salivary glands, the muscles of the jaws and the radula".

In addition to the review of Young (1971), more recently Wild et al. (2015) published a specialized monograph on the nervous system of six species of hatchling cephalopod using histology and 3D modelling.

5.10 Sensory System (Figs. 5.16 and 5.17)

Cephalopods have numerous sensory organs (Budelmann 1994; Budelmann and Tu 1997) such as large and well-developed eyes, a paired statocyst, a system similar to the fish lateral line, extraocular photoreceptor organs. Some octopuses are also sensitive to chemical and tactile stimuli.

5.10.1 The Visual System (Fig. 5.16)

All cephalopods possess eyes although there are differences in their morphology. The eyes are mostly spherical, but sometimes oval, telescopic or stalked (Wentworth and Muntz 1989; Young 1970, 1991). The Coleoidea eyes contain all the major components of a complex vertebrate eyes (Budelmann et al. 1997), namely: cornea (except those of *Todarodes*, *Illex* and *Ommastrephes*), iris, retina, pupil (which can be circular, horizontal or irregular in shape) and rigid lens that are suspended by ciliary muscles which allow for some near vision (Messenger 1981, 1991; Hartline and Lange 1984).

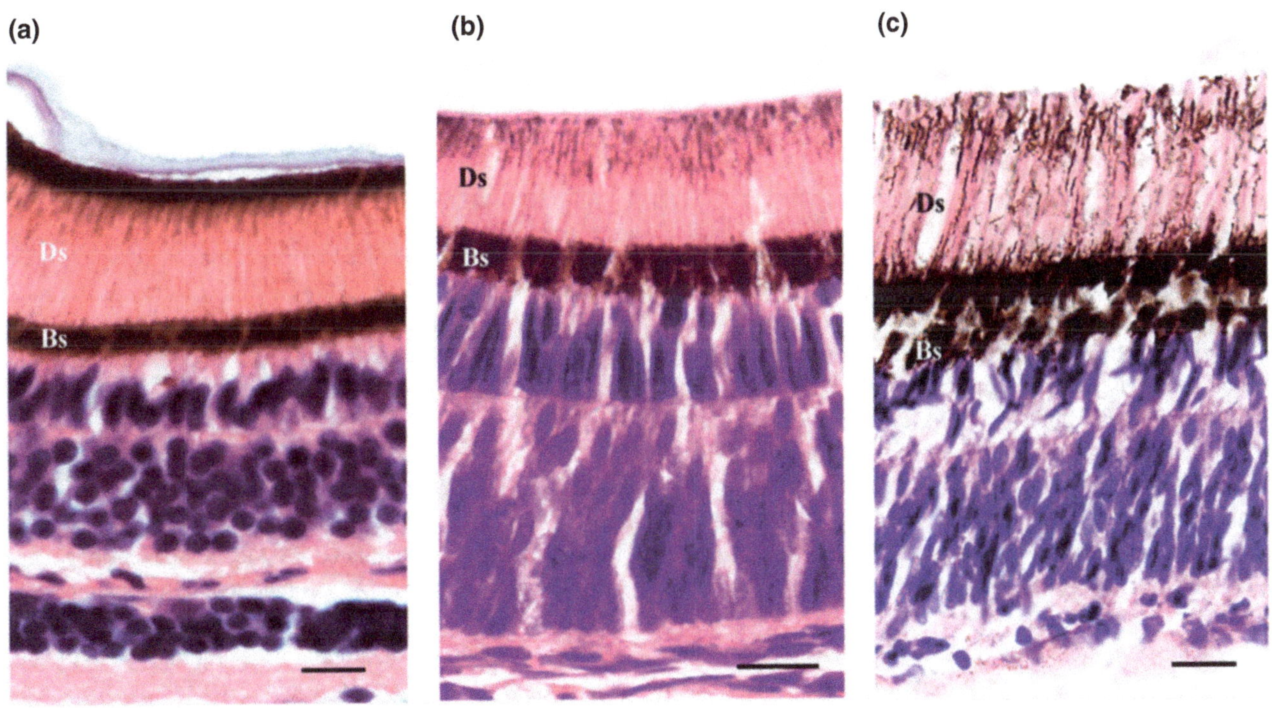

Fig. 5.17 Longitudinal section of the *O. vulgaris* retina (**a**). Longitudinal section of *L. vulgaris* retina (**b**). Longitudinal section of the *S. officinalis* retina (**c**). Bs, basal segment of the visual cell filled with pigment granules and Ds, distal photoreceptive segments bearing the rhabdomeres and pigment granules. **a–c** H&E stain. Scale bars: **a** 10 μm and **b–c** 20 μm

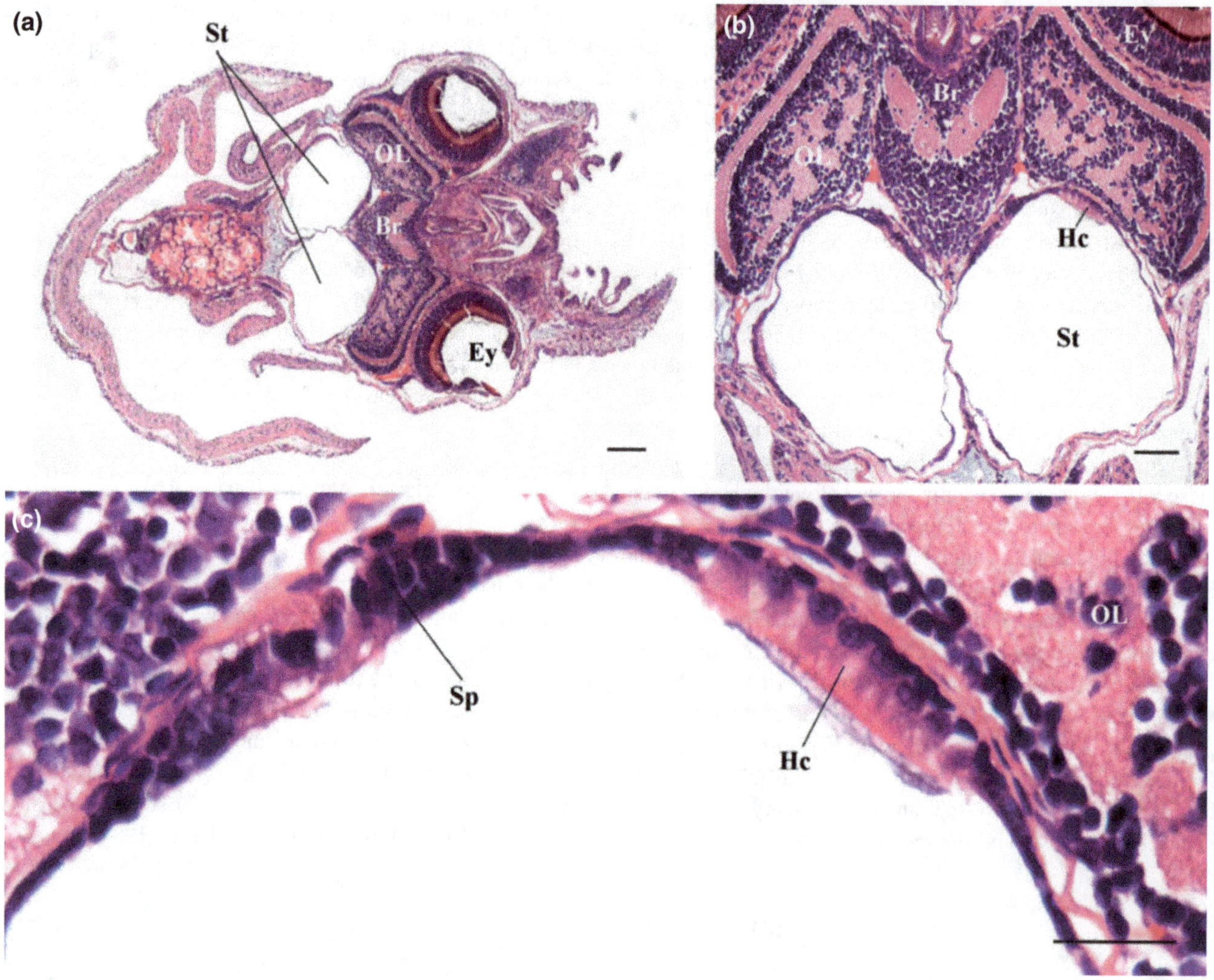

Fig. 5.18 Horizontal section of an *O. vulgaris* paralarva (**a**). Close view of statocysts (**b**). Detail of sensory areas of statocyst. Br, brain; Ey, eyes; Hc, hair cells; OL, optic lobes; Sp, supporting cells; St, statocyst. **a–c** H&E stain. Scale bars: **a** 100 μm; **b** 50 μm; and **c** 25 μm

The cephalopod iris is formed of five layers: external epithelium, chromatophore layer, iridophore layer, muscle and collagen fibre layer and pigment epithelium (Froesch 1973). The cephalopod retina is less developed than those in vertebrates. It is formed by receptor cells (primary sensory cells) and efferent fibres. The visual information from the retina runs to large optic lobes through the optic nerve (Budelmann 1994). The behaviour response of embryos to visual stimulus and their ability to learn visual features of potential prey indicate that the visual system, including the optic lobes, is functional before hatching (Darmaillacq et al. 2014).

In the hatchling octopus, squid and cuttlefish, the eyes are completely developed and have the same structure than in adults (Fig. 5.16). In some structures such as the retina, differences in the thickness or development of some of its layers are observed (Fig. 5.17). The plexiform layer is more developed in the first few days post-hatching. In *Loligo*, the pigmentary granules in the apical rhabdomere region are scarce (Fig. 5.17b).

5.10.2 The Statocysts (Fig. 5.18)

These structures are situated in the cranial cartilage and show a variety of forms in cephalopods (Budelmann et al. 1997). In octopus, this is a spherical sac (Fig. 5.18a, b) with a balance system and an angular acceleration system divided into nine segments (Young 1960). However, in decapods, this structure is irregularly shaped and has three gravity receptor systems and an angular acceleration system (Stephens and Young 1982). The equilibrium receptor organs provide information regarding body position. Different animals have different requirements for this organ depending on lifestyles and habitats. In general, fast-moving species orient themselves with respect to the direction of gravity (and other linear accelerations), as well as respond to rotatory body movements (angular accelerations) (Neumeister and Budelmann 1997). Consequently, the equilibrium receptor organs include two different receptor systems: a gravity receptor system for the detection of position relative to the direction of gravity and an angular acceleration receptor system for the detection of rotatory movements (Neumeister and Budelmann 1997).

Both receptor systems are formed by two types of cells, hair cells which are voluminous and have a large nucleus and microvillous supporting cells (Fig. 5.18c). The gravity receptor system comprises the macula epithelium and the accessory statolith. The hair cells of the macula are in different arrangements: concentric and half circles or in 360° or 180° radial fan-like. The other receptor system, an angular acceleration system, is formed by the crista epithelium with the cupula. This structure forms ridges that run inside the statocyst in the three dimensions of space.

The crista segments are composed of primary sensory hair cells and two types of secondary hair cells (Budelmann 1994). Along each crista segment, the hair cells are arranged in two or four regular rows. Just like in the macula, between the hair cells, there are supporting cells.

5.11 Concluding Remarks

The histological anatomy study of premature hatchlings of squid (*L. vulgaris*) and cuttlefish (*S. officinalis*) and of paralarvae of octopus (*O. vulgaris*) shows that most systems and their characteristic structures are present. However, comparing these structures with the adults of the same species it is possible to conclude that in general the level of development is lower. This lack of development is easily observed in digestive and circulatory systems. In the digestive system, the absence of glandular epithelia associated with the posterior part of the lateral lobes and the jaw during these stages of development is characteristic. It is also remarkable the low number of secretory cells in regions such as the caecum and intestine, where mucous secretions help the excretion of waste products resulting from digestion. Moreover, the octopus and squid intestines are the most underdeveloped organ in the digestive system. There are no folds or villi, the epithelium is simple squamous, and no secretory cells are present in the most part of the tube. In the circulatory system, a low level of development has been found in the branchial hearts and also in the systemic heart. In hatchling cephalopods, the branchial hearts present a large lumen that is absent in adults. Likewise, systemic a poorly developed wall is observed in the systemic heart of all the studied species. In paralarvae and juvenile, the systemic heart does not have the strong musculature observed in the systemic heart of adults.

In some instances, the degree of development in hatchling cephalopods is similar to that in adults. This happens, for example, in defensive systems, the ink complex, the structures that help in the prey capture and the visual system. In hatchling octopus, squid and cuttlefish, the eyes are completely developed. Only in the retina, differences in the thickness or development of some of its layers are observed.

Finally, there are tissues that change throughout the development to adapt to different habitats. This occurs in structures such as the *L. vulgaris* and *S. officinalis* epidermis where a large number of globet cells are observed differ from the characteristic epithelium of adults. Another example is the characteristic Kölliker cells that appear only in the epidermis of octopus paralarvae, disappearing after the first month of post-embryonic life.

The study of all tissues and systems in premature hatchling of squid (*L. vulgaris*) and cuttlefish (*S. officinalis*) and of paralarvae of octopus (*O. vulgaris*) allows us to conclude that although most systems are present, the majority of them show a lower degree of development than in adults. Some systems, mainly those related to sensory systems, present a similar development, and others change their morphological characteristics.

Acknowledgements We would like to thank Antonio Sykes (CCMAR–CIMAR) who generously donated the paraffin blocks from which the sections of *S. officinalis* were prepared.

References

Bidder AM (1950) The digestive mechanism of the European squids *Loligo vulgaris, Loligo forbesi, Alloteuthis media* and *Alloteuthis subulata*. Q J Microsc Sci 91:1–43

Bizikov VA (1987) New data on squid gladius structure. Zool Zhur 46 (2):177–184

Boletzky SV (1973) Structure and function of the Kölliker organs in young octopods (Mollusca, Cephalopoda). Z Morphol Tiere 75:315–327

Boletzky SV (1983) Sepia officinalis. In: Boyle PR (ed) Cephalopod life cycles, vol 2 Species accounts. Academic Press, San Diego, pp 31–52

Boletzky SV, Wiedmann J (1978) Schlup-Wachstum bei *Sepia officinalis* in Abhängigkeit von ökologischen Parametern. Neues Jahrb Geol P-A 157:103–106

Boucher-Rodoni R, Mangold K (1988) Comparative aspect of ammonia excretion in cephalopods. Malacology 29:145–151

Brocco SL, O'Clair R, Cloney RA (1974) Cephalopod integument: the ultrastructure of Kölliker's organs and their relationship to setae. Cell Tissue Res 151:293–308

Budelmann BU (1994) Cephalopod sense organs, nerves and the brain: adaptations for high performance and life style. Mar Freh Behav Physol 25:13–33

Budelmann BU, Tu Y (1997) The statocyst-oculomotor reflex of cephalopods and the vestibulo oculomotor reflex of vertebrates: a tabular comparison. Vie Milieu 47:95–99

Budelmann BU, Schipp R, Boletzky Sv (1997) Cephalopoda. In: Harrison FW, Kohn AJ (eds) Microscopic anatomy of invertebrates, Mollusca ii, vol 6a. Wiley-Liss, New York, pp 235–271

Derby DD (2014) Cephalopod ink: production, chemistry, functions and applications. Mar Drugs 12:2700–2730.

Dilly PN, Messenger JB (1972) The branchial gland: a site of haemocyanin synthesis in octopus. Z Zellforsch Mik An 2:192–221

Fernández-Gago R, Heb M, Gensler H. Rocha F (2017) 3D reconstruction of the digestive system in *Octopus vulgaris* Cuvier, 1797 embryos and paralarvae during the first month of life. Front Physiol 04 July 2017. https://doi.org/10.3389/fphys.2017.00462

Fiedler A, Schipp R (1987) the role of the branchial heart complex in circulation of coleoid cephalopods. Experientia 43(5):544–553

Fioroni P (1990) Our recent knowledge of the development of the cuttlefish (*Sepia officinalis*). Zool Anz 224:1–25

Froesch D (1973) On fine structure of the octopus iris. Z Zellforsch Mikrosk Anat 145:119–129

Frösch D (1971) Quantitative Untersuchungen am Zentralnervensystem der schlüpfstadien von zhen mediterranen Cephalopodenarte. Rev Suisse Zool 78:1069–1122

Furuya H, Ota M, Kimura R, Tsuneki K (2004) Renal organs of cephalopods: a habitat for dicyemids and chromidinids. J Morph 262:629–643

Hanlon RT, Messenger JB (1988) Adaptive coloration in young cuttlefish (*Sepia offcinalis* L.): the morphology and development of body patterns and their relation to behaviour. Phil Trans Roy Soc B Biol Sci 320:437–448

Hartline PH, Lange GD (1984) Visual systems of cephalopods. In: In Bolis L, Keynes RD, Maddrell SHP (eds) comparative physiology of sensory systems. Cambridge University Press, Cambridge, pp 335–355

Hopkins B, Boletzky Sv (1994) The fine morphology of the shell sac in the squid genus *Loligo* (Mollusca: Cephalopoda) features of a modified conchiferan program. Veliger 37:344–357

Iglesias J, Sánchez FJ, Bersano JGF, Carrasco JF, Dhont J, Fuentes L, Linares F, Muñoz JL, Okumura S, Roo J, van der Meeren T, Vidal EAG, Villanueva R (2007) Rearing of *Octopus vulgaris* paralarvae: present status, bottlenecks and trends. Aquaculture 266:1–15

Johnson FE (1987) The vasculature of the white bodies in the ommastrephid squid *Illex illecebrosus* (Lesueur, 1821): a proposed route for dissemination of newly formed haemocytes. Can J Zool 65:1607–1620

Kling G, Schipp R (1987) Comparative ultrastructural and cytochemical analysis of the cephalopod systematic heart and its innervation. Experientia 43(5):502–511

Laurie M (1888) The organ of Verril in *Loligo*. J Cell Sci s2–29: 97–100

Lemaire J, Richard A, Decleir W (1977) Le foie embryonnaire de *Sepia officinalis* L. (Mollusque Cephalopode). I. Organogenèse. Haliotis 6:287–296

Mangold K, Sv Boletzky, Frösch D (1971) Reproductive biology and embryonic development of *Eledone cirrosa* (Cephalopoda, Octopoda). Mar Biol 8:109–117

Mangold K, Bidder AM, Portmann A (1989) Structures cutaneés: la poche du noir. In: Grassé PP (ed) Céphalopodes. Traité de Zoologie 5/4. Masson, Paris, France, pp 154–162

Messenger JB (1973) Learning performance and brain structure: a study in development. Brain Res 58:519–528

Messenger JB (1981) Comparative physiology of vision in molluscs. In: Autrum H (ed) Comparative physiology and evolution of vision in invertebrates. Handbook of Sensory Physiology, vol vii/6c. Springer Verlag, Berlin, pp 93–200

Messenger JB (1991) Photoreception and vision in molluscs. In: Cronly-Dillon JR, Gregory RL (eds) Evolution of the eye and the visual system. McMillan, London, pp 364–397

Naef A (1923) Die Cephalopoden. Monographie 35, volume i, parts i and ii, Sistematik. Fauna und Flora der Golfo di Napoli

Neumeister H, Budelmann BU (1997) Structure and function of the nautilus statocyst. Phil Tran Roy Soc B Biol Sci 352:1565–1588

Nixon M, Mangold K (1996) The early life of *Octopus vulgaris* (Cephalopoda, Octopodidae) in the plankton and at settlement: a change in life style. J Zool 239:301–327

Portmann A (1933) Observations sur la vie embryonnaire de la pieuvre (*Octopus vulgaris* Lam.). Arch Zool Exp Gen 76:24–36

Schipp R (1987) General morphological and functional characteristics of the cephalopod circulatory system. An introduction. Experientia 43(5):474–477

Schipp R, Schäfer A (1969) Vergleichende elektronenmikroskopische untersuchungen an den zentralen herzorganen von cephalopoden (*Sepia officinalis*). Z Zellforsch Mikrosk Anat 101:367–379

Schipp R, Mollenhauer S, Sv Boletzky (1979) Electron microscopical and histochemical studies of differentiation and function of the cephalopod gill (*Sepia officinalis*). Zoomorphologie 93:193–207

Shigeno S, Tsuchiya K, Segawa S (2001) Embryonic and paralarval development of the central nervous system of the loliginid squid *Sepioteuthis lessoniana*. J Comp Neurol 437:449–475

Stephens PR, Young JZ (1982) The statocyst of the squid *Loligo*. J Zool 197:241–266

Sundermann G (1983) The fine structure of epidermal lines on arms and head of postembryonic *Sepia officinalis* and *Loligo vulgaris* (Mollusca, Cephalopoda). Cell Tissue Res 232: 669–677

Thompsett DH (1939) *Sepia*. Liverpool marine biological committee. Memoirs on typical British marine plants & animals, Universal Press of Liverpool 32, p 184

Villanueva R (1995) Experimental rearing and growth of planktonic *Octopus vulgaris* from hatching to settlement. Can J Fish Aqua Sci 52:2639–2650

Voss GL (1963) Function and comparative morphology of the funnel organ in cephalopods. In: Proceedings of the XVI International Congress of Zoology, Washington, DC, USA, 20–27 August 1963, vol 1, p 74

Wells MJ, Wells J (1982) Ventilatory currents in the mantle of cephalopods. J Exp Biol 99:315–330

Wentworth SL, Muntz WRA (1989) Asymmetries in the sense organs and central nervous system of the squid *Histioteuthis*. J Zool 219:607–619

Wild E, Wollesen T, Haszprunar G, Heb M (2015) Comparative 3d microanatomy and histology of the eyes and central nervous systems in coleoid cephalopod hatchlings. Org Divers Evol 15:37–64

Yamazaki A, Yoshida M, Uematsu K (2002) Post-hatching development of the brain in *Octopus ocellatus*. Zool Sci 19:763–771

Yun DK, No HK, Prinyawiwatkul W (2013) Preparation and characteristics of squid pen β-chitin prepared under optimal deproteinisation and demineralisation condition. Int J Food Sci Tech 48:571–577

Young JZ (1960) The statocyst of *Octopus vulgaris*. Proc Roy Soc B Biol Sci 152:3–29

Young JZ (1970) The stalked eyes of *Bathothauma* (Mollusca: Cephalopoda). J Zool 162:437–447

Young JZ (1971) The anatomy of the nervous system of *Octopus vulgaris*. Clarendon Press, Oxford

Young JZ (1977) Brain, behaviour and evolution of cephalopods. Symp Zool Soc London 38:377–434

Young JZ (1979) The nervous system of *Loligo*, V: the vertical lobe complex. Phil Trans Roy Soc B Biol Sci 285:311–354

Young JZ (1991) Light has many meanings for cephalopods. Visual Neurosci 7(1–1):2

Young RE, Harman RF (1988) "Larva", "paralarva" and "subadult" in cephalopod terminology. Malacologia 29:201–207

Part II
Pathogens and Related Diseases

Cephalopod Diseases Caused by Fungi and Labyrinthulomycetes

6

Jane L. Polglase

Abstract

This chapter describes infections of cephalopods by both the Labyrinthulomycetes (formerly fungi, now protists) and organisms still classified as fungi, with information on how to diagnose them. Both types of infection are rare, but those by Labyrinthulomycetes in captive cephalopod populations can increase with time and may last for three or more years, raising concerns about such ubiquitous organisms for cephalopod culture.

Keywords

Cephalopod diseases • Infection • Fungi • Labyrinthulomycetes • Labyrinthulomycota • Thraustochytrids • Aplanochytrids • Labyrinthula

6.1 Introduction

As well as considering the rare cephalopod infections by organisms currently recognised as being within the fungal kingdom, this chapter covers diseases caused by organisms known most commonly as Labyrinthulomycetes. As their name suggests, the Labyrinthulomycetes were originally thought to be fungi. However, these single-celled organisms, with unique "ectoplasmic nets", are now classified as protists. Bennet et al (2017) provide the most comprehensive, recent description of the group, while Moss (1986, Chap. 11) provides excellent images of diagnostic features of these organisms.

Labyrinthulomycetes are most commonly found as marine decomposers or remineralisers of complex organic material, but can be symbionts, parasites or pathogens. There are three major groupings within the Labyrinthulomycetes: the thraustochytrids and aplanochytrids (regularly found as opportunist pathogens or parasites of invertebrates, most commonly molluscs) and the labyrinthulids (not considered here but also opportunist pathogens of marine grasses and in land grasses in saline soils). The common factor that allows the Labyrinthulomycetes to become pathogenic is stress in the host.

6.2 Thraustochytrid/Aplanochytrid Infections in Cephalopods

In molluscs, thraustochytrids proper and aplanochytrids (collectively referred to here as thraustochytrids) are found as important pathogens or parasites of bivalves and also of nudibranchs (McLean and Porter 1982), octopus and squid.

Only one thraustochytrid infection has been described to date in European cephalopods. This was a fatal, progressive, ulcerative dermal necrosis of lesser or curled octopus, *Eledone cirrhosa* (Polglase 1980, 1981) found on the east coast of Scotland. The disease (originally spread from one individual) infected an entire research aquarium, despite stringent efforts to remove it, for over four years, during which a small number of other infected animals were also brought in from the wild. A similar condition had also been observed sporadically in the 1970s/80s in *Octopus vulgaris*, at the Stazione Zoologica, Naples, Italy (J. B. Messenger, pers. comm. to Polglase).

J. L. Polglase (✉)
Institute of Life and Earth Sciences, School of Energy, Geoscience, Infrastructure and Society, Heriot Watt University, Riccarton, Edinburgh, EH11 1QH, Scotland, UK
e-mail: JP44@hw.ac.uk

C. Gestal et al. (eds.), *Handbook of Pathogens and Diseases in Cephalopods*,
https://doi.org/10.1007/978-3-030-11330-8_6

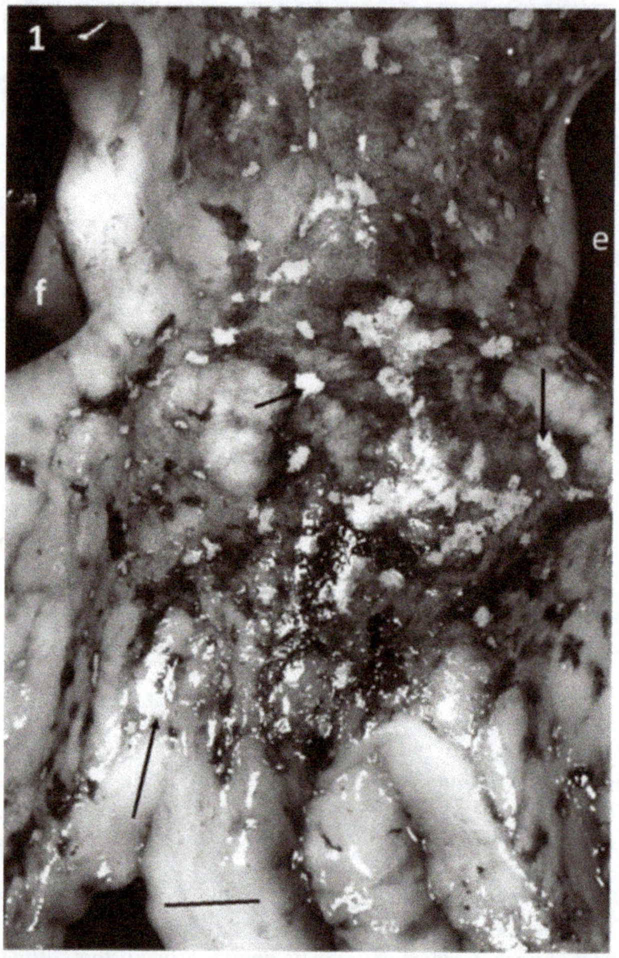

Fig. 6.1 *Eledone cirrhosa* showing symptoms of a rapidly progressing multi-lesion thraustochytrid infection. Arrows indicate lesions; e = eye; f = funnel. Scale bar: 12 mm

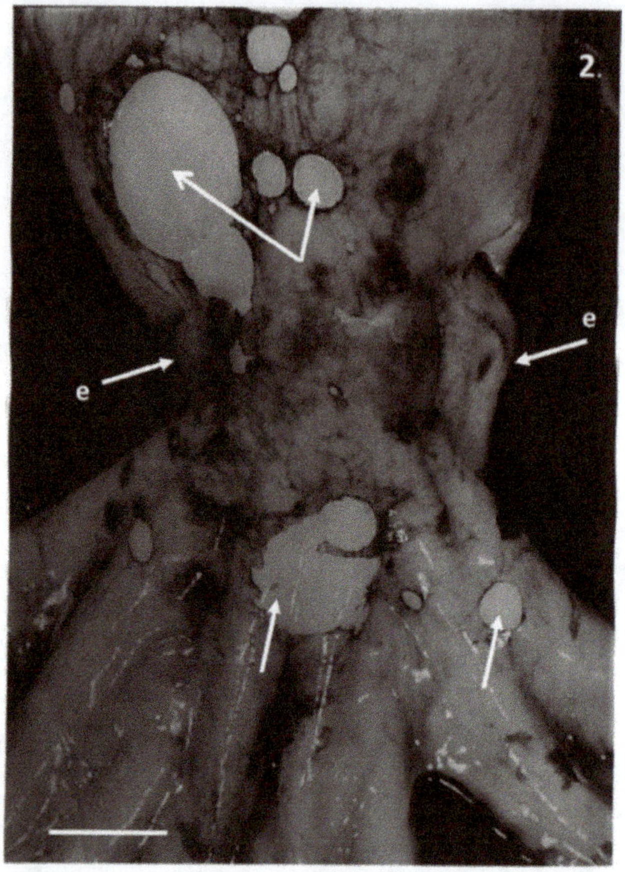

Fig. 6.2 Moribund *Eledone cirrhosa*, showing final stages of slow-progressing Labyrinthulomycete infection with major dermal lesions. Arrows indicate lesions; e = eye; f = funnel. Scale bar: 20 mm

Key signs were patches of inactive chromatophores, from which the epidermis was then lost (Fig. 6.1). Affected animals constantly rubbed their skin and shook their arms, as if itching. The lesions deepened, multiplied and spread, either rapidly or more slowly in individuals with fewer lesions, revealing the unpigmented connective tissue and muscle layers below (Fig. 6.2). The cause of the death was not clear but could have been metabolite imbalance (see Polglase 1980). In the light microscope, clear zones of tissue destruction were seen in the lesions around rounded cells approximately 6 μm in diameter (Figs. 6.3 and 6.4). The cells divided to produce diads, triads, tetrads and larger cell clusters, which point to thraustochytrid involvement (Figs. 6.3 and 6.4).

Only one organism was consistently seen in histological and electron microscope sections from all infected animals. This was a thraustochytrid tentatively identified from its life history in culture as *Ulkenia amoeboidea*, but more recent current work indicates that is a novel species and genus, with some metabolic differences from other thraustochytrids. In severe infections, small numbers of thraustochytrids were also seen in the gills and eyes (producing a cataract-like appearance) and in the lower dermis, but there was no evidence of a stage of systemic infection. Interestingly, labyrinthulids were also isolated from some of the lesions, but they appeared to be secondary to the thraustochytrid. Electron microscopy confirmed the diagnostic features of a thraustochytrid (see Fig. 6.8), but it was not possible to re-infect from cultures derived from the lesions.

Many haemocytes of infected animals responded by adopting the elongate "prefibroblast" morphology, seen in haemocytes moving towards the surface of mechanical wounds (Polglase et al. 1984). Groups of haemocytes were seen to produce incomplete capsules on the edge of the necrotic zones around the protists, but the thraustochytrids were never completely encapsulated and no dermal plug was ever formed across the lesion.

The condition appeared to be highly contagious (Polglase 1980) and made it extremely difficult to keep the Eledone in the aquarium for research purposes.

The only thraustochytrid infection in squid was found in the Northwest Atlantic. This is the gill disease in captive

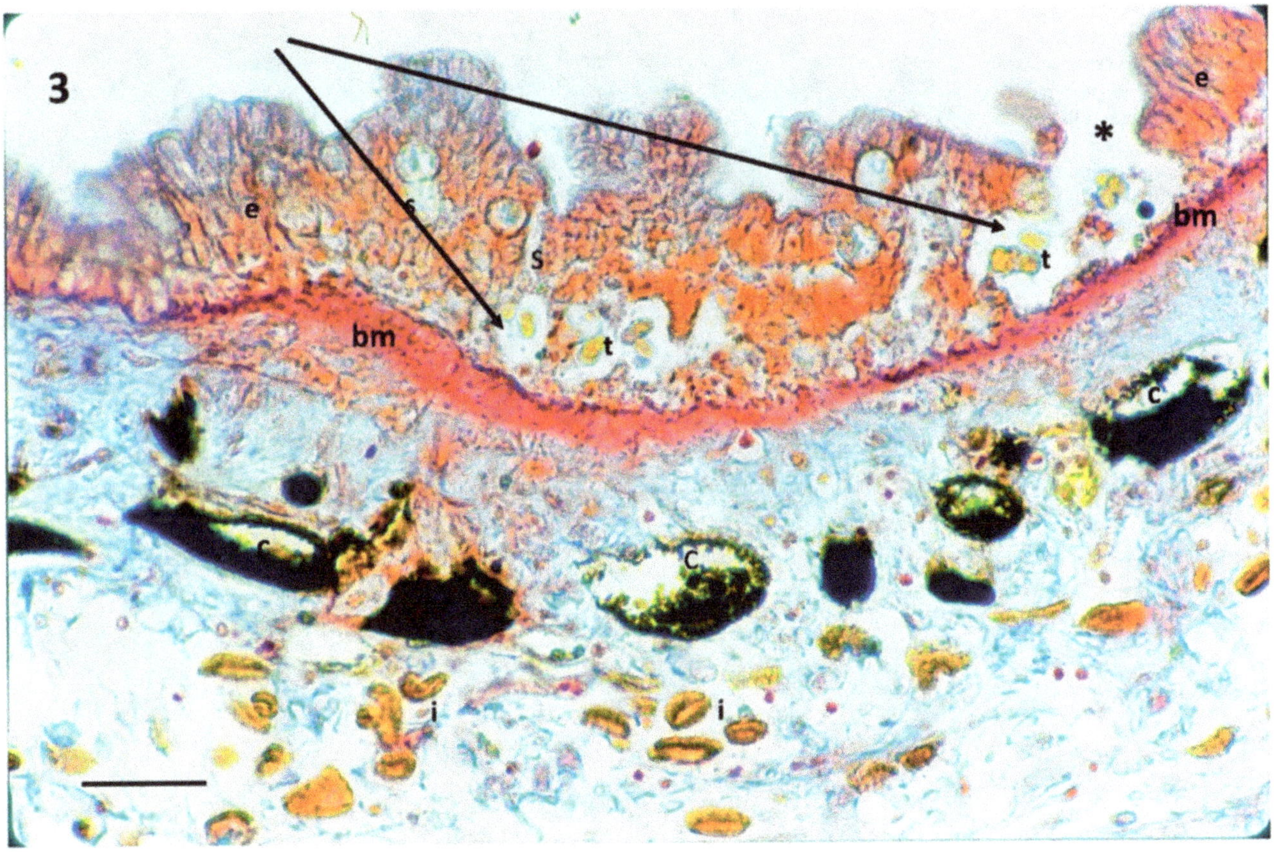

Fig. 6.3 Mallory's triple stained light microscope section showing thraustochytrids in the epidermis of *Eledone cirrhosa*. Arrows show clear zones where the host tissue has been dissolved by the lytic enzymes of the ectoplasmic net causing the cells to separate initially from the basal membrane (bm) and then be lost (asterisk). c = chromatophore; e = epidermis; i = iridophore; t = thraustochytrid. Scale bar: 40 µm

short-finned squids, *Illex illecebrosus*, reported by Jones (1981) and Jones and O'Dor (1983).

In 1977–79, this disease affected squid kept in a facility at Dalhousie University, Canada, designed to produce the best conditions possible for research on these delicate animals (the Aquatron). In 1977–78, only two or three animals died, atypically, before mating, while the others remained healthy. Those that died (Jones and O'Dor 1983) had a large number of small (1.5 mm) white nodule-like lesions in their gills (Figs. 6.5 and 6.6) and, in the later stages of heavy infections, also on the inside of the mantle; "sufficient numbers for these to be considered a likely cause of death" (Fig. 6.6). By the end of the 1979 squid "season", however, the lesions had become the main cause of mortality. They were never observed in animals in the wild and appeared after the animals had been kept for 3 weeks or longer in the Aquatron.

Light and electron microscopy again showed that only a single organism (spherical cells about 7 µm in diameter) could be identified in the lesions, often in large numbers (Fig. 6.7). Ultrastructural and semi-thin sections confirmed the organism was a thraustochytrid. In semi-thin sections, diads, triads and tetrads of cells could be seen beneath the gill epithelium, with evidence of substantial tissue damage from the activities of the lytic enzymes from the ectoplasmic net but not close to the cell bodies. In advanced infections, just as in *E. cirrhosa*, the overlying epithelium was disrupted, releasing the thraustochytrids into the mantle cavity.

Although some cells thought to be squid amoebocytes were found close to or even partially enclosing the thraustochytrids, there were no instances of complete encirclement or any degeneration of the thraustochytrids within the lesions. Jones and O'Dor were not able to isolate the thraustochytrid into pure culture for identification but speculated that it was a species of Schizochytrium. Lack of pure cultures also meant that re-infection experiments could not be undertaken, so there is no final proof that this was a pathogen.

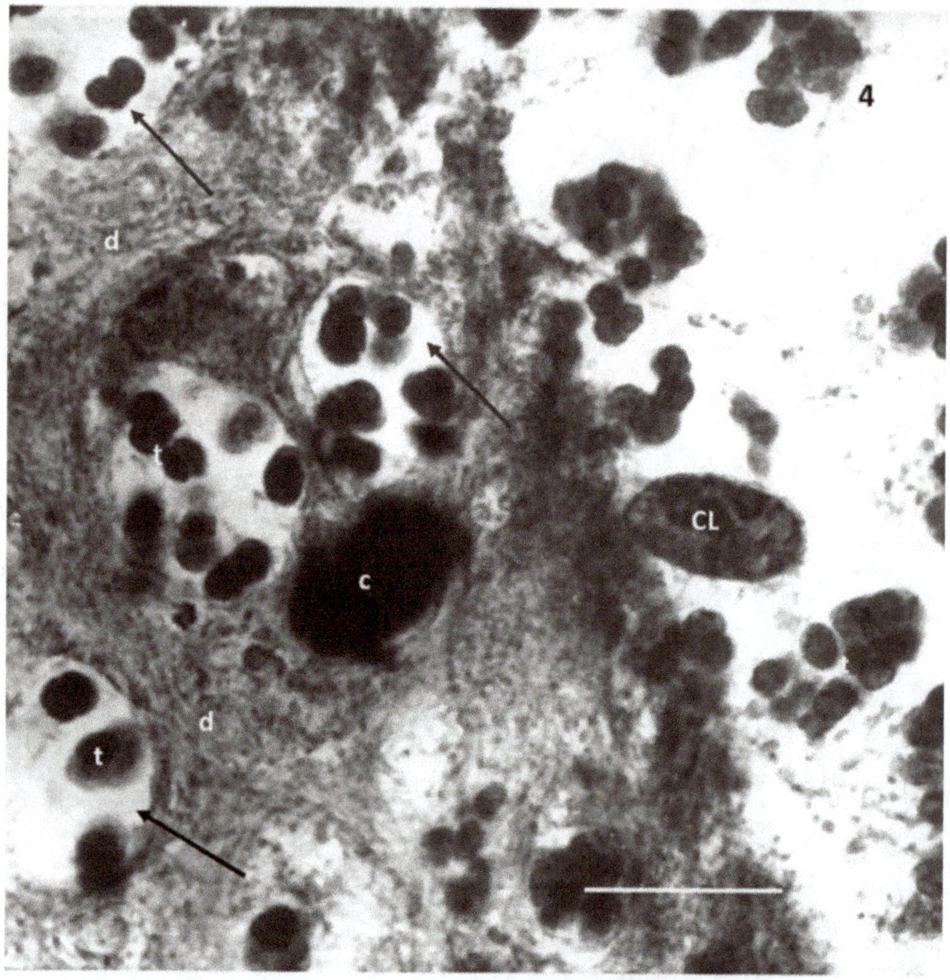

Fig. 6.4 Section of *Eledone cirrhosa* skin from which the epidermis has been lost, allowing the thraustochytrid (t) to move down into the dermal layer. Arrows indicate areas where tissue lysis is occurring surround the dividing thraustochytrid; c = chromatophore, CL = opportunist ciliate. Scale bar: 12 μm

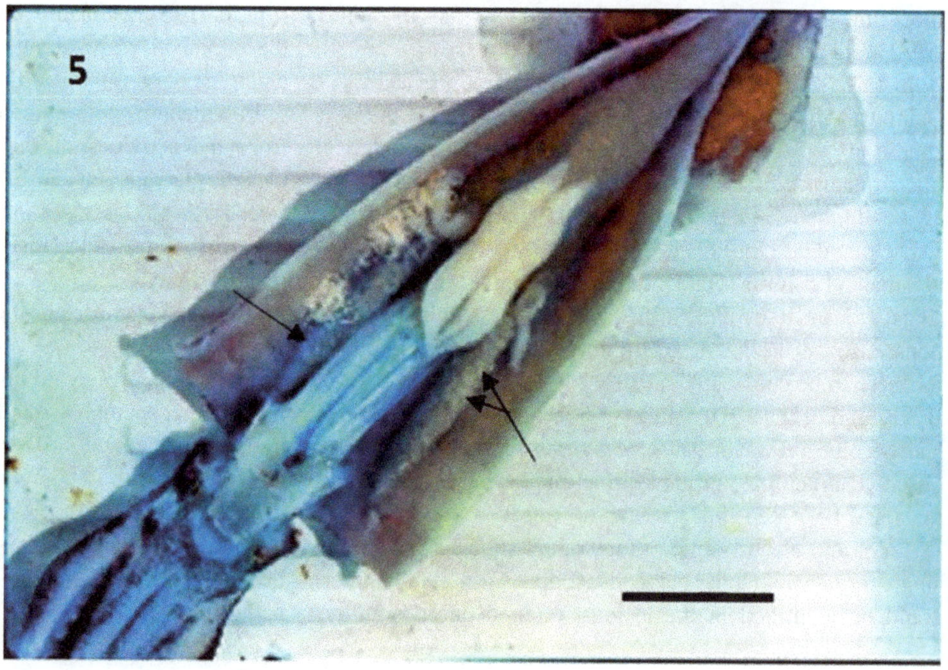

Fig. 6.5 Female northern short-finned squid, *Illex illecebrosus*, ventral dissection. Gills show small white lesions typical of the thraustochytrid disease. Scale bar ≈ 40 mm (Courtesy of Jones and O'Dor)

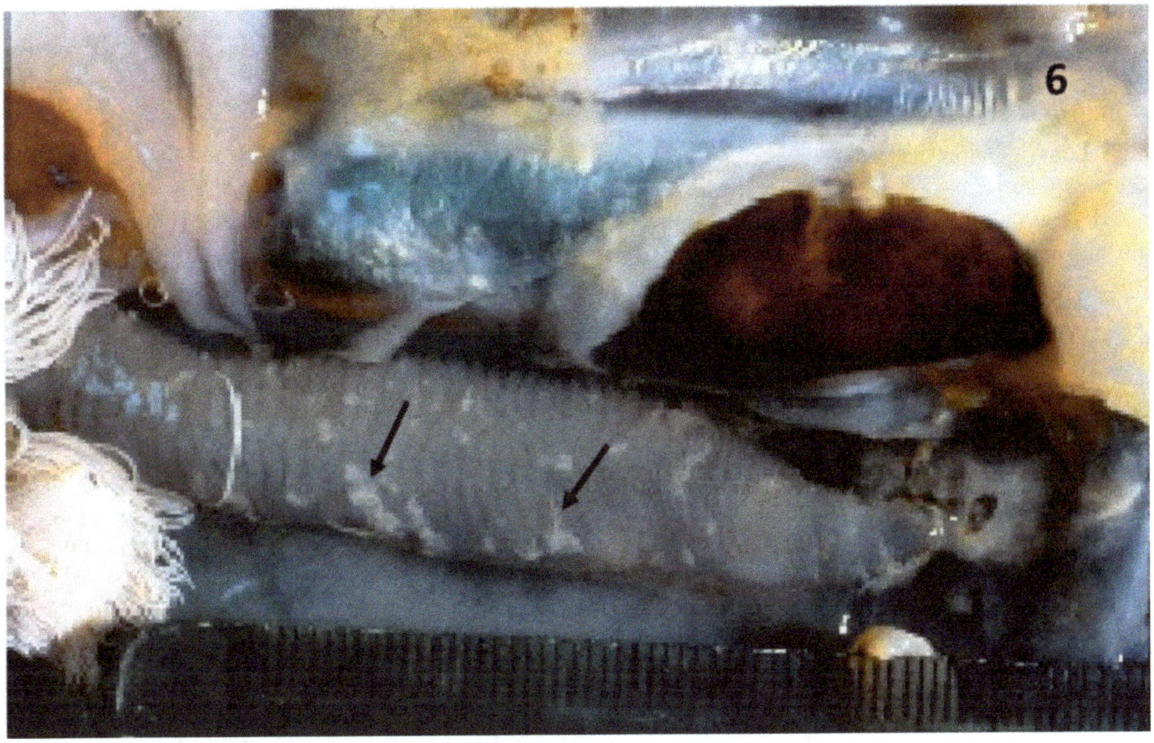

Fig. 6.6 *Illex illecebrosus* gill with scattered white lesions on filaments. Scale shows mm (Courtesy of Jones and O'Dor)

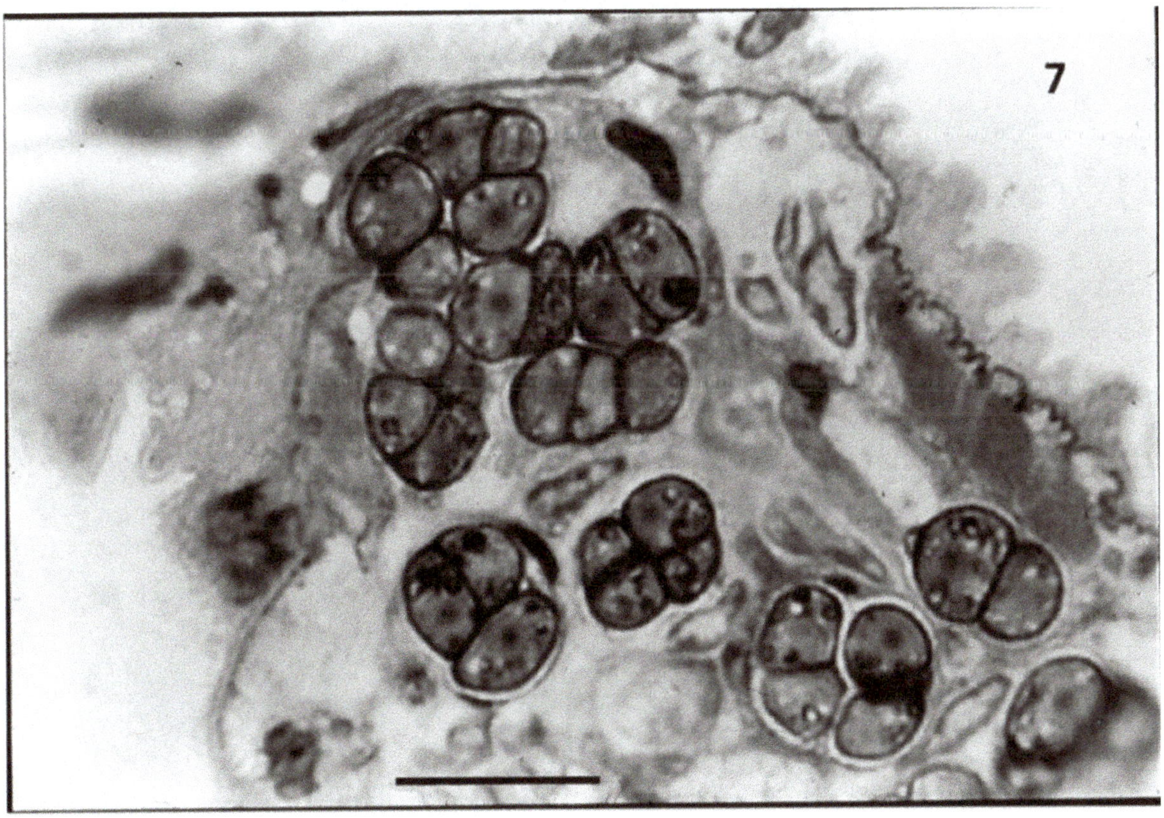

Fig. 6.7 Thraustochytrids within a lesion in the gill of *Illex illecebrosus*, note cells dividing to form diads, triads and tetrads. Scale bar ≈ 30 μm (Courtesy of Jones and O'Dor)

6.3 Diagnosing a Labyrinthulomycete Infection Using Electron and Light Microscopy

Almost all Labyrinthulomycetes have three unique, diagnostic features (see Bennett et al. (2017) and Moss (1986) for detailed descriptions). Electron microscopy shows all three, but high powered light microscopy generally reveals the ectoplasmic net and its effects.

- Unique, subcellular organelles, called sagenogenetosomes. These have been compared to spider spinnerets and secrete the ectoplasmic net system. They are positioned at the point at which the ectoplasmic net leaves the cell body and vary in structure between species. In all cases, however, ectoplasmic reticulum converges to become a dense array, which may have the appearance of a plug at the "top" of the net (Fig. 6.8).
- An ectoplasmic net. This consists only of unit membrane, continuous with that of the sagenogenetosome. It contains no organelles, only occasionally a few membranous structures. In thraustochytrids and aplanochytrids, the net takes the form of a root-like system and is known to secrete both digestive enzymes and transport nutrients

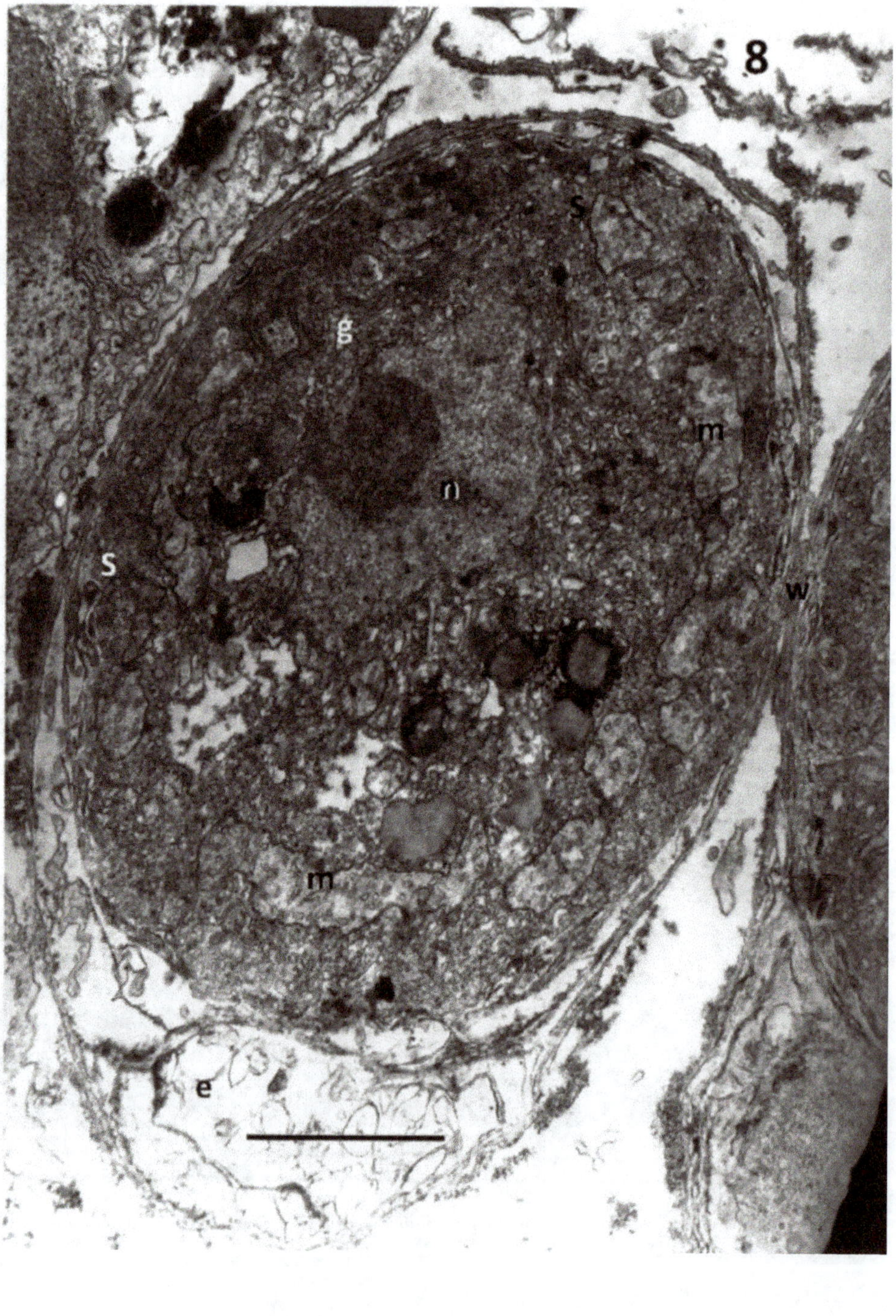

Fig. 6.8 Transmission electron micrograph of the thraustochytrid from *Eledone cirrhosa*, showing the sagenogenetosome (s); cell wall with layers of scales (w); the ectoplasmic net (e); n = nucleus; g = golgi; m = mitochondria with tubular cristae. Scale bar: 1.75 μm

back to the cell body. The net is also known to contain actin and myosin (Preston and King 2005), and in aplanochytrids, this allows the cells to move with a crawling motion, when observed by light microscope.

- The cell wall of the Labyrinthulomycetes (Moss 1986) consists of a unit membrane over which circular scales, 2–3 nm thick, are laid in layers in varying numbers, depending on the species and age of the cell. These scales are made either of fucose or galactose, again dependent on species (Honda et al. 1999).

Other features of Labyrinthulomycetes useful for diagnosis are the production of biflagellated zoospores, easily seen in culture. These are not always produced, but where they are, they swim with a "flipping" motion and have an anterior flagellum, which is covered with brush-like mastigonemes, and a posterior, shorter, "whiplash" flagellum (Moss 1986, Chap. 11). Thraustochytrids and aplanochytrids are, however, extremely plastic in the life stages they can present under different nutrient and environmental conditions (Fossier Marchan et al. 2018). It is therefore essential to sequence to identify to genus and species level. Mo et al. (2002) provide a comprehensive methodology, with details of appropriate primers.

6.4 Implications of Labyrinthulomycete Infections for Cephalopod Production

In the *E. cirrhosa* infection, one infected individual infected an entire aquarium, because of its reliance on brick-lined tanks. In both cases, the infection carried over from one year to the next and increased with severity with time. Treatments for thraustochytrid infections have only been tried with bivalves with limited success, with heat shock for QPX disease in hard clams being the most successful (Dahl et al. 2011). These observations are an indication that thraustochytrids could be a major, long-lasting problem in cephalopod rearing facilities, if the animals are stressed or mechanically damaged.

6.5 Infections Caused by Organisms Still Classified as Fungi

Only five infections of cephalopods by organisms classified as fungi have been observed to date. The same fungus is responsible for two infections, one in an octopus and one in squid. This is the deuteromycete, *Cladosporium sphaerospermum*. *Cladosporium* is a ubiquitous, salt-tolerant, generally saprobic fungus, which has a range of beneficial and deleterious habits (Bensch et al. 2012). It was first found as an opportunist infection of a mechanical wound in an aquarium kept lesser octopus, *E. cirrhosa* (Polglase et al. 1984), (Figs. 6.9 and 6.10), but these authors reported that it could be cultured on agar plates and would re-infect wounds (Fig. 6.11). Almost complete healing of the original wound was observed, except where fungal hyphae ran though the dermal connective tissue out to the exterior. No marked necrosis or oedema was associated with the hyphae (pics), but the connective tissue stained less deeply and had an attenuated appearance. Increased numbers of rounded haemocytes were present, but no encapsulation of the hyphae was observed.

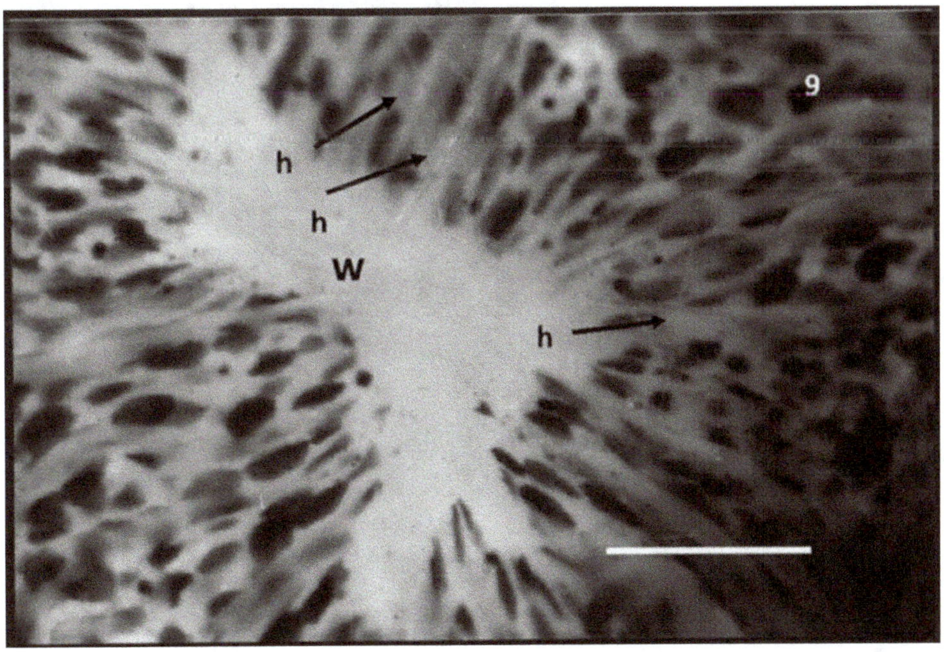

Fig. 6.9 *Eledone cirrhosa*; skin wound (w) infected with *Cladosporium sphaerospermum*. Arrows indicate transparent mycelium. Scale bar: 100 µm

Fig. 6.10 *Cladosporium sphaerospermum* mycelium growing from dermis of a wound in *Eledone cirrhosa*, c = chromatophores. Scale bar: 25 μm

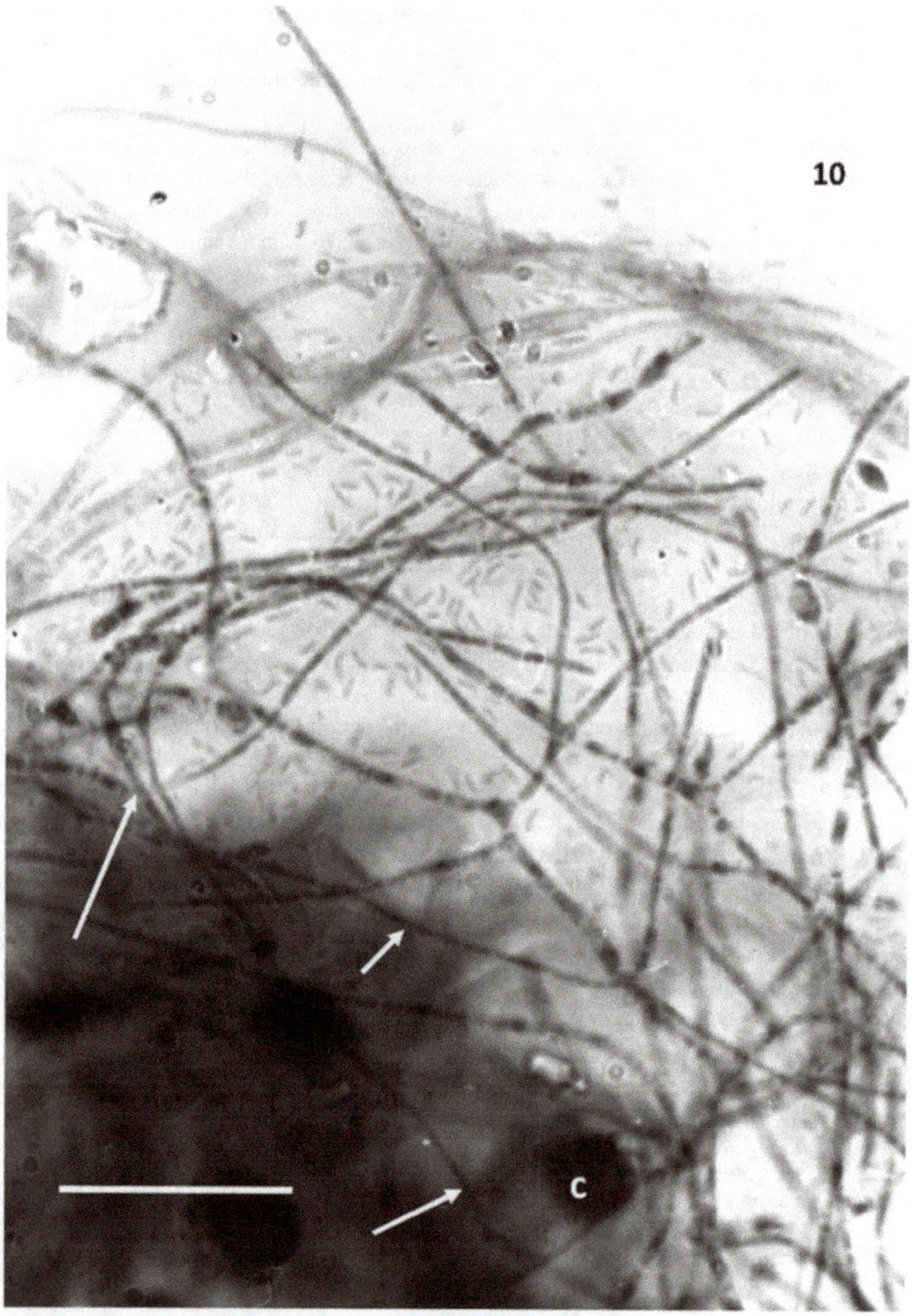

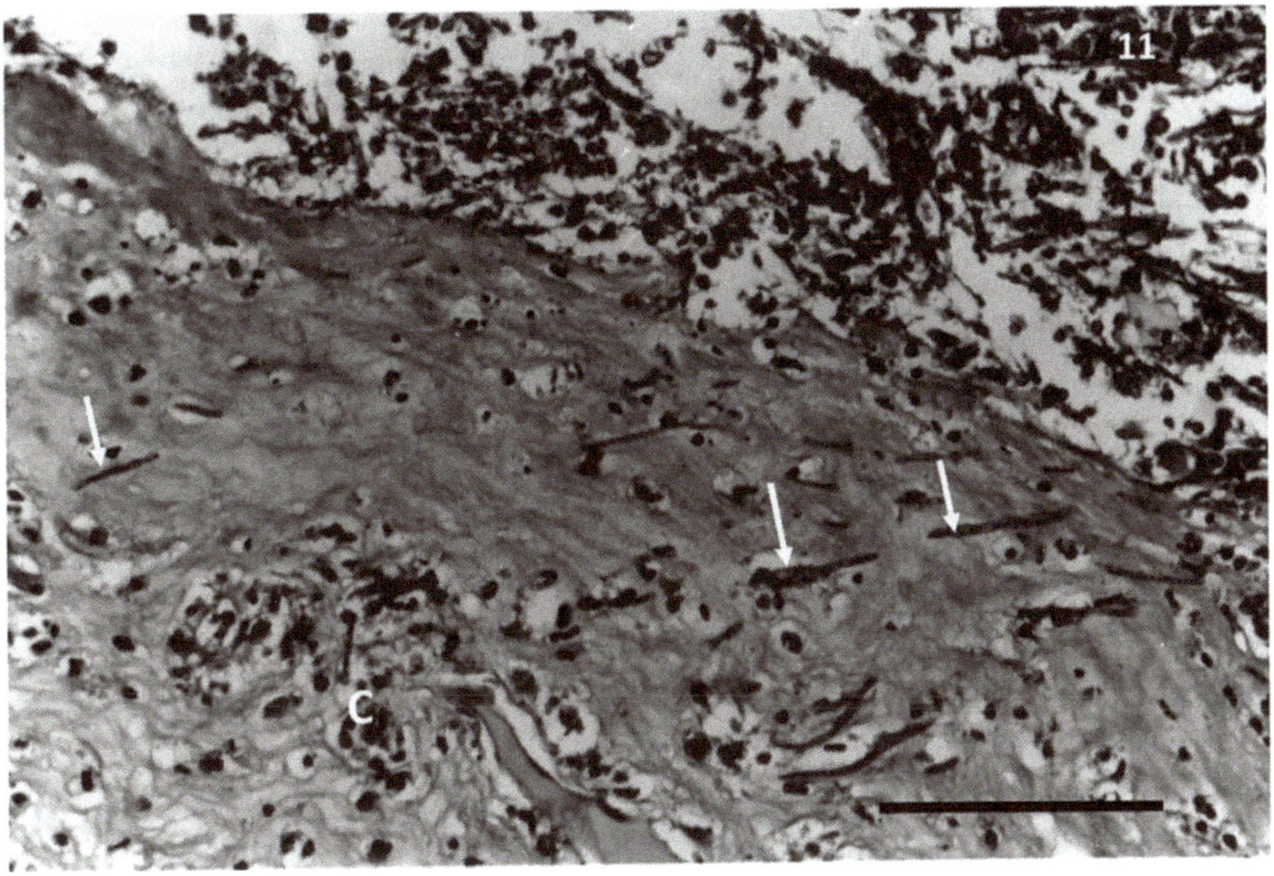

Fig. 6.11 Hyphae (arrowed) of *Cladosporium sphaerospermum* growing back into *Eledone cirrhosa* dermis after re-inoculation. Arrows indicate hyphae. c = chromatophore. Scale bar: 50 µm

Harms et al. (2006) reported a case in which a European cuttlefish, *Sepia officinalis*, developed an eruptive skin lesion of the dorsal mantle, which biopsy and subsequent culture revealed contained haemocyte granulomas, again induced by a *Cladosporium* sp. infection. The lesion was successfully treated by excision under anaesthesia, but the animal died two months later and was found to have a multi-systemic fungal infection.

Scimeca (1994) provides a previously unpublished, brief report of a *Fusarium* infection of the mantle of a nautilus. The fungus was identified using an indirect fluorescent antibody test for hyphae of the Fusarium group. In this case, the hyphae extended from the deep ulcer, which was the focus of the investigation, into the musculature of the mantle.

Finally, Scimeca and Oestmann (1995) mention a fungal infection, presumably therefore by a mycelial organism, in the hood of *Nautilus pompilius*. The abstract of this conference presentation does not give any further details.

6.6 Concluding Remarks

All these infections, both by the Labyrinthulomycetes and organisms still classified as fungi, have been reported in captive animals, so stress and/or mechanical damage from handling are again likely to have been contributory factors, allowing the infections to establish and develop. There are, however, still very small numbers of these reports and none to date of true fungal infections in cephalopods from the wild raising the question, “What is it about cephalopods that keeps them free from attack by the fungi commonly found in the sea, which infect other invertebrates and vertebrates to a much higher degree?”.

Acknowledgements Jane Polglase thanks Dr. Gwyneth M. Jones, Seatech Ltd., Halifax, Nova Scotia, Canada, and Dr. Ronald O’Dor, Dalhousie University, Halifax, Nova Scotia, Canada, for kind permission to reproduce their images.

References

Bennett RM, Honda D, Beakes GW, Thines M (2017) Labyrinthulomycota. In: Archibald J, Simpson A, Slamovits C (eds) Handbook of the protists. Springer, Cham, Switzerland, pp 507–542

Bensch K, Braun U, Graenewald JZ, Crous PW (2012) The genus *Cladosporium*. Stud Mycol 72(1):1–401

Dahl SF, Perrigault M, Liu Q, Collier JL, Barnes DA, Allam D (2011) Effects of temperature on hard clam (*Mercenaria mercenaria*) immunity and QPX (Quahog Parasite Unknown) disease development: I. Dynamics of QPX disease. J Invert Pathol 106(2):314–321

Fossier Marchan L, Lee Chang KJ, Nichols PD, Mitchell WJ, Polglas JL, Gutierrez JT (2018) Taxonomy, ecology and biotechnological applications of thraustochytrids: a review. Biotech Adv 36(1):26–46

Harms CA, Lewbart GA, McAlarney R, Christian LS, Geissler KA, Lemons C (2006) Surgical excision of mycotic (*Cladosporium* sp.) granulomas from the mantle of a cuttlefish (*Sepia officinalis*). J Zoo Wildlife Med 37(4):524–530

Honda D, Yokochi T, Nakahara T, Raghukumar S, Nakagiri A, Schaumann K, Nigashihara T (1999) Molecular phylogeny of labyrinthulids and thraustochytrids based on the sequencing of the 18S ribosomal RNA gene. J Eukaryot Microbiol 46(6):637–647

Jones G (1981) Thraustochytrid pathogens. Bull Brit Mycol Soc 16 (suppl 1):5–6

Jones G, O'Dor RK (1983) Ultrastructural observations on a thraustochytrid fungus parasitic on the gills of squid (*Ilex illecebrosus* Lesueur). J Parasitol 69: 903–911

McLean N, Porter D (1982) Yellow spot disease of *Tritonea diomedea* Bergh (Mollusca: Gastropoda: Nudibranchia): encapsulation of the thraustochytriaceous parasite by host amoebocytes. J Parasitol 68:243–252

Mo C, Douek J, Rinkevich B (2002) Development of a PCR strategy for thraustochytrid identification based on 18S rDNA sequences. Mar Biol 140:883–889

Moss ST (1986) Biology and phylogeny of the labyrinthulales and thraustochytriales. In: Moss ST (ed) The biology of the marine fungi. Cambridge University Press, Cambridge, pp 105–130

Polglase JL (1980) A preliminary report on the thraustochytrid(s) and labyrinthulid(s) associated with a pathological condition in the lesser octopus, *Eledone cirrhosa*. Bot Mar 23:699–706

Polglase JL (1981) Thraustochytrids as potential pathogens of marine animals. Abstract published in Bull Br Mycol Soc 16(suppl 1):5 (Full manuscript now available on Research gate)

Polglase JL, Dix NJ, Bullock AM (1984) Infection of skin wounds in the lesser octopus, *Eledone cirrhosa*, by *Cladosporium sphaerospermum*. Trans Brit Mycol Soc 82:577–580

Preston TM, King CA (2005) Actin-based motility in the net slime mould Labyrinthula: evidence for the role of myosin in gliding movement. J Eukaryot Microbiol 52(6):461–475

Scimeca JM (1994) The cephalopods in invertebrate medicine (2nd edn). Wiley, pp 112–125

Scimeca JM, Oestmann D (1995) Selected diseases of captive and laboratory-reared cephalopods. Poster presented to a meeting of the International Association for Aquat Ani Med 26:79. Recorded in online proceedings at https://www.vin.com/apputil/content/defaultadv1.aspx?id=3977208&pid=11257&

7 Virus and Virus-like Particles Affecting Cephalopods

María Prado-Álvarez and Pablo García-Fernández

Abstract

This chapter compiles the information available to date regarding virus affecting different species of cephalopods. A clear evidence of a virus-related disease on cephalopods was not stablished yet. However, the first description of a virus-like in *Octopus vulgaris* was observed in nodular tumors that finally caused the death of the animal. It is noteworthy that not too much effort has been focused on this area to date. However, the incidence of viruses in cephalopods might be further investigated since the attention on these species as an alternative to the aquaculture sector is increasing rapidly over last years and huge efforts are being made to stablish new cultures.

Keywords

Cephalopod diseases • Virus • Octopus • Cuttlefish • Nautilus • Squid

7.1 Introduction

Virus-like descriptions on cephalopods are rather scarce and quite spread over time. However, the incidence of viral diseases on bivalve and gastropod mollusks has been extensively studied (Arzul et al. 2017). Since first descriptions in 1971 in *Octopus vulgaris* and *Sepia officinalis*, only three more observations were reported in cephalopods in more species of the genus *Octopus* and *Nautilus* and in the squid *Loligo pealei* (Table 7.1).

Family classification was initially made based on similarities to viral mammalian diseases caused by virus (Farley 1978). In more recent studies, molecular diagnosis was applied to amplify genomic material and search for homology in public databases. However, it is important to remark that classification made on this chapter is based only on the information available to date which in most cases were made based on morphology observed under transmission electron microphotographs. Further analysis would be necessary to deepen on the effect caused by virus on these animals, especially considering the increasing interest on these animals as an alternative product to satisfy the global demand on the aquaculture sector. However, advances in this scope become a big challenge to the scientific community in part due to the difficulty to obtain specific cell lines and culture systems.

7.2 Iridoviridae

First observation of virus-like particles affecting a cephalopod was made in 1971 in *O. vulgaris* (Rungger et al. 1971). Nodular tumors on tentacles of 1 mm diameter were observed at early stages. However, these tumors can develop and grow up to 5–10 mm and be extended to the ventral surface and also the siphon. The progress of the infection leads to self-mutilation of affected areas, and death occurred after 3–5 months in captivity. Electron micrographs of tumor tissues at early stage showed organized virus-like particles that appeared in groups of 300 particles with hexagonal and electrodense internal cores and 120 nm diameter. It was also observed an envelope surrounding these particles in disaggregated tissues. Mortality was

M. Prado-Álvarez (✉) · P. García-Fernández
Aquatic Molecular Pathobiology Group, Institute of Marine Research, Spanish National Research Council (CSIC), 36208 Vigo, Pontevedra, Spain
e-mail: mprado@iim.csic.es

P. García-Fernández
e-mail: pablo.garcia@iim.csic.es

C. Gestal et al. (eds.), *Handbook of Pathogens and Diseases in Cephalopods*,
https://doi.org/10.1007/978-3-030-11330-8_7

Table 7.1 Summary of descriptions of viruses and virus-like particles in cephalopods

Year	*Cephalopod* sp.	Virus family	Reference
1971	*Octopus vulgaris*	Iridoviridae	Rungger et al. (1971)
1971	*Sepia officinalis*	Reoviridae	Devauchelle and Vago (1971)
1988	*Loligo pealei*	–	Pers. Comm. to authors (Hanlon and Forsythe 1990)
1988	*Octopus* spp.	–	Pers. Comm. to authors (Hanlon and Forsythe 1990)
2006	*Nautilus* spp.	Iridoviridae	Gregory et al. (2006)
2015	*O. vulgaris*	Nodaviridae	Fichi et al. (2015)
2018	*O. vulgaris*	Malacoherpesviridae	Prado-Álvarez et al. (in preparation)

described to be due to starvation, self-mutilation, or the presumed viral infection associated with these tumors. In 1978, Farley classified this virus particle as Iridoviridae (Farley 1978). The family Iridoviridae comprises icosahedral double-stranded DNA viruses and mainly affects ectothermic vertebrates, insects, and crustaceans (Chinchar et al. 2017).

Morphology similar to an Iridovirus was found in renal tubular epithelial cells of *Nautilus* spp. (Gregory et al. 2006). Viral particles were enveloped and measured 176 nm in diameter. Moreover, this was the first characterization that included molecular identification and sequencing to confirm the similarity to an amphibian Iridovirus.

7.3 Reoviridae

Devauchelle and Vago (1971) reported a no-pathogenic incidence of a virus in the European cuttlefish, *Sepia officinalis*. These non-enveloped particles were observed on epithelial cells on the stomach and were 75 nm in diameter. Initial studies suggested that these particles could correspond to the family Reoviridae. Reoviridae are viruses with icosahedral symmetry and double-stranded RNA. However, they could be spherical and infect a wide number of hosts including vertebrates, invertebrates, plants, protists, and fungi (Lefkowitz et al. 2018).

7.4 Nodaviridae

Finally, a betanodavirus (family Nodaviridae) was described affecting *O. vulgaris* (Fichi et al. 2015) particularly in white lesions observed in the skin, and also in eye and branchial heart tissues. Molecular detection by PCR and quantitative PCR confirmed the incidence of betanodavirus. However, one animal showing similar symptom seemed to be affected by a nodavirus-like particle. Virions belonging to this family are non-enveloped, 30 nm in diameter, and single-stranded RNA (Artimo et al. 2012).

7.5 Unclassified Viruses

Hanlon and Forsythe revised in 1990 the descriptions of virus-like particles in cephalopods made to date (Hanlon and Forsythe 1990). Apart from the two descriptions detailed

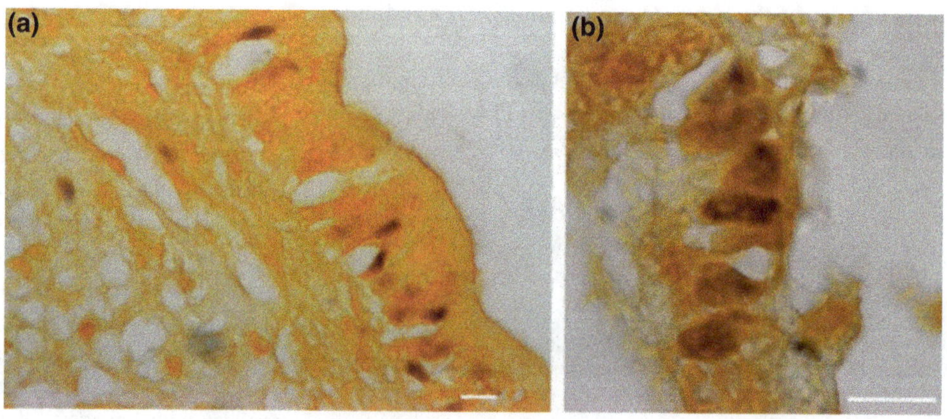

Fig. 7.1 In situ hybridization labeling of ostreid herpesvirus. Positive cells are labeled in blue. Gill tissue of adult *O. vulgaris* (**a**). Detailed area at higher magnification (**b**). Scale bar = 10 μm

above, two more annotations were made based on personal communications to the authors. One was in the squid *Loligo pealei* on which cytoplasmic inclusions were found in the digestive gland and the other on different species of octopus in New Zealand and the east and west coasts of USA.

More recently, an interspecific study of the incidence of the ostreid herpesvirus demonstrated that the virus was widely spread in oyster-culturing areas. This virus belongs to the family Malacoherpesviridae and caused massive mortalities in spat and juvenile oysters (Prado-Álvarez et al. 2016). This family comprised of enveloped double-stranded DNA viruses, 150–200 nm in diameter, and affects to mollusks (Davison et al. 2009). A collection of samples of *O. vulgaris* including paralarvae at different stages and adult animals were analyzed by molecular techniques. Homology searches on positive results showed the highest similarity to the ostreid herpesvirus-1 μVar (unpublished data). Moreover, ostreid herpesvirus-specific probes for in situ hybridization were positively labeled on epithelial cells of the gills (Fig. 7.1). Further analysis should be carried out to decipher if this virus could be the causative agent of any pathology in these animals.

7.6 Concluding Remarks

Several virus and virus-like particles were described on cephalopods. However, a clear incidence associated with a virus-related disease was not well described to date. It deserves to be further investigated as cephalopods could be considered as an alternative to be aquacultured and satisfy the global demand.

References

Artimo P, Jonnalagedda M, Arnold K et al (2012) ExPASy: SIB bioinformatics resource portal. Nucleic Acids Res 40:W597–W603

Arzul I, Corbeil S, Morga B, Renault T (2017) Viruses infecting marine molluscs. J Invertebr Pathol 147:118–135

Chinchar VG, Hick P, Ince IA et al (2017) ICTV report consortium. ICTV virus taxonomy profile: Iridoviridae. J Gen Virol 98:890–891

Davison AJ, Eberle R, Ehlers B et al (2009) The order Herpesvirales. Arch Virol 154:171–177

Devauchelle G, Vago C (1971) Particles of viral asepct in stomach cells of the cuttle-fish *Sepia officinalis L.* (Mollusca, Cephalopoda). C R Acad Sci Hebd Seances Acad Sci D 272(6):894–6

Farley C (1978) Viruses and viruslike lesions in marine mollusks. Mar Fish Rev 40:18–20

Fichi G, Cardeti G, Perrucci S et al (2015) Skin lesion-associated pathogens from *Octopus vulgaris*: first detection of *Photobacterium swingsii*, *Lactococcus garvieae* and betanodavirus. Dis Aquat Organ 115:147–156

Gregory CR, Latimer KS, Pennick K, Benson K, Moore T (2006) Novel Iridovirus in a *Nautilus* (*Nautilus* Spp.). J Vet Diagnostic Investig 18:208–211

Hanlon RT, Forsythe JW (1990) Diseases of Mollusca: Cephalopoda. Diseases caused by microorganisms. In: Kinne O (ed) Diseases of marine animals, vol III. Biologische Anstalt Helgoland, Hamburg, Germany, pp 23–46

Lefkowitz EJ, Dempsey DM, Hendrickson RC, Orton RJ, Siddell SG, Smith DB (2018) Virus taxonomy: The database of the International Committee on Taxonomy of Viruses (ICTV). Nucleic Acids Res 46: D708–D717

Prado-Álvarez M, Darmody G, Hutton S, O'Reilly A, Lynch SA, Culloty SC (2016) Occurrence of OsHV-1 in *Crassostrea gigas* Cultured in Ireland during an exceptionally warm summer. Selection of less susceptible oysters. Front Physiol 7:492

Rungger D, Rastellt M, Braendle E, Malsberger RG (1971) A viruslike particle sssociated with lesions in the muscles of *Octopus vulgaris*. J Invertebr Pathol 17:72–89

8 Bacteria-Affecting Cephalopods

Rosa Farto, Gianluca Fichi, Camino Gestal, Santiago Pascual, and Teresa Pérez Nieto

Abstract

Bacterial pathogens contribute to obtain an unsuccessful production of cephalopods. An updated overview of the knowledge of these pathogens must be a valuable tool to improve their aquarium maintenance and aquaculture. The present work provides a description of the main bacterial pathogens associated with larval stages of cultured *Octopus vulgaris,* and juvenile and adults of several cephalopods. *Vibrio* species, reported with ability to cause vibriosis in aquaculture, are the main bacteria associated with skin lesions in adults. Different species of *Pseudomonas* and *Aeromonas,* among others, have also been detected. Furthermore, gram-positive bacteria such as *Bacillus* have been also described. Among them, *V. alginolyticus, V. carchariae, V. parahaemolyticus, V. splendidus* and *V. lentus* have also been isolated from sterile organs or fluids of animals and their potential as invaders proved. However, only *V. alginolyticus* or *V. lentus* has the ability to cause lesions, and, in addition, the last one is proved as the causative agent of death in octopuses. Other organs such as eyes of squids are also colonized by *Vibrio* species or *Micrococcus* sp., and recently *Photobacterium swingsii* and *Lactococcus garvieae* have been reported associated with a retrobulbar lesion in octopus. Rickettsial-like organisms (RLO) are also detected in the gills of the octopus, having a detrimental effect on the respiratory gaseous exchange of the animals. Cultures of octopus paralarvae show a genetically diverse community comparable to those reported previously from other marine hatcheries. Bacteria included in the Splendidus clade is the dominant group in all conditions, except in one of them, where *V. alginolyticus, V. proteolyticus* or *Pseudomonas*

R. Farto (✉) · T. P. Nieto
Marine Research Centre (CIM-UVIGO), University of Vigo, 36331 Vigo, Pontevedra, Spain
e-mail: rfarto@uvigo.es

T. P. Nieto
e-mail: mtperez@uvigo.es

G. Fichi
Istituto Zooprofilattico Sperimentale delle Regioni Lazio e Toscana, 56123 Pisa, Italy
e-mail: Gianluca.fichi@gmail.com

C. Gestal
Aquatic Molecular Pathobiology Group, Institute of Marine Research, Spanish National Research Council (CSIC), 36208 Vigo, Pontevedra, Spain
e-mail: cgestal@iim.csic.es

S. Pascual
Ecology and Biodiversity Department, Institute of Marine Research, Spanish National Research Council (CSIC), 36208 Vigo, Pontevedra, Spain
e-mail: spascual@iim.csic.es

C. Gestal et al. (eds.), *Handbook of Pathogens and Diseases in Cephalopods*,
https://doi.org/10.1007/978-3-030-11330-8_8

fluorescens are the main detected groups. Furthermore, *Shewanella* or *Pseudoalteromonas undina* have also been identified. All this shows that pathogenic bacteria are frequent microorganisms associated with aquarium maintenance and culture of cephalopods, and special attention on maintaining a well-balanced community of microorganisms should be applied.

Keywords
Cephalopod diseases • Paralarvae • Microbial community • Pathogenic bacteria • Splendidus clade • Rickettsia-like organisms

8.1 Introduction

Incidence of diseases, several of them caused by bacteria, is one of the most important problems which avoid obtaining a successfully production in the aquaculture of cephalopods or its suitable maintenance in captive conditions (García--Fernández et al. 2016; Sykes and Gestal, 2014).

Knowledge on bacterial species associated with cephalopods culture and its ecological role would be essential for improving industrial culture production. Seawater have a variable microscopic population density (Harder 2009), and it contains a high microbial diversity depending on physico-chemical and geographic factors such as the temperature of the water, latitude and salinity. The ability of bacteria to colonize surfaces (epibiotic bacteria) is very well documented, and they comprise well-organized bacterial communities associated with marine organisms, which are influenced by temporal changes in the environment. However, some bacteria are specifically and persistently associated with particular marine animals, and they are not found in seawater or on other animals (Thakur et al. 2004; Sharp et al. 2007). This can explain the species-specific vulnerability to pathogens previously suggested for *Octopus bimaculoides* and *O. maya* (Hanlon and Forsythe 1990). These 'microepibionts' are multi-functional and are involved in obtaining nutrients, acquiring new genetic traits and providing some measure of chemical defence against pathogens (Wahl et al. 2012). In these epiphytic communities, developing biofilms is the most common, and quorum sensing modulates behaviour of many biofilm-associated bacteria, affecting symbiotic relationships and host interactions (Maximilien et al. 1998; Parsek and Greenberg 2005). Co-infection is another important factor affecting bacterial diseases, in fact in previous studies parasite infection enhanced bacterial invasion in fish (Rodríguez-Quiroga et al. 2016).

Differences in culturable bacteria most frequently isolated from skin of apparently healthy, wild or laboratory-maintained adult squids have been previously found. In fact, a higher diversity is shown in the former ones (Hanlon and Forsythe 1990). Similar data are observed in the gastrointestinal microbiome of wild octopus paralarvae with respect to that of reared ones (Roura et al. 2017). Although aquaculture systems are designed to imitate the natural environment, the maintenance of adequate conditions during all culture production is problematic. Furthermore, diets provided are less diverse than in natural media. Therefore, it can produce alterations in microbial community of seawater and/or surface (external or internal) of cephalopods. This provides an opportunity for the dominance of bacteria, which show the ability to invade the host, and in the end, to cause a fatal infection. On the other hand, this is also facilitated when the surface of the animal is injured.

In 1990, Hanlon and Forsythe described the main bacterial pathogens associated with juvenile and adults. In fact, they included data from published literature, and their own data collected from analyses resultant of 14 species of different cephalopods for 13 years. Species of *Vibrio*, mainly, but also members of the genera *Pseudomonas, Aeromonas, Staphylococcus* or *Streptococcus*, among others, have been associated with healthy octopuses or squids in nature. Some of these genera have also been associated with the ulcerated skin of octopuses and squids from their natural environment or laboratory-maintained, being this, their route of entrance in animals, and progressing later until a fatal infection. Furthermore, a possible food-borne was the suggested route of entrance for *V. carchariae*, which was associated with sudden death of laboratory-maintained octopuses, which showed lack of any external of behavioural symptoms. Similarly, an unknown route of entrance, not associated with ulcerated skin, was proposed for cuttlefish which suffered a highly virulent systemic infection. Squids with eye damage associated with bacteria were also reported, but no further information on the route of infection was given. However, it is unknown if bacteria are the initial cause of infection, with the exception of one study, where *V. alginolyticus* was proved as causation of lesions in octopus. Similarly, there is a lack of information on culturable bacteria associated to different stages of cephalopods in reared conditions.

In attempting to be comprehensive, we reviewed the knowledge about bacterial disease in the most representative European cephalopod species to date, detailing the main bacterial pathogens associated with juvenile or adults.

Furthermore, data from bacterial associated with larval stages of cultured octopuses (unpubl.), recently qualitatively sampled 'in situ' by us were also included.

The common signs caused by bacteria on cephalopods, and, when possible, images, are shown. In addition, it is included a brief description of characteristics of bacteria, diagnostic and treatments used against bacteria.

8.2 Potential Pathogenic Bacteria for Larval Development Stages

Bacterial septicaemia was occasionally observed in paralarvae (13–15 days old) of *O. vulgaris* reared in aquaculture tanks, which could be causative of the dead of the paralarvae (Fig. 8.1a, b). The identification of the aetiological agent was not established by the authors. Seawater quality, and maintenance and cleaning precautionary measures were suggested as factors that could facilitate the growth of pathogenic bacteria that as a result caused the infection. Previous studies have revealed that uncontrolled factors in the culture have an important impact on the establishment and evolution of the microbial community in the culture tanks of *Artemia* (Verschuere et al. 1997). Similar results were also found for culture of clams (Kwan and Bolch 2015). It was also shown that an effective balance of microbial populations included in the same community ensures the final rearing success (Verschuere et al. 1997; Kwan and Bolch 2015; Shi et al. 2017).

Recently, it has been proved that the intestinal microbiome, highly diverse, of octopus paralarvae reared in captivity and feed with *Artemia* is rapidly become less diverse and is mainly suggested as a consequence of culture conditions (Roura et al. 2017). However, to date, there is an absence of published data available on diversity of bacteria from cephalopod hatcheries. Recent qualitative preliminary analysis of seawater associated with different stages of *O. vulgaris* hatchery culture has focused to characterize and identify the culturable bacteria.

8.2.1 Microbial Community Counts

8.2.1.1 Water Samples

Culturable bacteria was isolated on three different dates corresponding to Experiment 1, 2 and 3 from seawater associated with different stages of an *O. vulgaris* culture in Galicia (Table 8.1). After 13–15 days of paralarvae culture, samples were taken on the same day in all stages of each Experiment. Seawater inside the hatchery was filtered until 1 μm for all experiments, but in addition, a high wattage UV treatment was also applied for *Artemia* (*Artemia salina*) culture. Moreover, seawater filtered until 20 μm and treated with low wattage UV was analysed for comparative purposes (Experiment 4). Standard conditions of natural photoperiod, seawater temperature (19–23 °C) and salinity of 33‰ were maintained.

Larval tanks (1000 L) containing 5 larvae l^{-1} were reared following the protocol described by Iglesias et al. (2004). In this study, paralarvae were fed with *Artemia* nauplius or *Artemia* nauplius complemented with *Maja brachydactyla* zoeas or freeze-dried feed (made from different species of crustaceans).

Water samples (1 ml) were serially diluted in sterile seawater and spread out (0.1 mL) over plates of Tryptic Soy Agar supplemented up to 1% (w/v) NaCl (TSA-1) and Thiosulphate-Citrate-Bile-Sucrose (TCBS) in duplicate. Colonies were counted after 4 days of incubation at 22 °C, and the results expressed in colony-forming units (CFU) per ml. Whereas TSA-1 was used for total heterotrophic bacteria counts, TCBS was for presumptive *Vibrio* ones. The last one was used since *Vibrio* species are a significant component of culturable marine bacterial populations (Thompson et al. 2004; Montes et al. 2006; Beaz-Hidalgo et al. 2008; Guisande et al. 2008).

Colonies of each morphology from TSA-1 or TCBS were picked off and spread on TSA-1 to obtain pure cultures, and then inoculated on Tryptic soy broth with 1% (w/v) NaCl and 15% (v/v) of glycerol for their conservation at −80 °C.

8.2.1.2 Microbial Counts

Total heterotrophic bacteria associated with the octopus cultures are shown in Table 8.1. The results showed that

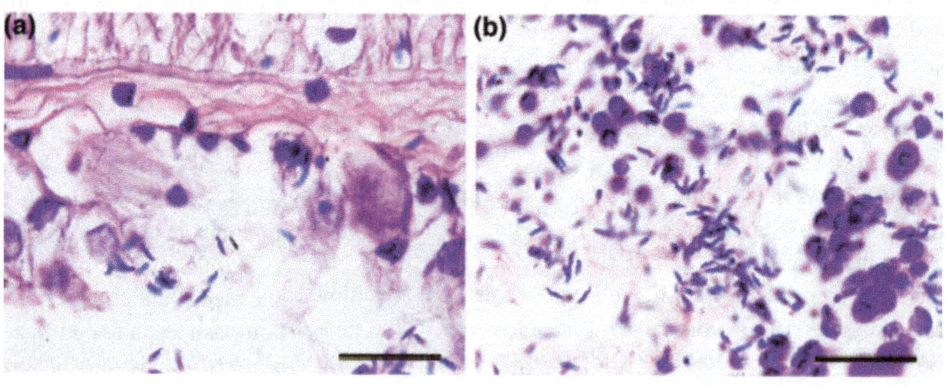

Fig. 8.1 *O. vulgaris* paralarvae reared in aquarium conditions. **a** Histological section of the connective tissue of paralarvae infected by bacteria (arrow). **b** Detail showing the strong septicemia observed in the whole paralarvae. H&E stain. Images **a** and **b** by courtesy of Dr. R. Fernández-Gago. *Scale bars* **a**, **b** 20 μm

Table 8.1 Bacterial counts and species identified in different paralarval stages of *O. vulgaris* hatchery

	Experiment 1					Experiment 2			Experiment 3		Experiment 4
	WIH1	WOA	ATW	ZTW	PTW + AZ	PTW + DA	PTW + DAZ	DAWT	PTW + A	PTW + ACF	WIH2
Culturable bacteria counts											
Total heterotrophic (TSA-1) (CFU/ml)	7×10^2	–	1×10^4	1.3×10^4 ($\pm 7 \times 10^3$)	2×10^4 ($\pm 5 \times 10^3$)	4×10^2 ($\pm 3 \times 10^2$)	1.5×10^2 ($\pm 5 \times 10^1$)	1×10^1	7.5×10^5 ($\pm 2 \times 10^5$)	4×10^6 ($\pm 7 \times 10^3$)	1.8×10^4 ($\pm 7 \times 10^3$)
Presumptive Vibrios (TCBS) (CFU/ml)	–	–	4.8×10^2 ($\pm 2.1 \times 10^2$)	2.5×10^2 ($\pm 1.5 \times 10^2$)	9×10^2 ($\pm 1 \times 10^2$)	1.9×10^2 ($\pm 1 \times 10^2$)	1×10^2	1×10^1	5.8×10^4 ($\pm 1.5 \times 10^3$)	7×10^5 ($\pm 5 \times 10^4$)	4.8×10^3 ($\pm 2 \times 10^3$)
Species identified											
Splendidus Clade											
V. atlanticus/V. tasmaniensis						+(32)	+(23)		+(1, 2, 3, 8, 13)	+(4, 5, 7)	+(25, 38)
V. gigantis/V.crassostreae/V.pomeroyi					+(34)	+(31, 35, 36)	+(33)		+(6, 14)	+(11)	
V. gallaecicus				+(39)							
V.hemicentroti/V.lentus									+(10)		+(26, 28, 29)
V. alginolyticus			−(27)								
V. neptunius					+(30)						
V. proteolyticus			+(18, 19)	+(21)	+(12)						
P. fluorescens			+(17, 20)		+(16)						
Pa. undina										+(24)	
Sh. marinintestina/Sh. sairae/Sh. schelegeliana									+(9, 22)	+(15)	

In brackets SE for bacteria counts and strain for species identified. *WIH1* seawater inside the hatchery filtered until 1 µm; *WOA*: seawater outside *Artemia* culture; *ATW Artemia* tank water; *ZTW* Zoeae tank water; *PTW + AZ* octopus paralarvae tank water mixed with *Artemia* and zoeae; *PTW + DA* octopus paralarvae tank water mixed with disinfected *Artemia*; *PTW + DAZ*: octopus paralarvae tank water mixed with disinfected *Artemia* and zoeae; *DAWT* disinfected *Artemia* water tank; *PTW + A* octopus paralarvae tank water mixed with *Artemia; PTW + ACF* octopus paralarvae tank water mixed with *Artemia* and freeze-dried food; *WIH2* seawater inside the hatchery filtered until 20 µm and treated with low wattage UV there are strong evidences that the food (live or freeze-dried) supplied to the larvae constitutes the main source of the bacteria associated to the cultures of the octopus larvae.

A significant percentage (50–75%) of total heterotrophic bacteria grew in TCBS, and as it was confirmed in this study, most of them were included in genus *Vibrio* (Table 8.1). Their counts remained uniform in most of the culture conditions studied. The lowest value was detected in the cultures treated with disinfectant, whereas the highest was detected in that containing *Artemia* mixed with freeze-dried feed. These results are in agreement with those of scallop larval culture, where concentrations of *Vibrio* varied only between 10^2 and 10^3 cels ml^{-1} (Nicolas et al. 1996). However, higher counts from a culture water of *Artemia* (10^3–10^4 cfu ml^{-1}) were detected in early times of the culture period (Verschuere et al. 1997). Variations in *Vibrio* counts are frequent in hatcheries. In fact, an increase of *Vibrio* counts associated to clam's hatchery was previously found after the rise of environmental temperature (Mechri et al. 2012).

Finally, in Experiment 4, the total heterotrophic bacteria and the presumptive *Vibrio* were increased in 2-log or 3-log units, respectively, with respect at those from water inside the hatchery used for larval culture. Variations in the treatment of the seawater (mainly due to filtration) could explain these results.

8.2.2 Characterization of Culturable Bacteria Associated with Octopus Paralarvae Culture

To carry out the characterization of bacteria associated with the different culture conditions studied, a total of 38 strains corresponding to the colonies that had different morphologies on TSA-1 or TCBS were selected. For their characterization, primary and secondary identification biochemical tests and PCR with specific primers were performed, but the final identification and/or assignation to closely related species was performed by sequencing of 16S rRNA gene.

All strains were characterized by phenotypical tests and only 30 by sequencing of 16S rRNA gene. The closest-neighbouring species, which shared a similarity value in the 16S rRNA sequences of $\geq 98\%$, were used to identify the isolates. Molecular identification was assigned to the remaining strains (8), when the strains identified by 16S rRNA and the unidentified ones shared the same phenotypical profile.

8.2.2.1 Phenotypical Characterization

Firstly, the strains were phenotypically characterized by using a set of primary identification tests: gram staining, motility, oxidase, catalase, oxidative or fermentative glucose metabolism on O/F Basal Medium (O/F), growth ability at 0% NaCl or in TCBS and susceptibility to O129 vibriostatic agent (2, 4-diamino-6, 7-di-isopropylpteridine phosphate; 150 μg/disc).

These assays indicated that all the strains were gram-negative motile rods and that they were positive for all tests except for being able to grow at 0% NaCl and the glucose metabolism. The two last tests allowed discriminating three groups of strains; (1) strains showing aerobic/anaerobic glucose metabolism, being all of them unable to grow at 0% NaCl (facultative anaerobes); (2) strains without aerobic/anaerobic glucose metabolism, being all of them unable to grow at 0% NaCl; (3) strains without oxidative/fermentative glucose metabolism (aerobes), but with ability to grow at 0% NaCl.

All these tests presumptively grouped all facultative anaerobes in genus *Vibrio*. All of them were able to grow well on TCBS and allowed discriminating between strains with ability to use sucrose (Table 8.2). Although, this medium is used for the isolation of *Vibrio* spp., it is also possible, but with poor growth, for other genera (Guisande et al. 2004). In fact, this was the case for our bacteria identified as *P. fluorescens*.

In order to confirm this presumptive identification, secondary biochemical tests were performed for the anaerobic facultative group by using the commercial phenothypic test API 20E (BioMerieux) (Table 8.2). This system is frequently used for the identification of fish pathogens, since its database includes an important number of them. However, it is well known that several reactions, among them decarboxylases [arginine dehydrolase (ADH), lysine decarboxylase (LDC), ornithine decarboxylase (ODC)], must be compared with conventional biochemical tests, since if there are differences, data from the last are preferable as reference (Buller 2004; Popovic et al. 2007). In addition, they were also included in this study, and they were determined as described by Montes et al. (1999). Presence of *Vibrio* was confirmed by the system, and its database allowed determining that the strains were closely related to *V. alginolyticus, V. proteolyticus* and *V. splendidus*.

It is well known that *V. splendidus* is phylogenically closely related to other species all of them termed as *V. splendidus*-related group (Splendidus clade), which is the most diverse among *Vibrionales* (Sawabe et al. 2007). API 20E was unable to discriminate these species since strains included in the same group showed variable biochemical profiles (Table 8.2). It is also difficult by using numerical taxonomy or molecular methods (Lago et al. 2009; Revised by Oden et al. 2016).

8.2.2.2 Molecular Characterization

In a previous study, the combined specificity of *V. tasmaniensis* (VTS/VT) and *V. splendidus* (VTS/VS) primer sets offered the best coverage (86%) in terms of separating

Table 8.2 Characterization and Identification of *Vibrio* strains associated with of *Octopus vulgaris* hatchery

	Groups identified by sequencing assignment[a]						
	Splendidus clade				*V. alginolyticus*	*V. neptunius*	*V. proteolyticus*
	V. atlanticus/ V. tasmaniensis	*V. gigantis/ V. crassostreae/ V. pomeroyi*	*V. gallaecicus*	*V. hemicentroti/ V. lentus*			
Tests to identify strains							
Sequence (16S rRNA) identity (%) with the closest neighbour	≥98.7%	≥99.5%	99.8%	>98.5%	99.9%	99.9%	99.9%
Amplification with specific primers							
VTS/VT (*V. tasmaniensis*)	+(10/12)	+(4/8)	+	+(1/4)	−	−	−
VTS/VS (*V. splendidus*)	+(4/12)	+(4/8)	−	−	−	−	−
VN1/VN2 (*V. neptunius*)	−	−	−	−	−	+	−
Biochemical characteristics							
TCBS (sucrose +)[b]	+(8/12)	+(4/8)	−	−	+	+	−
TCBS (sucrose −)[b]	+(4/12)	+(4/8)	+	+(4/4)	−	−	+(3/3)
Arginine dihydrolase (ADH)[b]	+	+	+	+	−	+	+
Lysine decarboxylase (LDC)[b]	−	−	−	−	+	−	+
Ornithine decarboxylase (ODC)[b]	−	−	−	−	+	−	−
ß-galactosidase[c]	+(4/8)	+(7/8)	−	+	−	−	−
Gelatinase[c]	+(5/8)	+	−	+	+	+	+
Citrate utilization[c]	−(5/8)	−	−	−	−	+	+
Voges Proskauer[c]	−	−	−	−	+	−	+
NO_2 production[c]	+	+	+	+	+	−	+
Fermentation/Oxidation[c]							
Amygdalin	+	+(5/8)	+	+(1/2)	+	+	−
Arabinose	−(7/8)	−	−	−	−	−	−
Inositol	+	+(7/8)	+	+	+	−	+
Melibiose	−(6/8)	−(7/8)	−	−	−	−	−
Rhamnose	+(5/8)	−(5/8)	−	−	+	−	−
Sorbitol	+(7/8)	+(6/8)	−	+(1/2)	+	−	+
Sucrose	+(5/8)	+(6/8)	−	−	+	+	+(2/3)

[a]Multiple alignment of sequences was created by ClustalW in Genious Editor version 12.0.6 (Biomatters; http://www.geneious.com/). This included 1.138 positions after the removal of ambiguous ones. A phylogenetic tree was constructed using Molecular Evolutionary Genetics Analysis (MEGA) version 6 (Tamura et al. 2013). This was performed using the neighbour-joining method and Tamura–Nei distance model, with the calculation of cluster stability by bootstrap analysis with 1000 replicates. All available species of each genus closest to studied strains were selected

[b]Tests performed by using conventional biochemical tests

[c]Tests performed by using API 20E. All strains were negative for H_2S production, hydrolysis of urea or presence of tryptophane deaminase; and they were positive for indole production and fermentation/oxidation of D-glucose or D-mannitol (all of them performed by using API 20E). In brackets number of positive or negative strains of all assayed

several of the species included in the Splendidus clade, and from other *Vibrio* species (Lago et al. 2009). In this study, a positive amplification was shown in all strains which were characterized in the Splendidus clade, except in six (13, 26, 28, 29, 31, 33). In fact, from the positive ones, 84% (16/19) and 42% (8/19) of strains reacted with VTS/VT and VTS/VS primer sets, respectively (Table 8.2). Negative amplification was shown by the remaining strains characterized as *Shewanella* (*Sh.*) or *Pseudomonas*; on the contrary, a positive amplification with the primer set VTS/VT was shown by strain 24, which was identified by 16S rRNA gene analyses as *Pseudoalteromonas* (*Pa.*) *undina*. Furthermore, a

V. neptunius primer set was highly specific, showing only cross-reaction with *V. parahaemolyticus* species from 44 tested species (Lago et al. 2009). Similarly, in this study only one strain, which was identified by 16S rRNA gene analyses as *V. neptunius*, was positive (Table 8.2). Since these primer sets were developed, the number of species included in the Splendidus clade has increased (revised by Oden et al. 2016). In this study, it is shown that they have cross-reaction with them. Nevertheless, these results revealed that the primer sets are a valuable tool for a fast detection of Splendidus clade, and to separate this clade from other *Vibrio* species.

Additionally, a sequencing of 16S rRNA gene analyses was performed according to the method described by Guisande et al. (2008), in order to confirm all these results. The strains assigned to each phylogenetic group are shown in Table 8.1, and the sequence identity (%) with the closest neighbour in Table 8.2. These results allowed to confirm that 81% (31 of a total of 38 strains) of strains were facultative anaerobes, and the remaining was aerobic. Among facultative anaerobic bacteria, the dominant genus identified was *Vibrio* (100%). The highest number (63.2%) of *Vibrio* strains was included in Splendidus clade, and they were assigned to different groups depending on their closest similarity with species (Table 8.2). In addition, one strain was identified as *V. gallaecicus*.

The 16S rRNA gene analyses allowed a more complete identification since *V. gallaecicus, V. neptunius, V. proteolyticus, Pa. undina* and *P. fluorescens* were identified. Furthermore, several strains were shown more closely related to specific species of Splendidus clade, *V. alginolyticus* or *Shewanella*.

8.2.3 Pathogenicity of Culturable Bacteria Associated with Octopus Paralarvae Culture

The Splendidus clade is the most abundant in marine samples associated with several marine animals, water column, occurring in bacterioplankton and sediments (revised by Pérez-Cataluña et al. 2016), and also are part of regular components of farmed aquatic animal microbiota (Montes et al. 2003; Guisande 2004; Baez et al. 2008; Kwan and Bolch 2015; Oden et al. 2016).

In this study, these strains were the most abundant in all culture conditions analysed, except in the conditions of Experiment 1, where dominant groups were strains identified as *V. proteolyticus, V. alginolyticus* or *P. fluorescens*. Similarly, *V. alginolyticus* was also the predominant species associated with clam or gilthead sea bream hatcheries (Snoussi et al. 2006; Mechri et al. 2012); *P. fluorescens* was also found associated with the sea bream hatchery, and it was one of the autochthonous denitrifying bacterium isolated from marine biofilters at a recirculation aquaculture system (Snoussi et al. 2006; Borges et al. 2008). Other species of *Pseudomonas* were also associated with oyster larvae (Farto et al. 2006) and with *Artemia* culture (Verschuere et al. 1997). Finally, *Shewanella* or *Pa. undina* were also identified associated with culture water containing octopus paralarvae and commercial feed or *Artemia* of this study. These groups were also previously found from healthy oyster cultures (Farto et al. 2006).

It is well known that several of the groups isolated in this study may have a role in larval mortality in cultures. In fact, several bacterial included in the Splendidus clade are considered pathogenic for bivalve molluscs (oyster, clam, scallop, mussel) (Revised by Beaz-Hidalgo et al. 2009; Revised by Kwan and Bolch 2015; Vanhove et al. 2015; Cheikh et al. 2016) and also cephalopod molluscs (Farto et al. 2003; Iehata et al. 2016). Similarly, *V. alginolyticus* was pathogenic for carpet shell clam larval and juvenile (Gómez-León et al. 2005; Mechri et al. 2015), fish (Liu et al. 2004; Zheng et al. 2017), crustacean (Jayaprakash et al. 2006; Xu et al. 2013), scallop (Riquelme et al. 1996), red abalone (Anguiano-Beltrán et al. 1998), associated with infected Chilean octopus eggs (Iehata et al. 2016), with ability to cause skin lesions to young octopus (Hanlon and Forsythe 1990), and isolated from skin ulcers and/or different organs of cultured cuttlefish (Sangster and Smolowitz 2003). *V. proteolyticus* has been previously identified as part of the *Vibrio* consortium isolated from diseased corals (Cervino et al. 2008), and were identified as pathogens of *Artemia* spp. (Verschuere et al. 2000). Another pathogen described for *Artemia* sp. is *V. neptunius* (Verschuere et al. 2000; Austin et al. 2005), being also for oyster (Prado et al. 2005; Guisande et al. 2008). There are several strains of *Pa. undina* described as biological controllers of virus (Maeda et al. 1997), however, other were pathogens for gilthead sea bream or scallop (Pujalte et al. 2007; Sandaa et al. 2008). The genus *Pseudoalteromonas* was also previously found associated with infected Chilean octopus eggs (Uriarte et al. 2011; Iehata et al. 2016).

Then, although there is an absence of published data available from octopus hatcheries, the culturable species observed are comparable to those reported previously from other marine hatcheries. This diversity resembles that of coastal seawater (Thompson et al. 2005), and several of them can cause mortality in hatchery production. Previous studies have shown that differences in dominance of a specific group can be explained by variations in interactions within the total bacterial community due to alterations in environmental conditions of cultures. Those changes can encourage dominance and diversity of more virulent species (Kwan and Bolch 2015). So, in our study, all cultures of octopus larvae analysed showed similar levels of mortality, and also a genetically diverse community, but different between Experiment 1 and Experiments 2–3.

Further studies are needed to understand the equilibrium among a community of microorganisms, and how changes in husbandry practices select for more virulent genotypes.

8.3 Potential Pathogenic Bacteria for Juvenile and Adults

Several bacteria have been associated with diseased cephalopods (octopuses, squids and cuttlefish). Although most of them have been isolated from skin lesions, they were also from sterile organs or fluids (gill heart, reproductive organs, haemolymph) and others (eye). Particularly, mainly several species of *Vibrio*, such as *V. alginolyticus, V. parahaemolyticus, V. splendidus* or *V. lentus*, and recently *Photobacterium (Ph.) swingsii* and *L. garvieae* have been reported. This fact confirms their potential as invaders, and also the positive septicaemia described in several cases, which is associated with advanced stages of infection. The halting of disease progression and the promotion of healing, after antibiotic treatment of several animals, also show a role of bacteria in diseases of animals (Hanlon and Forsythe 1990; Sherrill et al. 2000; Sangster and Smolowitz 2003). However, most of bacteria were not confirmed as the cause of death of animals, and it is uncertain if they were the initial cause of infection. In this section, a brief reference to those bacteria not confirmed as the causative agent of death and/or the initial cause of infection are included.

8.3.1 Miscellaneous Bacteria Associated with Skin Lesions

There are several studies showing a variety of bacteria with ability to colonize skin lesions in octopus maintained in captivity. Crowding and increased contact among cultured octopus are proposed as the more probable cause of physical injury, developing into ulcerations due to colonization of bacteria, which would induce a fatal infection affecting multiple organs in the same individual, if untreated. Similarly, this would be the process for wild-caught squids maintained in the laboratory or cuttlefish maintained during a 12-year period in exhibition aquariums. Furthermore, several captured wild octopuses displayed skin lesions, which became worse under laboratory conditions (Hanlon and Forsythe 1990; Sherrill et al. 2000; Farto et al. 2003).

The clinical signs most frequently described for octopus include skin ulcers in the head through which bacteria penetrate, progressing into an advanced infection stage showing deep wounds in arms or head mantle of octopus (Hanlon and Forsythe 1990; Farto et al. 2003).

Previously, until 36 bacteria species had been isolated from skin ulcers of diseased octopuses or squids, most of them from cultured conditions. Particularly, the majority corresponded to gram-negative bacteria. From these, the mainly ones were different species from the genus *Vibrio* with ability to cause vibriosis such as *V. anguillarum, V. alginolyticus, V. parahamolyticus and V. splendidus*. Different species of *Pseudomonas* and *Aeromonas*, and presumptive *Cytophaga*-like strains were also detected. Furthermore, gram-positive bacteria were also detected such as *Bacillus* and *Staphylococcus* (Hanlon and Forsythe 1990; Farto et al. 2003; Tsai et al. 2012; Fichi et al. 2015). However, only *V. alginolyticus* or *V. lentus* have been confirmed with ability to cause lesions in octopus (Hanlon and Forsythe 1990; Farto et al. 2003). All these studies have also shown that is frequent that skin lesions contain different species of bacteria simultaneously.

A brief description of several bacteria indicated in this section is shown below.

<u>*Vibrio alginolyticus* and *Vibrio parahaemolyticus*</u>

Both *V. alginolyticus* and *V. parahamolyticus* are motile gram-negative bacteria in *Vibrionaceae* family, Gammaproteobacteria class, which have been isolated frequently from marine and coastal waters throughout the world. Particularly, in a clam hatchery located in the Mediterranean coast has been shown that *V. alginolyticus* strains were the most dominant, and *V. parahaemolyticus* strains represent only 2% of all *Vibrionaceae* isolated (Mechri et al. 2012). Both have been associated with marine organism's diseases, and molluscs among them. This is detailed for *V. alginolyticus* in Sect. 8.2 (Pathogenicity). Furthermore, an exhaustive description of infection stages of this species was previously reported for cultured sepoids, suggesting, in addition to skin lesion, other routes of entrance in animals (Sangster and Smolowitz 2003). On the other hand, in diseases affecting small abalone, Spanish toothcarp and shrimp was isolated *V. parahaemoyticus* (Alcaide et al. 1999; Liu et al. 2000; Choi et al. 2017).

Both species were also isolated from skin ulcers of *O. joubini*, but only *V. alginolyticus* was proved with ability to produce ulcers in this species (1 g) at concentrations of 10^6 CFU ml^{-1}, after performing an incision on mantle in order to provide an invasion site for bacteria (Hanlon and Forsythe 1990). Furthermore, both species were also isolated from skin lesions of cultured *O. vulgaris* (Fichi et al. 2015). Small and larger lesions were detected (Fig. 8.2), showing a white appearance similar to those previously described (Hanlon

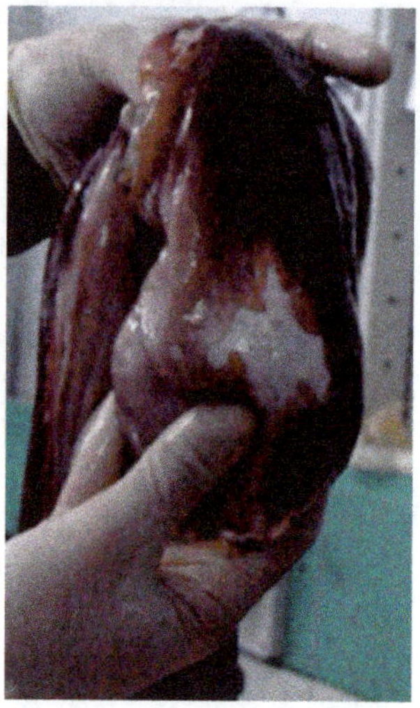

Fig. 8.2 White skin lesion on head in an adult female of *O. vulgaris* cultured in Italy

and Forshyte 1990; Farto et al. 2003). Moreover, it was also isolated from gill heart, evidencing their potential as invader. Similarly, it was shown for *V. parahaemolyticus* in squids and cuttlefish being isolated from haemolymph and other organs (Hanlon and Forshyte 1990; Sangster and Smolowitz 2003). In addition, to bacterial species, *Aggregata octopiana* oocysts and betanodavirus were also found in the same skin lesion (Fichi et al. 2015). Co-infection was previously shown as an enhancing factor for bacterial invasion in fish (Rodríguez-Quiroga et al. 2016).

Additionally, both species can infect humans. Whereas, the infections of *V. alginolyticus* are frequently associated with wound infections, external otitis or cellulitis, acute gastroenteritis are caused by *V. parahamolyticus*. The strains of *V. parahaemolyticus* affecting humans have the ability to produce a thermostable direct haemolysin (TDH) and/or a thermostable-related haemolysin (TRH). To date, these toxins have not been produced by most of strains associated with diseases in aquatic animals. On the other hand, there are limited studies on ability of human clinical isolates to cause diseases in marine organisms, but was proved that human clinical or environmental strains were infectious for both humans and abalones (Lee et al. 2003). On the contrary, recently, the lack of effectiveness in causing disease in a shrimp host was proved for human clinical strains (Choi et al. 2017). Differences between strains of *V. alginolyticus* affecting humans or marine organisms are still unavailable.

Both species swarm across TSA-1% and completely covers the plate in 24 h at 22 °C. Differences in colour of colonies are shown in TCBS, and they are yellow and green for *V. alginolyticus* and *V. parahaemolyticus*, respectively. Photographs of culture and microscopic appearance of organisms are detailed in texts such as Buller (2004).

They are also halophilic. Although most of them show an optimum growth with NaCl concentrations of 2–4% of NaCl, particularly, *V. alginolyticus* is more tolerant to higher and lower concentrations. In fact, there is a well growth up to 8% of NaCl and 40% of strains were described with ability to grow also at 10% NaCl. On the contrary, *V. parahamolyticus* exhibits poor growth in media with 6% NaCl and 10% NaCl is inhibitory (Mechri et al. 2015). Moreover, both are able to growth between 15 and 42 °C. Although they can live in a wide range of temperatures their growth is favoured by the increase of temperatures, and for example, in *V. parahamolyticus* their outbreak of diseases has been associated with thermal induction (Liu et al. 2000; Huang et al. 2001).

A fast preliminary identification is proposed through the number of steps described in Sect. 8.2 (Characterization of culturable bacteria). Other commercial identification systems (API ZYM, API 20NE, etc.) were also proposed for their identification. Although several of primers developed have cross-reaction with both species, specific primers were also proposed. Particularly, for *V. alginolyticus* that corresponding to the heat shock protein 40, and for *V. parahamoltycus* PCR that detects a fragment (including a non-coding region and a phosphatidylserine synthetase gene) termed R72H (Buller 2004; Mechri et al. 2015).

Sensitivity or resistance at the same antibiotic was shown by strains of both species depending on their origin. Both are resistant to a wide range of antibiotics commonly used in aquaculture (ampicillin, erythromycin, tetracycline, streptomycin and chloramphenicol). Flumequine and streptomycin are promising candidates for therapy against *V. alginolyticus* and *V. parahamolyticus*, respectively (Mechri et al. 2015). Alternative promising measures to antibiotics to prevent the diseases caused by these species such as the use of antibiofilm agents (palmitic acid, nanoparticles) were recently proposed (Chari et al. 2017; Santhakumari et al. 2017). Another hopeful treatment are the peptides produced by *Bacillus subtilis* which were proved with antimicrobial activity against both species, and in addition, had a protective effect against *V. parahaemolyticus* when they were incorporated into the diet of shrimps (Cheng et al. 2017). Water treatment by using photolysis therapy was effective in controlling *V. parahamolyticus* (Malara et al. 2017).

Vibrio splendidus-related group (Splendidus clade)

Splendidus clade, *Vibrionaceae* family, Gammaproteobacteria class, consists of a group of species phylogenically closely related with *V. splendidus*. To date, the species are: *V. artabrorum, V. atlanticus, V. crassostreae, V. celticus, V. cortegadensis, V. cyclitrophicus, V. chagasii, V. fortis, V. gallaecicus, V. gigantis, V. hemicentroti V. kanaloae, V. lentus, V. pomeroyi, V. pelagius, V. splendidus, V. tasmaniensis* and *V. toranzoniae*. Recently, it has been proposed the exclusion of 5 species (*V. atlanticus, V. cortegadensis, V. chagasii, V. fortis, V. pelagius*), but still they

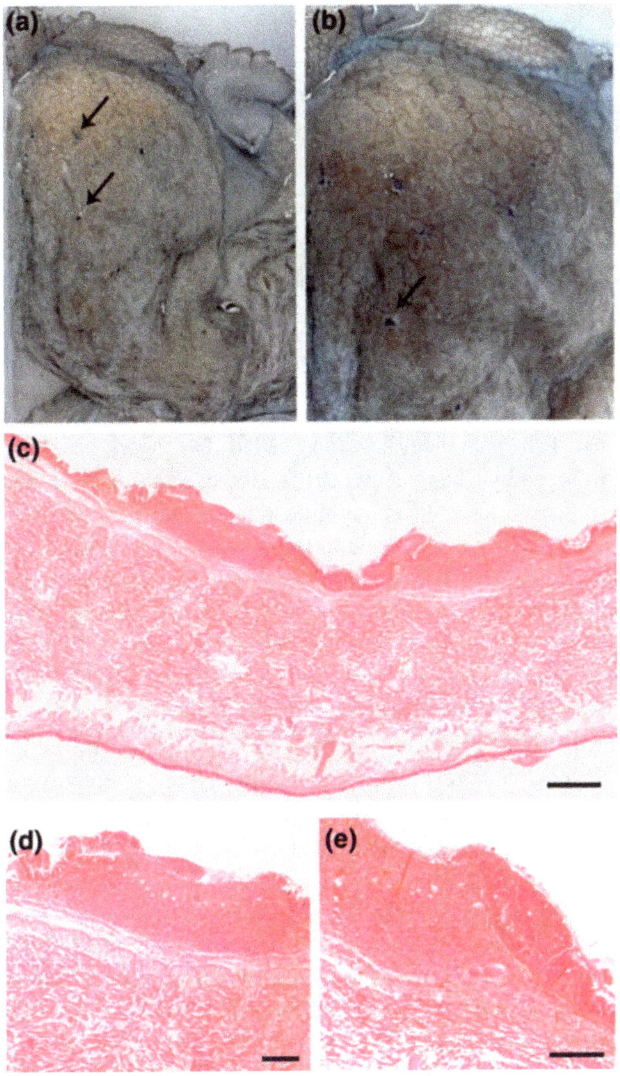

Fig. 8.3 *O. vulgaris* from maintained in aquarium conditions. **a** Macrophotography of the dorsal mantle showing small black spots on the skin. **b** Detail of small ulcers surrounding the black spots. **c–d**. Histological sections of the skin lesions showing ulceration and loss of skin epithelium (arrows) (**c**). Dense aggregations of bacteria, haemocyte infiltration and inflammation of the infected area (arrow heads) H&E stain. *Scale bars* **c**, 500 μm; **d**, **e** 200 μm

form a clade composed of at least 13 species (Oden et al. 2016).

Most of them have been associated with marine organism's diseases, including molluscs (Sect. 8.2). In wild-caught *O. vulgaris,* without apparent damage, we frequently detected small black spots on their dorsal mantle, and in some occasions small ulcers surrounding the spots (Fig. 8.3a, b). Bacteria isolated, which were identified by using sequencing of 16S rRNA gene, were closely related to *V. splendidus/V. atlanticus/V. kanlaloae*. However, when octopus were kept in the aquarium tanks, the ulcerations were much more evident and spread infection to head and arms, and also to other conspecifics sharing the tank. Death was not observed in any of animals at least for four months.

Histopathological lesions were characterized by dense aggregations of bacteria, ulceration, loss of skin epithelium, and haemocyte infiltration and inflammation of the infected area (Fig. 8.3c, d).

Splendidus clade includes gram-negative rods, motile and facultatively anaerobic bacteria with ability to growth on TCBS, ability to produce acid from a wide variety of substrates, and also with facility to grow by using an extensive number of substrates as sole carbon source. These lasts phenotypic features are the mainly basis to differentiate the species within Splendidus clade, but it is still difficult since variations in the same phenotypic test are reported among different strains included in the same species and different research groups.

A fast preliminary identification is proposed through the number of steps described in Sect. 8.2 (Characterization of culturable bacteria). Firstly, a phenotypical characterization with primary identification tests including the decarboxylases (ADH, LDC, ODC). Secondly, since Splendidus clade, is the most abundant in marine environment, the use primers VTS/VT and VTS/VS primer sets are a valuable tool for a fast detection of Splendidus clade. Finally, the 16S rRNA gene analyses are also a valuable tool to resolve distinct genera, but it is insufficient to discriminate closely related species such as those included in the Splendidus clade. If a final identification will be necessary, then a multilocus sequence analysis (MLSA) technique, which is based on the sequencing of multiple housekeeping genes, should be applied (Pérez-Cataluña et al. 2016; Oden et al. 2016).

The susceptibility of *V. splendidus* to several antibiotics was recorded (chloramphenicol, flumequine, nitrofurantoin, nifurpirinol, oxonic acid and potentiated sulphonamide), and their use was successful for the treatment of infection in fish (Revised by Austin et al. 2007). Chloramphenicol and gentamycin were also highly effective in the treatment of squids or cuttlefishes (Hanlon and Forsythe 1990). Recently, other alternative strategies to control an outbreak have been effective, such as the use of a combination of different phages (Li et al. 2016). Treatments to control disease caused by other species of Splendidus clade are still unavailable.

8.3.2 Miscellaneous Bacteria Associated with Eye Damages or Associated Tissues

Previously, several *Vibrio* species were proved as invaders of squid eyes, having hardly affected the cornea. Particularly, *V. anguillarum, V. charchariae* or *V. harveyi* were cultured from the posterior chamber of squids. Furthermore, *Micrococcus* sp. was also detected in the vitreous humour, the posterior lens surface and the haemolymph of affected

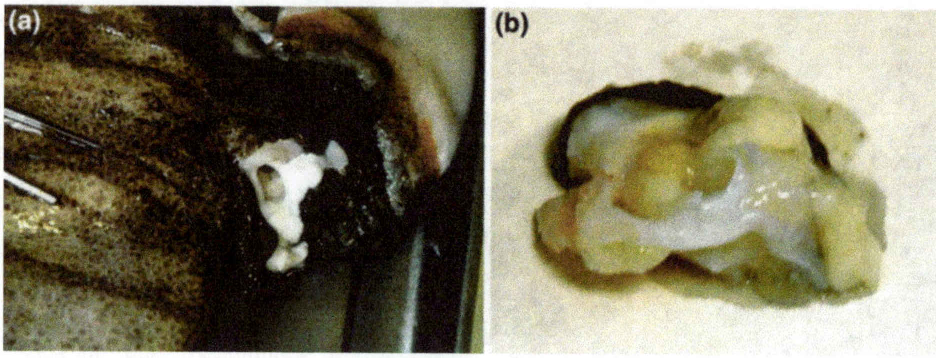

Fig. 8.4 Retrobulbar lesion in an adult male of *O. vulgaris* cultured in Italy: **a** White fluid material leaked from the retrobulbar lesion after the removal of the ocular bulb. **b** Retrobulbar-confined cavity (2–3 cm diameter) excised from the head

squids. Authors proposed a primarily involving damage to the cornea, which would be previous to the infection (Hanlon and Forsythe 1990). Recently, *Ph. swingsii* and *L. garvieae* were isolated from a white fluid material leaked from a retrobulbar lesion after the removal of the ocular bulb in an adult male common octopus. Until removing the ocular bulb, no gross lesion was observed. The lesion appeared as a confined cavity of 2–3 cm diameter (Fig. 8.4a, b).

Lactococcus garvieae

This is a gram-positive bacterium, which causes diseases in several aquatic and terrestrial animals (Tsai et al. 2012). In fish, it is responsible for hyperacute haemorrhagic septicaemia, but it has also been identified in bacterial outbreaks in aquatic invertebrates, such as the giant freshwater prawn, *Macrobrchium rosenbergii* (Vendrell et al. 2006; Tsai et al. 2012; Meyburgh et al. 2017). This bacterium has been reported in several species of fish, but it has also detected in other marine animals, such as a bottlenose dolphin, *Tursiops truncatus* (Evans et al. 2006) and a sea turtle, *Caretta caretta* (Fichi et al. 2016). Furthermore, it is considered an emerging pathogen related with handling or ingestion of raw fish and seafood for humans (Gibello et al. 2016). In cephalopods, *L. garvieae* was previously isolated in the muscle of a squid collected in a restaurant as the source of infection in a human endocarditis in Taiwan, but there was the possibility that the squid resulted positive for this bacterium due to a cross contamination with other raw fish (Wang et al. 2007).

L. garvieae, *Streptococcaceae* family, Bacilli class, is an ovoid coccus, not-motile, which grows from 4 to 45 °C, and at 6.5% NaCl (Meyburgh et al. 2017), on several common media. On blood agar and Columbia-colistin-nalixic acid (CNA) agar, the colonies are small, white, alpha haemolytic and catalase negative. Several commercial identification systems, such as API strips, BD Phoenix, the Vitek system or MicroScan are able to identify it, but some strains can be misidentified as *L. lactis* or *Enterococcus* spp. (Gibello et al. 2016). A selective medium to differentiate *L. garvieae*, from other fish pathogen bacteria, called LG agar, has been developed by Chang et al. (2014). However, some molecular techniques, such PCR amplification of the internal transcribed spacer (ITS) region, sequencing of the 16S rRNA gene, multiplex PCR and DNA microarray have been developed and allow to identify *L. garvieae* (Chang et al. 2014; Gibello et al. 2016; Meyburgh et al. 2017).

The treatment of *L. garvieae* infection in fish is based on lincomycin, oxytetracycline and macrolide antibiotics. A characteristic of this bacterium is the resistance to clindamycin, but resistance to erythromycin, streptomycin, tetracycline, oxytetracycline, florfenicol and some quinolones have also been reported (Gibello et al. 2016).

Photobacterium swingsii

This is a motile gram-negative small coccobacillus in *Vibrionaceae* family, Gammaproteobacteria class. It has been isolated and characterized for the first time from oysters during a vibriosis in Mexico and from the haemolymph of wild spider crabs collected in Canary Islands, Spain, by Gómez-Gil et al. (2011). It grows in TCBS agar, TSA supplemented up 2% NaCl (TSA-2), marine agar, and blood agar in the temperature range of 4–37 °C, and in the salt concentration range from 3 to 6% (Gómez-Gil et al. 2011, Fichi et al. 2015). In TCBS, the colonies of *Ph. swingsii* are green, small, round with smooth border, 2–3 mm diameter, while in TSA-2 and marine agar they are white (Gómez-Gil et al. 2011; Fichi et al. 2015). Some differences were observed among the six strains isolated by Gómez-Gil et al. (2011), regarding the growth conditions and the biochemical reactions.

The strain isolated from octopus grew from 22 to 37 °C and at the 3% salt concentration and it tested positive for oxidase and catalase, and it is possible the identification by API 20 E or API 20NE systems. The identification of *Ph. swingsii* was applied by the sequencing of 16S rRNA gene. By the fact that this bacterium has been isolated from oysters during a vibriosis outbreak and from a retrobulbar lesion in

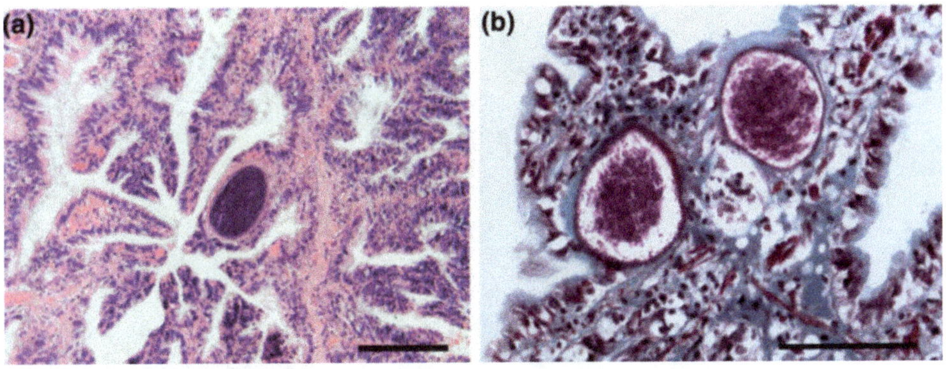

Fig. 8.5 *O. vulgaris* gills maintained in aquarium conditions. Histological sections of an adult showing rickettsiales-like organisms (arrows) at the base of the gill epithelium with distension of the basal membrane and hypertrophy of the infected cell. H&E stain. *Scale bars* **a** 100 µm; **b** 50 µm

the common octopus, there are strong evidences of its pathogenic role, but this should be confirmed by an experimental infection.

The isolated strain resulted susceptible to the vibrio static O129 at 10 and 150 µg, but no other antibiotic test susceptibility was performed.

8.3.3 Rickettsial-like Organisms (RLO)

RLO are gram-negative bacteria, which have been associated with infection and mass mortalities in several aquatic animals. Particularly, cases of molluscs bivalves have increased since the first description in clams was reported (Azevedo et al. 2006; revised by Romalde and Barja 2010; Ceuta and Boehs 2012; revised by Gollas-Galván et al. 2014). These organisms have been found mainly within the epithelial cells of the mantle, gills digestive gland, connective tissue and hepatopancreas of several molluscs (revised by Gollas-Galván et al. 2014).

Similarly, they were detected in the gills of the common octopus *O. vulgaris*. They were observed like basophilic intracytoplasmatic microcolonies of about 102 µm (70–150) infecting the epithelial cells of the gills (Fig. 8.5a). Invaded host cells became hyperthophic (Fig. 8.5b) and necrosis were occasionally observed (Gestal et al. 1998). No significant harm or signs of disease have been observed in the hosts, since usually a few cells were affected. However, conditions of stress, high animal density or crowding system under intensive rearing increased the occurrence of diseases. Under these conditions, RLO were able to have a detrimental effect on the respiratory gaseous exchange of the octopus and special attention and controls were needed.

RLO are obligate intracellular organisms, highly fastidious, non-motile, non-spore-forming and highly pleomorphic. Unfortunately, artificial media to isolate these organisms are still unavailable for most of them, being difficult their isolation and characterization. To date, only one species was able to grow on agar plates or broth (revised by Gollas-Galván et al. 2014).

Light microscopic examinations of paraffin sections or indirect immunofluorescence with specific immune serum are the methods used for their identification. Sequencing of 16S, internal transcribed spacer (ITS) or 23S ribosomal DNA sequencing are also strategies used to characterize these bacteria. Moreover, some specific primers set have been developed to identify Rickettsia in salmonids (Mauel et al. 1996).

Limited studies about treatment of RLO to control disease are published. The supply of medicated feed (oxytetracycline and florfenicol) was effective for the treatment against the necrotizing hepatopancreatitis bacterium (NHPB), which is a RLO-affecting crustaceans (Gollas-Galván et al. 2014).

8.4 Pathogenic Bacteria for Adults

In this section, a brief reference to those bacteria confirmed as the causative agent of diseases and mortality in octopus are included.

8.4.1 *Vibrio lentus*

This is a gram-negative bacterium, which was firstly described as an environmental species being associated to reared Mediterranean oyster (Macián et al. 2001), and later also associated with larvae cultures of scallops, and turbot (Le Roux et al. 2004). Studies to assess the diversity of bacteria based on 16S rRNA showed that this species seems to be also associated with mussel or adult turbot hatcheries, and surface of algae (Montes et al. 2006; Wang et al. 2009; Kwan and Bolch et al. 2015). Moreover, it is one of the intestinal autochthonous bacteria from the intestinal tract of the common carp (Chi et al. 2014), and recently it was revealed as a protective agent against vibriosis caused by *V. harveyi* in gnotobiotic sea bass larvae (Schaeck et al. 2016). On the contrary, this species was also associated with lesions in lobsters (Chistoserdov et al. 2005) or octopus. Particularly, in octopus, *V. lentus* was isolated from skin lesions and the gill heart of diseased individual captured from their

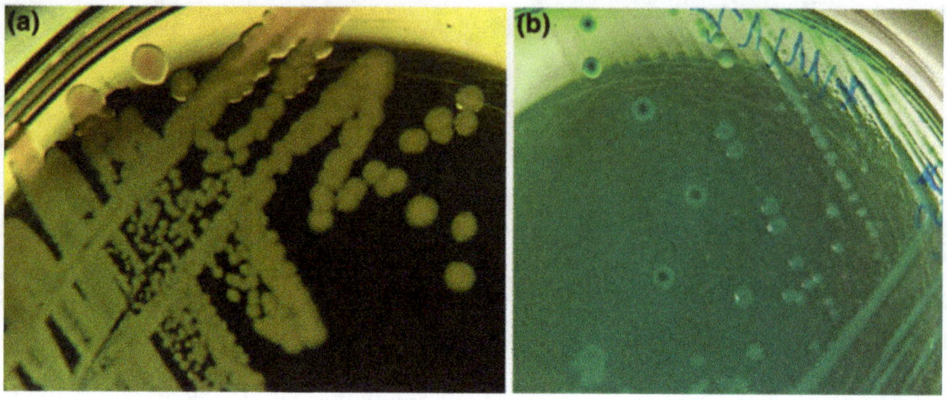

Fig. 8.6 *V. lentus* on plates, 48 h, 22 °C. **a** TSA-2. **b** TCBS

natural marine environment, and it was able to induce both skin lesions and mortality in healthy octopuses (0.5–1 kg) maintained in the laboratory (Farto et al. 2003).

The signs caused by bacteria in octopuses were round hard lesions in the arm or head mantle, which can evolve to skin losing and muscle beneath exposition when the time is advancing. These symptoms were similar to those of stages 3 and 4 of the disease described by Hanlon and Forsythe (1990) for *O. joubini*. In addition, the bacteria was able to colonize gill heart, and induce lesions and mortality after 72 h of exposition, depending on immunity of each individual (Farto et al. 2003).

V. lentus, Vibrionaceae family, Gammaproteobacteria class, is a rod-shaped bacteria, motile, unable to growth at 37 °C or with 7% of NaCl. It shows 0.2–0.4 mm colonies, which are, round, transparent, non-pigmented and unable to swarm after 48 h on TSA-2 at 22 °C (Fig. 8.6a); on TCBS, the colonies are green (Fig. 8.6b). Other phenotypical characteristics were previously described in detail (Macián et al. 2001; Farto et al. 2003).

This species is closely related to other species, which are all included in the Splendidus clade. Specific primers have not been developed, and the number of steps described in Sect. 8.2.1 (Splendidus clade) is suggested for their identification.

V. lentus showed a wide antimicrobial susceptibility pattern, having the highest, with amoxicyllin, cefotaxime, chloramphenicol or piperacillin (Farto et al. 2003). Safer strategies, such as probiotics or others, are still unavailable, for the treatment of infection in octopus.

8.5 Concluding Remarks

To date, different species of *Vibrio* and new potential pathogens (most of them previously reported as causal agents of high losses in hatcheries as well as in natural beds in aquaculture of molluscs) have been shown associated with different stages of cultured or aquarium-maintained cephalopods. However, it is still unknown if most of them are the initial cause of infection.

To understand the equilibrium among a community of microorganisms, and how changes in husbandry practices select for more virulent genotypes are important targets to be addressed in the future.

Prevention techniques are needed to avoid bacterial infections in cephalopods maintained in aquarium systems, which include good welfare practices, cleaning of tanks and control of water and food quality supplied. However, once the presence of the pathogen is confirmed, treatments to combat the infection are needed. To date, most of treatments to control diseases caused by bacteria-affecting cephalopods are based on applying antibiotics. This therapy is becoming more restrictive as a consequence of generating multi-drug resistant pathogens and accumulation of toxic compounds in farmed organisms, causing long-term adverse health effect to humans and other animals. Therefore, special attention should be focussed on the use of alternative methods in order to protect larvae, juvenile and adult cephalopods against pathogens and improve their survival, and also safeguard human health and environment.

Acknowledgements Authors would like to thank Raquel Fernández-Gago (University of Vigo) who has generously donated images (Fig. 8.1a, b) and tissue sections of bacterial-infected *O. vulgaris* paralarvae, and María Gómez-Costas (University of Vigo) who has collaborated in Sect. 8.2.

References

Alcaide E, Amaro C, Todolí R, Oltra R (1999) Isolation and characterization of *Vibrio parahaemolyticus* causing infection in Iberian toothcarp *Aphanius iberus*. Dis Aquat Org 35:77–80

Anguiano-Beltrán C, Searcy-Bernal R, Lizárraga-Partida M (1998) Pathogenic effects of *Vibrio alginolyticus* on larvae and postlarvae of the red abalone *Haliotis rufescens*. Dis Aquat Org 33:119–122

Austin B, Austin D, Sutherland R, Thompson F, Swings J (2005) Pathogenicity of vibrios to rainbow trout (*Oncorhynchus mykiss*, Walbaum) and *Artemia* nauplii. Environ Microbiol 7:1488–1495

Azevedo C, Conchas RF, Tajdari J, Montes M (2006) Ultrastructural description of new Rickettsia-like organisms in the commercial abalone *Haliotis tuberculata* (Gastropoda: Haliotidae) from the NW of Spain. Dis Aquat Org 71:233–237

Beaz-Hidalgo R, Cleenwerck I, Balboa S, De Wachter M, Thompson F, Swings J, DeVos P, Romalde JL (2008) Genomic diversity amongst *Vibrio* isolates associated with clam culture in Galicia (NW of Spain). Syst Appl Microbiol 31:215–222

Beaz-Hidalgo R, Doce A, Pascual J, Toranzo AE, Romalde JL (2009) *Vibrio gallaecicus* sp. nov. isolated from cultured clams in north-western Spain. Syst Appl Microbiol 32:111–117

Borges MT, Sousa A, De Marco P, Matos A2, Hönigová P, Castro PML (2008) Aerobic and anoxic growth and nitrate removal capacity of a marine denitrifying bacterium isolated from a recirculation aquaculture system. Microb Ecol 55:107–118

Buller NB (2004) Bacteria from fish and other aquatic animals: a practical identification manual. CABI Publishing, UK

Cervino JM, Thompson FL, Gomez-Gil B, Lorence EA, Goreau TJ, Hayes RL, Winiarski-Cervino KB, Smith GW, Hughen K, Bartels E (2008) The *Vibrio* core group induces yellow band disease in Caribbean and Indo-Pacific reef-building corals. J Appl Microbiol 105:1658–1671

Ceuta L, Boehs G (2012) Parasites of the mangrove mussel *Mytella guyanensis* (Bivalvia: Mytilidae) in Camamu Bay, Bahia, Brazil. Braz J Biol 72:421–427

Chang C-I, Lee C-F, Tsai J-M, Wu C-C, Chen L-H, Chen S-C, Lin K-J (2014) Development of a selective and differential medium for capsulated *Lactococcus garvieae*. J Fish Dis 37:719–728

Chari N, Felix L, Davoodbasha M, Sulaiman Ali A, Nooruddin T (2017) In vitro and in vivo antibiofilm effect of copper nanoparticles against aquaculture pathogens. Biocatal Agric Biotechnol 10:336–341

Cheikh YB, Travers MA, Morga B, Godfrin Y, Rioult D, Le Foll F (2016) First evidence for a *Vibrio* strain pathogenic to *Mytilus edulis* altering hemocyte immune capacities. Dev Comp Immunol 57:107–119

Cheng A-Ch, Lin H-L, Shiu Y-L, Tyan Y-Ch, Ch-H (2017) Isolation and characterization of antimicrobial peptides derived from *Bacillus subtilis* E20-fermented soybean meal and its use for preventing *Vibrio* infection in shrimp aquaculture. Fish & Shellfish Immunol 67:270–279

Chistoserdov AY, Smolowitz R, Mirasol F, Hsu A (2005) Culture-dependent characterization of the microbial community associated with epizootic shell disease lesions in american lobster, *Homarus americanus*. J Shellfish Res 24:741–747

Choi M, Stevens AM, Smith SA, Taylor DP, Kuhn DD (2017) Strain and dose infectivity of *Vibrio parahaemolyticus*: the causative agent of early mortality syndrome in shrimp. Aquacult Res 48:3719–3727

Evans JJ, Pasnik DJ, Klesius PH, Al-Ablani S (2006) First report of *Streptococcus agalactiae* and *Lactococcus garvieae* from a wild bottlenose dolphin (*Tursiops truncates*). J Wild Dis 42:561–569

Farto R, Armada SP, Montes M, Guisande JA, Pérez MJ, Nieto TP (2003) *Vibrio lentus* associated with diseased wild octopus (*Octopus vulgaris*). J Invertebr Pathol 83:149–156

Farto R, Montes M, Guisande JÁ, Armada SP Prado S, Nieto TP (2006) An improved and rapid biochemical identification of indigenous aerobic culturable bacteria associated with Galician oyster production. J Shellfish Res 25:1059–1066

Fichi G, Cardeti G, Perrucci S, Vanni A, Cersini A, Lenzi C, De Wolf T, Fronte B, Guarducci M, Susini F (2015) Skin lesion-associated pathogens from *Octopus vulgaris*: first detection of *Photobacterium swingsii, Lactococcus garvieae* and betanodavirus. Dis Aquat Org 115:147–56

Fichi G, Cardeti G, Cersini A, Mancusi C, Guarducci M, Di Guardo G, Terracciano G (2016) Bacterial and viral pathogens detected in sea turtles stranded along the coast of Tuscany, Italy. Vet Microbiol 185:56–61

García-Fernández P, Castellanos-Martínez S, Iglesias J, Otero JJ, Gestal C (2016) Selection of reliable reference genes for RT-qPCR studies in *Octopus vulgaris* paralarvae during development and immune-stimulation. J Invertebr Pathol 138:57–62

Gestal C, Abollo E, Pascual S (1998) Rickettsiales-like organisms in the gills of reared *Octopus* vulgaris (Mollusca, Cephalopoda). Bull Eur Ass Fish Pathol 18:13–14

Gibello A, Galán-Sánchez F, Mar Blanco M, Rodríguez-Iglesias M, Domínguez L, Fernández-Garayzábal JF (2016) The zoonotic potential of *Lactococcus garvieae*: An overview on microbiology, epidemiology, virulence factors and relationship with its presence in foods. Res Vet Sci 109:59–70

Gollas-Galván T, Avila-Villa LA, Martínez-Porchas M, Hernández-López J (2014) Rickettsia-like organisms from cultured aquatic organisms, with emphasis on necrotizing hepatopancreatitis bacterium affecting penaeid shrimp: An overview on an emergent concern. Rev Aquacult 6:256–269

Gómez-Gil B, Roque A, Rotllant G, Peinado L, Romalde JL, Doce A, Cabanillas-Beltra H, Chimetto LA, Thompson FL (2011) *Photobacterium swingsii* sp. nov., isolated from marine organisms. Int J Syst Evol Microbiol 61:315–319

Gómez-León J, Villamil L, Lemos ML, Novoa B, Figueras A (2005) Isolation of *Vibrio alginolyticus* and *Vibrio splendidus* from aquacultured carpet shell clam (*Ruditapes decussatus*) larvae associated with mass mortalities. Appl Environ Microbiol 71:98–104

Guisande JA, Lago EP, Prado S, Nieto TP, Farto R (2008) Genotypic diversity of culturable *Vibrio* species associated with the culture of oysters and clams in Galicia and screening of their pathogenic potential. J Shellfish Res 27:801–809

Guisande JA, Montes M, Farto R, Armada SP, Pérez MJ, Nieto TP (2004) A set of test for the phenoypic identification of culturable bacteria associated with Galician bivalve mollusc production. J Shellfish Res 23:599–609

Hanlon RT, Forsythe W (1990) Diseases of Mollusca: Cephalopoda. 1.1. Diseases caused by microorganisms. In: Kinne O (ed) Diseases of marine animals, vol III. Hamburg, Biologische Anstalt Helgoland, pp 21–46

Harder T (2009) Marineepibiosis: concepts, ecological consequences and host defence. Mar Ind Biofouling 4:219–231

Huang C-Y, Liu P-C, Lee K-K (2001) Withering syndrome of the small abalone, *Haliotis diversicolor supertexta*, is caused by *Vibrio parahaemolyticus* and associated with thermal induction. Z Naturforsch (C) 56:898–901

Iehata S, Valenzuela F, Riquelme C (2016) Evaluation of relationship between Chilean octopus (*Octopus mimus* Gould, 1852) egg health condition and the egg bacterial community. Aquacult Res 47:649–659

Iglesias J, Otero JJ, Moxica C, Fuentes L, Sánchez FJ (2004) The completed life cycle of the octopus (*Octopus vulgaris*, Cuvier) under culture conditions: paralarval rearing using *Artemia* and zoeae, and first data on juvenile growth up to 8 months of age. Aquacult Int 12:481–487

Jayaprakash NS, Pai SS, Philip R, Singh ISB (2006) Isolation of a pathogenic strain of *Vibrio alginolyticus* from necrotic larvae of *Macrobrachium rosenbergii* (de Man). J Fish Dis 29:187–191

Kwan TN, Bolch CJS (2015) Genetic diversity of culturable *Vibrio* in an Australian blue mussel *Mytilus galloprovincialis* hatchery. Dis Aquat Org 116:37–46

Lago EP, Nieto TP, Farto R (2009) Fast detection of *Vibrio* species potentially pathogenic for mollusc. Vet Microbiol 139:339–346

Le Roux FL, Gay M, Lambert Ch, Nicolas JL, Gouy M, Berthe F (2004) Phylogenetic study and identification of *Vibrio splendidus*-related strains based on *gyrB* gene sequences. Dis Aquat Org 58:143–150

Lee KK, Liu P-C, Huang C-Y (2003) *Vibrio parahaemolyticus* infectious for both humans and edible mollusk abalone. Microbes Infect 5:481–485

Li Z, Xiaoyu L, Jiancheng Z, Xitao W, Lili W, Zhenhui C,Yongping X (2016) Use of phages to control Vibrio splendidus infection in the juvenile seacucumber *Apostichopus japonicas*. Fish Shellfish Immunol 54:302–311

Liu P-C, Chen Y-C, Huang C-Y, Lee K-K (2000) Virulence of *Vibrio parahaemolyticus* isolated from cultured small abalone, *Haliotis diversicolor supertexta*, with withering syndrome. Lett Appl Microbiol 31:433–437

Liu PC, Ji-Yang L, Pei-Tze H, Kuo-Kau L (2004) Isolation and characterization of pathogenic *Vibrio alginolyticus* from diseased cobia *Rachycentron canadum*. J Basic Microbiol 44:23–28

Macián MC, Ludwig W, Aznar R, Grimont PA, Schleifer KH, Garay E, Pujalte MJ (2001) *Vibrio lentus* sp. nov., isolated from Mediterranean oysters. Int J Syst Evol Microbiol 51:1449–1456

Maeda M, Nogami K, Kanematsu M, Hirayama K (1997) The concept of biological control methods in aquaculture. Hydrobiologia 358:285–290

Malara D, Mielke Ch, Oelgemöller M, Senge MO, Heimann K (2017) Sustainable water treatment in aquaculture—photolysis and photodynamic therapy for the inactivation of *Vibrio* species. Aquacult Res 48:2954–2962

Mauel MJ, Giovannoni SJ, Fryer JL (1996) Development of polymerase chain reaction assays for detection, identification, and differentiation of *Piscirickettsia salmonis*. Dis Aquat Org 26:189–195

Maximilien R, de Nys R, Holmström C, Gram L, Givskov M (1998) Chemical mediation of bacterial surface colonisation by secondary metabolites from the red alga *Deliseapulchra*. Aqua Microb Ecol 15:233–246

Mechri B, Salem IM, Medhioub A, Medhioub MN, Aouni M (2012) Diversity of *Vibrionaceae* associated with *Ruditapes decussatus* hatchery in Tunisia. Ann Microbiol 61:597–606

Mechri B, Salem IM, Medhioub A, Medhioub MN, Aouni M (2015) Isolation and genotyping of potentially pathogenic *Vibrio alginolyticus* associated with *Ruditapes decussatus* larva and juvenile mass mortalities. Aquacult Int 23:1033–104

Meyburgh CM, Bragg RR, Boucher CE (2017) *Lactococcus garvieae*: an emerging bacterial pathogen of fish. Dis Aquat Org 123:67–79

Montes M, Farto R, Pérez MJ, Armada SP, Nieto TP (2006) Genotypic diversity of *Vibrio* isolates associated with turbot (*Scophthalmus maximus*) culture. Res Microbiol 157:487–495

Montes M, Farto R, Pérez MJ, Nieto TP, Larsen JL, Christensen H (2003) Characterization of *Vibrio* Strains Isolated from turbot (*Scophthalmus maximus*) culture by phenotypic analysis, ribotyping and 16S rRNA gene sequence comparison. J Appl Microbiol 95:693–703

Montes M, Pérez MJ, Nieto TP (1999) Numerical taxonomy of Gram-negative, facultative anaerobic bacteria isolated from skin of Turbot (*Scophthalmus maximus*) and surrounding water. System Appl Microbiol 22:604–618

Nicolas JL, Corre S, Gauthier G, Robert R, Ansquer D (1996) Bacterial problems associated with scallop *Pecten maximus* larval culture. Dis Aquat Org 27:67–76

Oden E, Burioli EAV, Trancart S, Pitel PH, Houssina M (2016) Multilocus sequence analysis of *Vibrio splendidus* related-strains isolated from blue mussel *Mytilus* sp. during mortality events. Aquaculture 464:420–427

Parsek MR, Greenberg EP (2005) Socio Microbiol: the connections between quorum sensing and biofilms. Trends Microbiol 13:27–33

Pérez-Cataluña A, Lucena T, Tarazona E, Arahal DR, Macián MC, Pujalte MJ (2016) An MLSA approach for the taxonomic update of the Splendidus clade, a lineage containing several fish and shellfish pathogenic *Vibrio* spp. System Appl Microbiol 39:361–369

Popovic NT, Coz-Rakovac R, Strunjak-Perovic I (2007) Commercial phenotypic tests (API 20E) in diagnosis of fish bacteria: a review. Vet Med 52:49–53

Prado S, Romalde JL, Montes J, Barja JL (2005) Pathogenic bacteria isolated from disease outbreaks in shellfish hatcheries. First description of *Vibrio neptunius* as an oyster pathogen. Dis Aquat Org 67:209–215

Pujalte MJ, Ariadna Sitjà-Bobadilla A, Macián MC, Álvarez-Pellitero P, Garay E (2007) Occurrence and virulence of *Pseudoalteromonas* spp. in cultured gilthead sea bream (*Sparus aurata L.*) and European sea bass (*Dicentrarchus labrax L.*). Molecular and phenotypic characterisation of *P. undina* strain U58. Aquaculture 271:47–53

Riquelme C, Toranzo AE, Barja J, Vergara N, Araya R (1996) Association of *Aeromonas hydrophila* and *Vibrio alginolyticus* with larval mortalities of scallop (*Argopecten purpuratus*). J Invertebr Pathol 67:213–218

Rodríguez Quiroga JJ, Ferreiro A, Iglesias R, García Estévez JM, Farto R, Nieto TP (2016) Susceptibility of turbot to *Aeromonas salmonicida* subsp. *salmonicida* during a mixed experimental infection with *Philasterides dicentrarchi*. Bull Eur Ass Fish Pathol 36:118–125

Romalde JL, Barja JL (2010) Bacteria in molluscs: good and bad guys. In: Méndez-Vilas A (ed) Current research, technology and education topics in applied microbiology and microbial biotechnology, pp 136–147. Formatex Research Center, Badajoz

Roura A, Doyle S R, Nande M, Strugnell JM (2017) You Are What You Eat: A Genomic Analysis of the Gut Microbiome of Captive and Wild *Octopus vulgaris* Paralarvae and Their Zooplankton Prey. Front Physiol 8:Article 362

Sandaa R, Laila B, Thorolf M, Øivind B (2008) Monitoring the opportunistic bacteria *Pseudoalteromonas* sp. LT-13 in a great scallop, *Pecten maximus* hatchery. Aquaculture 276:14–21

Sangster CR, Smolowitz RM (2003) Description of *Vibrio alginolyticus* infection in cultured *Sepia officinalis*, *Sepia apama*, and *Sepia pharaonic*. Biol Bull 205:233–234

Santhakumaria S, Nilofernishaa NM, Ponrajb JG, Pandiana SK, Ravia AV (2017) In vitro and in vivo exploration of palmitic acid from *Synechococcus elongatus* as an antibiofilm agent on the survival of *Artemia franciscana* against virulent vibrios. J Invertebr Pathol 150:21–31

Sawabe T, Kita-Tsukamoto K, Thompson FL (2007) Inferring the evolutionary history of Vibrios by means of multilocus sequence analysis. J Bacteriol 189:7932–7936

Schaeck M, Duchateau L, Van den Broeck W, Van Trappen S, De Vos P, Coulombet C, Boon N, Haesebrouck F, Decostere A (2016) *Vibrio lentus* protects gnotobiotic sea bass (*Dicentrarchus labrax L.*) larvae against challenge with *Vibrio harveyi*. Vet Microbiol 185:41–48

Sharp KH, Eam B, Faulkner DJ, Haygood MG (2007) Vertical transmission of diverse microbes in the tropical sponge *Corticium* sp. Appl Environ Microbiol 73:622–629

Sherrill J, Spelman LH, Reidel CL, Montali RJ (2000) Common cuttlefish (*Sepia officinalis*) mortality at the national zoological park: Implications for clinical management. J Zoo Wildlife Med 31:523–531

Shi L-y, Liang S, Luo X, Ke C-h, Zhao J (2017) Microbial community of Pacific abalone (*Haliotis discus hannai*) juveniles during a disease outbreak in South China. Aquacult Res 48:1080–1088

Snoussi M, Chaieb K, Mahmoud R, Bakhrouf A (2006) Quantitative study, identification and antibiotics sensitivity of some *Vibrionaceae* associated to a marine fish hatchery. Ann Microbiol 56:289–293

Tamura K, Stecher G, Peterson D, Filipski A, Kumar S (2013) MEGA6: molecular evolutionary genetics analysis version 6.0. Mol Biol Evol 30:2725–2729

Sykes AV, Gestal C (2014) Welfare and diseases under culture conditions. In: Iglesias J, Fuentes L, Villanueva R (eds) Cephalopod culture. Springer, Dordrecht, pp 97–112

Thakur NL, Anil AC, Müller WEG (2004) Culturable epibacteria of the marine sponge *Ircinia fusca*: temporal variations and their possible role in the epibacterial defense of the host. Aquat Microb Ecol 37:295–304

Thompson FL, Lida T, Swings J (2004) Biodiversity of vibrios. Microbiol Mol Rev 68:403–431

Thompson JR, Pacocha S, Pharino C, Klepac-Ceraj V, Hunt DE, Benoit J, Sarma-Rupavtarm R, Diste DL, Polz MF (2005) Genotypic diversity within a natural coastal bacterioplankton population. Science 307:1311−1313

Tsai MA, Wang PC, Liaw LL, Yoshida T, Chen SC (2012) Comparison of genetic characteristics and pathogenicity of *Lactococcus garvieae* isolated from aquatic animals in Taiwan. Dis Aquat Org 102:43–51

Uriarte I, Iglesias J, Domingues P, Rosas C, Viana MT, Navarro JC, Seixas P, Vidal E, Ausburger A, Pereda S, Godoy F, Paschke K, Farías A, Olivares A, Zuñniga O (2011) Current status and bottle neck of octopod aquaculture: the case of American species. J World Aquacult Soc 42:735–752

Vanhove AS, Duperthuy M, Charrière GM, Le Roux F, Goudenège D, Gourbal B, Kieffer-Jaquinod S, Couté Y, Wai SN, Destoumieux-Garzón D (2015) Outer membrane vesicles are vehicles for the delivery of *Vibrio tasmaniensis* virulence factors to oyster immune cells. Environ Microbiol 17:1152–1165

Vendrell D, Balcàzar JL, Ruiz-Zarzuela I, de Blas I, Gironés O, Múzquiz JL (2006) *Lactococcus garvieae* in fish: a review. Comp Immunol Microbiol Infect Dis 29:177–198

Verschuere L, Dhont J, Sorgeloos P, Verstraete W (1997) Monitorin Biolog patterns and *r/K*-strategists in the intensive culture of *Artemia* juveniles. J Appl Microbiol 83:603–612

Verschuere L, Heang H, Criel G, Sorgeloos P, Verstraete W (2000) Selected bacterial strains protect *Artemia* spp. from the pathogenic effects of *Vibrio proteolyticus* CW8T2. Appl Environ Microbiol 66:1139–1146

Wahl M, Goecke F, Labes A, Dobretsov S, Weinberger F (2012) The second skin: ecological role of epibiotic biofilms on marine organisms. Front Microbiol 3:1–21

Wang CY, Shie HS, Chen SC, Huang JP, Hsieh IC, Wen MS, Lin FC, Wu D (2007) *Lactococcus garvieae* infections in humans: possible association with aquaculture outbreaks. Int J Clin Pract 61:68–73

Wang Z, Xiao T, Pang S, Liu M, Yue H (2009) Isolation and identification of bacteria associated with the surfaces of several algal species. Chin J Oceanol Limnol 27:487–492

Xu SL, Dan-Li W, Chao-Yan J, Shan J, Chun-Lin W, Xiu Z (2013) Effects of *Vibrio alginolyticus* infection on immune-related enzyme activities and ultrastructure of *Charybdis japonica* gills. Aquaculture 396–399:82–88

Zheng F, Liu H, Zhang Y, Xu Z, Wang B (2017) Identification and characterization of pathogens associated with fin erubescence and ulceration of cultured *Scophthalmus maximus*. Aquacult Res 48:521–530

Check for updates

9 Protist (Coccidia) and Related Diseases

Sheila Castellanos-Martínez, Camino Gestal, Santiago Pascual, Ivona Mladineo, and Carlos Azevedo

Abstract

Coccidia of the genus *Aggregata* is the most widely distributed coccidian in cephalopods. Damages caused to the hosts include mechanical (tissue injury), biochemical (malfunction of digestive enzymes), and molecular (affects cellular immune response) effects. However, coccidiosis is not a fatal disease to the cephalopod host; it severely weakens its innate immunity making it vulnerable to secondary infections. Therefore, coccidia of the genus *Aggregata* are considered the most dangerous parasite for cephalopods affecting wild species of notable economic importance for fishery and aquaculture activity. The pathology caused by coccidiosis to the most important European cephalopod species is the subject of the present chapter.

Keywords

Cephalopods • Diseases • Histopathology • Ultrastructure • Coccidian • Apicomplexa

9.1 Introduction

Cephalopods are hosts for several parasitic organisms. Although most of them are known for scientific community, gaps with respect to their entire biology remain. Coccidian protozoans of the phylum Apicomplexa are among the commonest parasites infecting the digestive tract of cephalopods; however, a limited number of species have been described worldwide. All of them are included in the genus *Aggregata*. Their life cycle requires an intermediary host, a crustacean, and a definitive host, the cephalopod, where the parasite develops into the infective stage, the esporozoites, which are contained inside the sporocysts that are released to the ocean in the feces of the cephalopod host. The apparent simplicity of coccidia becomes a challenge to clarify very basic aspects that are not yet clear such as taxonomy, phylogeny, life cycle, distribution or effects on their hosts. Two coccidia species, *Aggregata octopiana* and *Aggregata eberthi*, both infecting European hosts are the best know species to date. Coccidiosis

S. Castellanos-Martínez (✉)
Instituto de Investigaciones Oceanológicas, UABC, Ensenada, 22860, Mexico
e-mail: mixtly2000@hotmail.com

C. Gestal
Aquatic Molecular Pathobiology Department, Institute of Marine Research, Spanish National Research Council (CSIC), 36208 Vigo, Pontevedra, Spain
e-mail: cgestal@iim.csic.es

S. Pascual
Ecology and Biodiversity Group, Institute of Marine Research, Spanish National Research Council (CSIC), 36208 Vigo, Pontevedra, Spain
e-mail: spascual@iim.csic.es

I. Mladineo
Institute of Oceanography and Fisheries, 21000 Split, Croatia
e-mail: mladineo@izor.hr

C. Azevedo
Laboratory of Cell Biology, Institute of Biomedical Sciences (ICBAS/uP), University of Porto, 4050-013 Porto, Portugal
e-mail: azevedoc1934@gmail.com

C. Gestal et al. (eds.), *Handbook of Pathogens and Diseases in Cephalopods*,
https://doi.org/10.1007/978-3-030-11330-8_9

is highly prevalent in most of the studied cephalopod hosts and reaches severe levels of infection that compromise the host well-being at functional, biochemical, and molecular levels. Traditional techniques of detection are still used until advanced protocols are being designed. Detection of coccidiosis is particularly important in species of aquaculture relevance such as *Octopus vulgaris* and *Sepia officinalis*, both caught from the wild for rearing and naturally infected by *Aggregata* spp. Hence, the study of coccidiosis in cephalopods including characterization, detection, and eradication of the parasite is under research. The mentioned protistan that infects cephalopods hosts is far from being well known. However, the up-to-date knowledge regarding biological aspects of the parasites and histopathological damage caused to the cephalopod host is presented in this chapter.

9.2 Etiology and Epidemiology

Coccidiosis is caused by an obligate, intracellular protozoa classified in the phylum Apicomplexa, family Aggregatidae. To date, 10 species have been described worldwide in octopus, squid, and cuttlefish, being *Aggregata* the single genus recognized (Table 9.1), and all the species known are parasites causative of coccidiosis (Hochberg 1983). The intensity of infection can be as high as 82×10^6 sporocyst/digestive tissue of the cephalopod host (Pascual et al. 1996; Gestal 2000). The prevalence of infection varies among the cephalopod species. The highest prevalence (98–100%) is recorded in *O. vulgaris* and *S. officinalis* (Pascual et al. 1996). In contrast, the lowest prevalence of infection (3%) has been recorded in the flying squid, *Todarodes sagittatus* and all of them in the NE Atlantic (Gestal et al. 2000). In the wild *O. vulgaris* from Adriatic and Ionian seas, 100% of prevalence were observed, whereas 98% were recorded in octopuses from Tyrrhenian Sea with no mortalities associated with coccidiosis reported from both localities (Tedesco et al. 2017).

Identification of *Aggregata* spp. relies on the morphological characterization of sporogonial stages (size, shape, number of sporozoites per sporocyst and ornamentation sporocyst) and parasite–host specificity. To date, the best known species are *A. octopiana*, parasite of *O. vulgaris*, and *A. eberthi*, which infects *S. officinalis*. *A. octopiana* characterizes because of the spiny sporocyst and eight sporozoites inside each. In contrast, smooth sporocysts harboring three sporozoites characterize *A. eberthi* (Fig. 9.1) (Dobell 1925; Gestal et al. 1999). The *Aggregata* species from the

Table 9.1 *Aggregata* species recorded worldwide in cephalopod hosts. (–) denotes not available

Aggregata sp.	Hosts	Localities	Cyst wall	Sporozoites number	GenBank accession number	References
octopiana	*O. vulgaris*	Mediterranean	Spiny/smooth	8	LC186909-LC186925	Tedesco et al. (2017)
		NW Atlantic	Spiny	8	KC188342	Gestal et al. (1999); Castellanos-Martínez et al. (2013)
		Adriatic Sea	–	–	DQ096837	Kopečná et al. (2006)
eberthi	*S. officinalis*	NE Atlantic	Smooth	3	KC188343	Labbé (1895); Castellanos-Martínez et al. (2013)
		Adriatic Sea	Smooth	–	DQ096838	Kopečná et al. (2006)
bathytherma	*Vulcanoctopus hydrothermalis*	NE Pacific	Smooth	14–17	–	Gestal et al. (2010)
andresi	*Martialia hyadesi*	SW Atlantic	Smooth	3	–	Gestal et al. (2005)
patagonica	*Enteroctopus megalocyatus*	SW Atlantic	Smooth	8	–	Sardella et al. (2000)
valdesensis	*Octopus tehuelchus*	SW Atlantic	–	4–8	–	Sardella et al. (2000)
sagittata	*T. sagittatus*	NE Atlantic	Smooth	4–8	–	Gestal et al. (2000)
dobelli	*Enteroctopus dofleini*	NE Pacific	Smooth	9–22	–	Poynton et al. (1992)
millerorum	*Octopus bimaculoides*	NE Pacific	Smooth	8–10	–	Poynton et al. (1992)
kudoi	*Sepia elliptica*	NW Indian	Smooth	6–12	–	Narasimhamurti (1979)

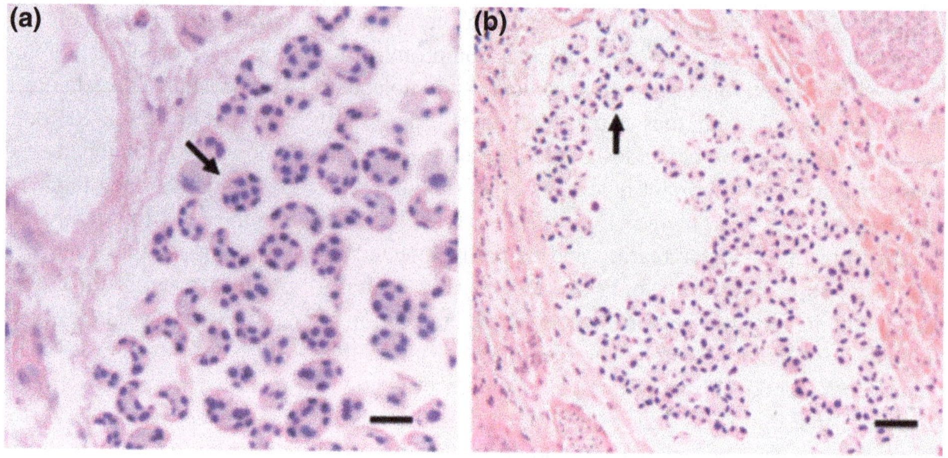

Fig. 9.1 Comparison of the number of sporozoites per sporocyst. **a** Histological section of *O. vulgaris* cecum showing eight sporozoites of *A. octopiana*. **b** Histological section of *S. officinalis* cecum showing three sporozoites of *A. eberthi*. *Scale bars* **a** 15 µm; **b** 20 µm

Adriatic differs morphologically from those in the NE Atlantic, Tyrrhenian, and Ionian seas in the appearance of the cyst wall (smooth in the former, spiny in the latter) and some minor variations in the size of oocysts and sporocysts (Tedesco et al. 2017). All the species show the same number of sporozoites (being eight), and the characterization of the SSU rRNA gene that complements morphological and morphometric descriptions provides molecular support that distinguish among *Aggregata* species from NE Atlantic, Adriatic, Ionian, and Tyrrhenian seas (Kopečná et al. 2006; Castellanos-Martínez et al. 2013; Tedesco et al. 2017). Phylogeny indicates three lineages of which Adriatic isolates significantly separated from those of the Ionian and Tyrrhenian seas although being more related to Ionian isolates than the rest. These observations all together evidence the existence of different *Aggregata* species or subspecies complex in octopuses from different seas (Tedesco et al. 2017).

9.3 Pathogenesis

Coccidiosis is a disease that affects the digestive tract of cephalopods. The *Aggregata* spp. life cycle is heteroxenous; asexual merogonial stages develop inside the gut of the intermediate host, which is a crustacean (Fig. 9.2). The infective stage called merozoite invades the intestinal mucosa of the crustaceans and develops intracellularly into meronts that remains awaiting until the intermediate host is eaten by the cephalopod. Merogonial stages ingested by the cephalopod are able to infect the whole digestive tissue tract of the mollusk and epithelial cells in additional tissues. Unusual organs of infection such as the connective tissue of gills, mantle, arms, visceral mass and mesentery of the host have been recorded when it harbor an intense infection. It is named extraintestinal coccidiosis, and most of the time, it is macroscopically identified because the presence of white oocysts on the tissue (Figs. 9.3 and 9.4) simply opening gently the mantle cavity of the cephalopod (Sykes and Gestal 2014). Extraintestinal infection has been recorded in cephalopods reared in floating cages from the NE Atlantic. Either the site of extraintestinal infection, the parasite causes hypertrophy of invaded cells, hemocytic infiltration and activates phagocytosis by hemocytes (Fig. 9.5) (Gestal et al. 2002a; Pascual et al. 2006). In the Adriatic Sea, *Aggregata* spp. has been also identified in experimentally reared *O. vulgaris* (250–500 g) fished from wild (Island of Brač, Adriatic Sea) and held individually in 4 m^2 concrete tanks. After 8 months of rearing without expected weight gain, animal ceased the feeding, became excitated and aggressive, lacked the capacity of camouflage, and developed epidermal lesions on the mantle and arms (Fig. 9.5), with visible miliary protozoan oocysts (Mladineo and Jozić 2005). Extraintestinal gamogonial and sporogonial *Aggregata* stages infecting arms and gills triggered notable infiltrated hemocytes and replacement of the host tissue (Mladineo and Bočina 2007).

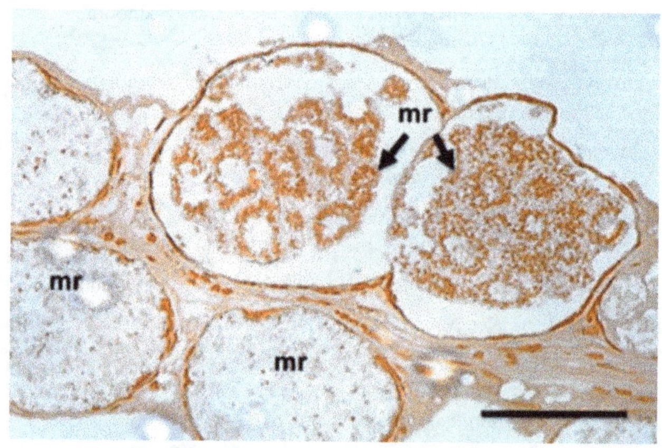

Fig. 9.2 Merogonial (mr) stages of *A. octopiana* infecting the gut of *Palaemon serratus* (Bismark brown stain). *Scale bars* 100 µm

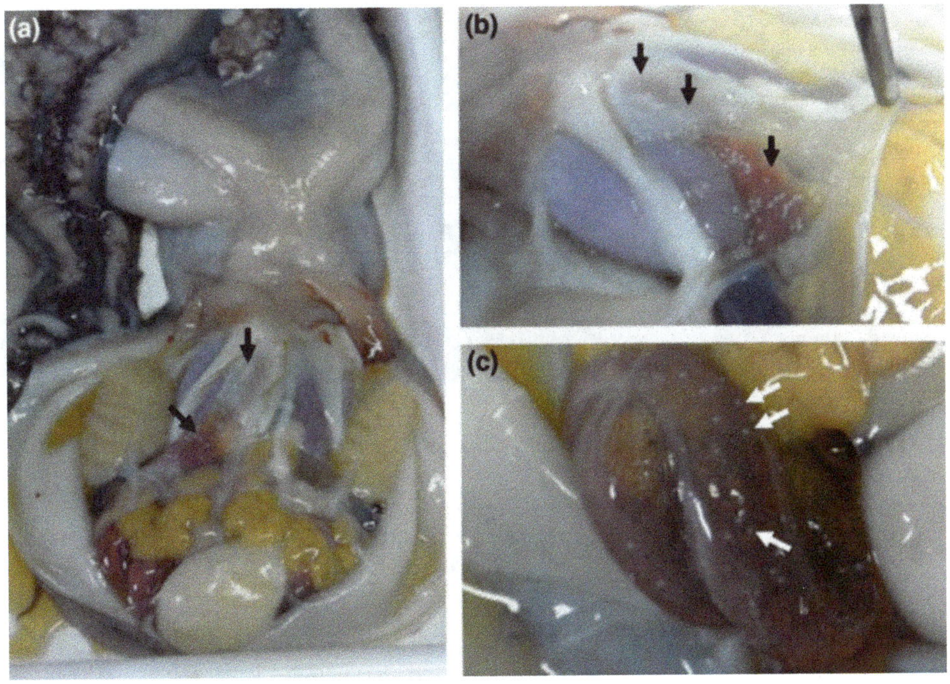

Fig. 9.3 Macroscopical detection of *A. octopiana* in *O. vulgaris*. **a** Gross observation of white oocysts (arrows) on the muscle of the siphon and visceral mass. **b** Detail of white round and ovoid oocysts observed infecting the visceral mesentery. **c** White round oocyst (arrows) observed infecting the serosa on the octopus gut

After merogonial stages are ingested by the cephalopod, the establishment of the infection inside the mollusk takes place. The infection initiates with gamogony, the formation of gametes, which occurs by unequal fission of merozoites inside the cephalopod digestive tract. Macrogametes (♀) and microgametes (♂) are formed. The macrogamete is the most conspicuous one due to their round to ovoid in shape, central nucleus, and large nucleolus that stains darker than the rest of the cell when H&E is used (Fig. 9.6). Although the infection can be recorded in the whole digestive tract of the mollusk, no infection is recorded in the stomach because the lumen is covered by a wide cuticle that reduces the nutrient intake (Garri and Lauria de Cidre 2013). A similar but thick cuticle covers the crop and esophagus (Garri and Lauria de Cidre 2013) that make nutrients and space available for infection, although in low frequency (Gestal et al. 2002a). Therefore, the target organs of infection are the non-cuticularized cecum, a tubular, spiraled organ and the gut of the cephalopod (Gestal et al. 2002a). In these tissues, the macrogamete once fertilized by a microgamete produces a zygote that in turn suffers from multiple fission, and gives rise to the sporogonial stage where oocysts, sporocysts and the infective sporozoites are formed (Gestal et al. 2002a) (Fig. 9.7). The ultrastructural analysis by transmission electron microscopy (TEM) of the sporoblast formation shows the presence of multiple nuclei inside each oocyst (Fig. 9.8), while each sporoblast has a single nucleus and a thin sporoblast cover (Fig. 9.9). The development of each sporoblast into sporocyst results in the formation of the sporozoites inside (the specific number is species specific) and a thickening of the sporocyst wall (Fig. 9.10). The infection by macrogametes and initial sporogonial stages induces a strong hemocytic infiltration, distention and rupture of the tissue infected (Fig. 9.11). The cecum wall is covered by longitudinal folds lined with cylindrical, simple, and ciliated epithelium (Garri and Lauria de Cidre 2013) that can be totally replaced by the parasite (Fig. 9.12). The infection by coccidia triggers hemocytic defensive activities such as phagocytosis of sporogonial stages, encapsulation of oocysts and gametes by flattened hemocytes and then connective tissue (Fig. 9.12) in order to isolate the parasite (Castellanos-Martínez and Gestal 2013). Mature sporocysts

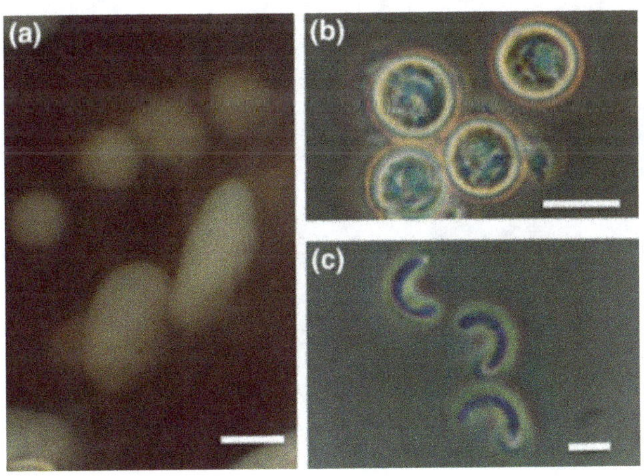

Fig. 9.4 Detailed macroscopic observation of *A. octopiana* oocysts. **a** White round and ovoid oocysts of *A. octopiana*. **b** Purified sporocyst of *A. octopiana* observed by light microscopy. **c** Sporozoites of *A. octopiana* free from the sporocyst. *Scale bars* **a** 0.4 mm; **b** 15 μm; **c** 5 μm

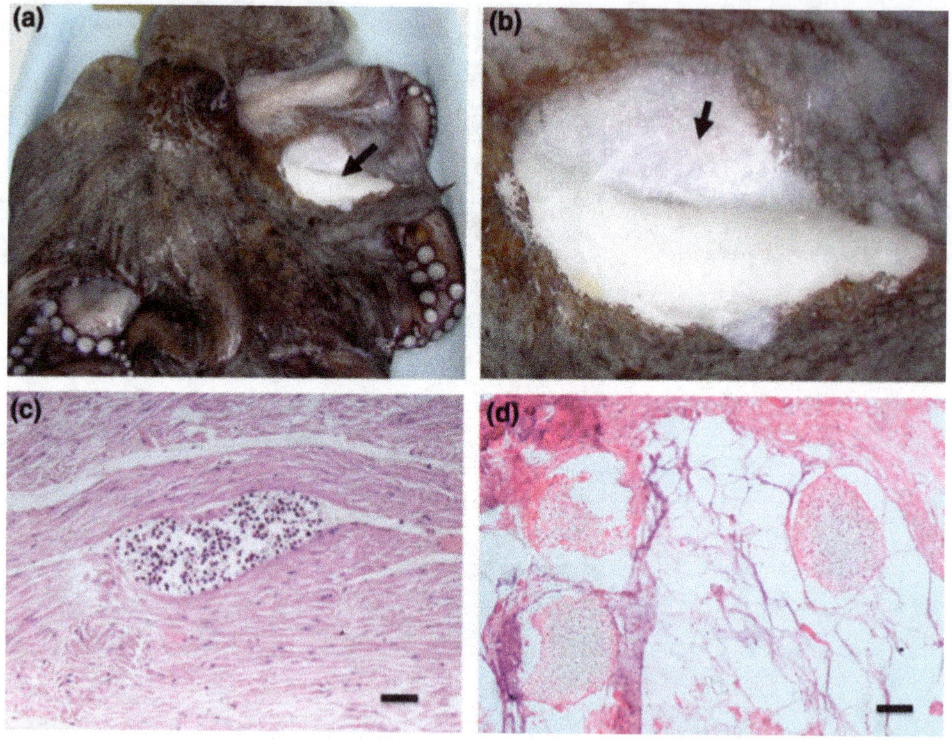

Fig. 9.5 Extraintestinal infection of *A. octopiana*. **a** Epidermal lesions on the arms of *O. vulgaris* showing visible infection by protozoan oocysts (arrow). **b** Detail of epidermal lesion showing numerous white oocysts of coccidia (arrow). **c** Connective tissue of *O. vulgaris* infected by oocyst. **d** Connective tissue of the octopus arm destroyed by sporogonial stages of *A. octopiana* and after parasite release. *Scale bars* **c**, **d** 200 μm

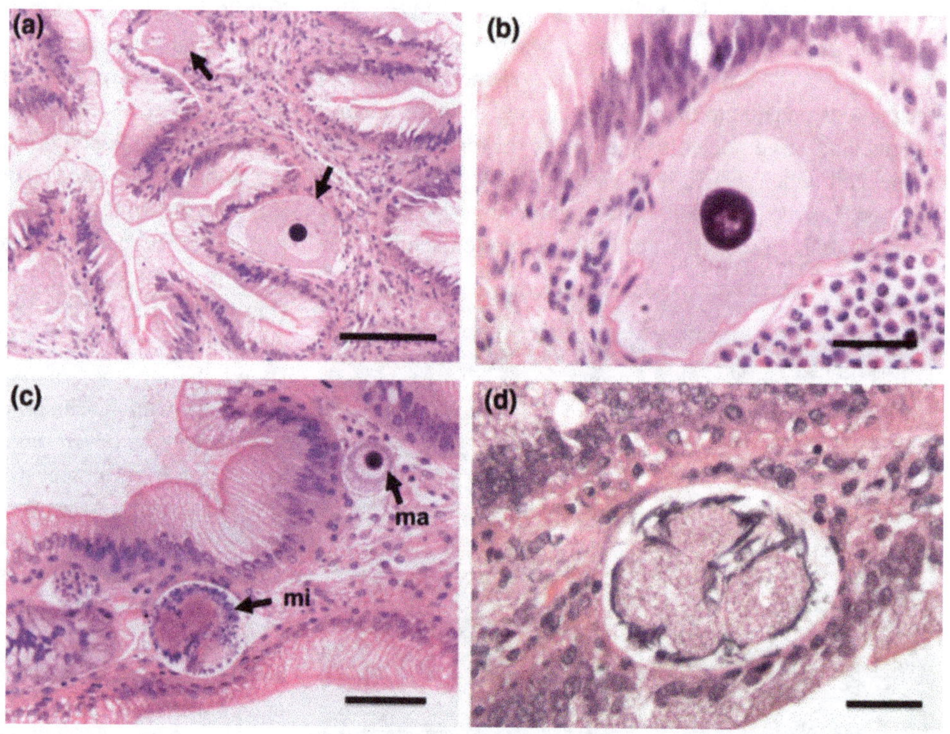

Fig. 9.6 Gamogonial stages infecting *O. vulgaris* cecum. **a** Macrogametes (arrows) infecting the folds of the cecum epithelium. **b** Detail of macrogamete infecting the fold of *O. vulgaris* cecum **c** Comparative view of macrogametes (ma) and microgametes (mi) infecting the cecum epithelium. **d** Detail of microgametes infecting digestive epithelia and surrounded by hemocytes. *Scale bars* **a** 100 μm; **b**, **d** 30 μm; **c** 60 μm

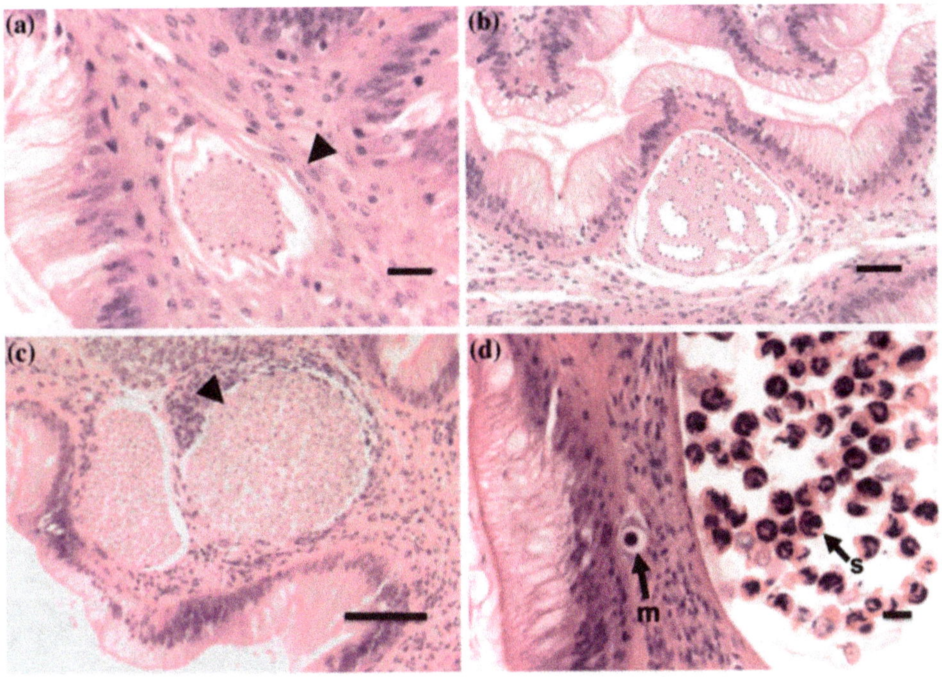

Fig. 9.7 Sporogonial development of coccidia *Aggregata* spp. **a** Zygote after starting multiple division in cecum epithelium of *O. vulgaris*. Note numerous hemocytes (arrowhead) that surround the parasites. **b** Advanced multiple division toward the formation of sporocyst. The nuclei observed in the periphery will give rise to sporozoites enclosed in sporocyst. **c** Oocyst containing immature sporocysts (arrowhead) and surrounded by hemocytes. **d** Oocyst with mature sporocysts of *A. octopiana*. Note macrogamete (m) close to the oocyst and sporozoites (s) inside sporocysts. *Scale bars* **a**, **b** 100 μm; **c** 200 μm; **d** 10 μm

are released to the lumen of the cephalopod digestive tract in order to discharge the parasite to the aquatic medium in the feces of the mollusk and make them available for infecting a crustacean intermediate host (Hochberg 1983). The release of the parasite causes detachment of the epithelial cells and rupture of the connective tissue. As a result, the mucosal folds atrophy and ulcers in the digestive tissue tract of the host appear (Fig. 9.13). Coccidiosis originates acidification of the mucosal lumen that affects the stability of the digestive enzymes and nutrient absorption. It is exacerbated by the destruction of the mucosal intestinal epithelium after parasite release that also impedes the nutrient uptake of the cephalopod host (Gestal et al. 2002b). Signs of coccidiosis in cephalopods include malabsorption syndrome, decrease of cephalopod condition, the number of hemocytes, plasmatic protein, and even the concentration of copper, the respiratory pigment of hemocyanine in the hemolymph, is affected (Gestal et al. 2002b, 2007). Intense coccidiosis also alters the cephalopod immune response. Immune genes involved in pathogen recognition and regulation are up-regulated in the cecum of highly infected hosts indicating active detection of parasite-derived ligands (Castellanos-Martínez et al. 2014a). The antioxidant gene peroxiredoxin, responsible to protect the host against oxidative stress, is up-regulated in the cecum of cephalopod with high parasite load. However, peroxiredoxin is weakly expressed in hemocytes of such hosts, suggesting that coccidia might suppress the respiratory burst and, thus, affect the octopus cellular immune response (Castellanos-Martínez et al. 2014a, b).

9.4 Diagnosis

Signs of infection are not easily visible in the infected cephalopod hosts. Gross detection of coccidia can be realized by direct observation of macroscopic white cysts when the host is highly infected (Mayo-Hernández et al. 2013), and small pieces of digestive epithelia can be observed in feces as a result of severe infection (Dobell 1925; Hochberg 1990). Fecal oocyst count is a common method for detecting coccidia, although it is not yet standardized in cephalopods. Oocyst and sporocyst detection in feces is being under standardization as a diagnostic approach in *O. vulgaris*. Presently, the challenge is focused on the design of molecular probes for detecting coccidia in the cephalopod feces that avoid the need to sacrifice the host, as is currently done, and provide certainty on experiments that uses

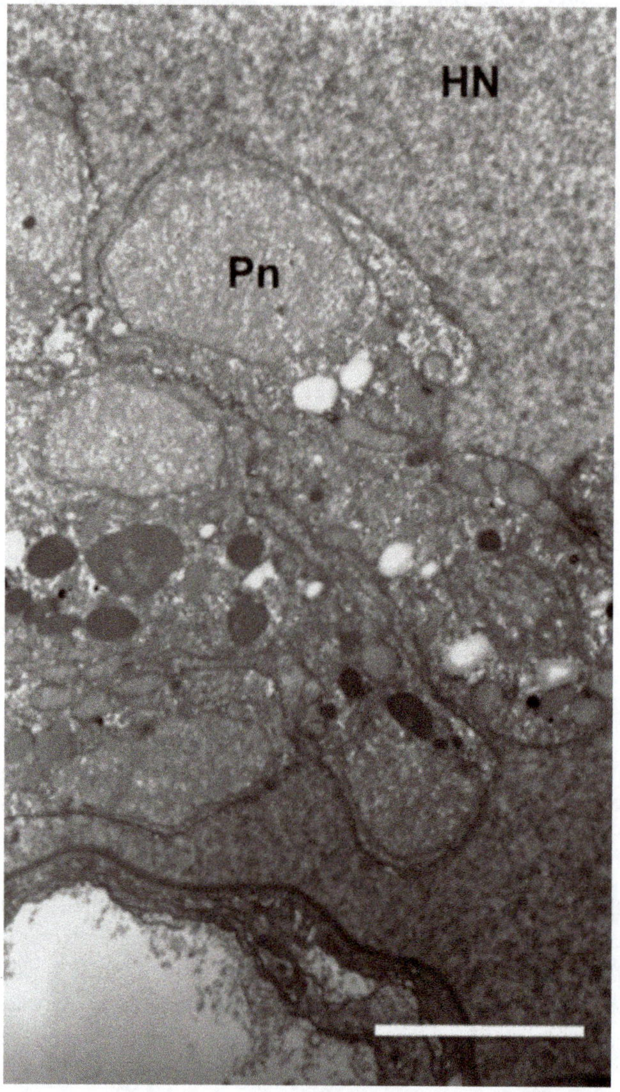

Fig. 9.8 Formation of sporoblast showing multiple nuclei inside each oocyst. Ultrastructural aspects by TEM. HN: host nucleus, Pn: parasite nucleus *Scale bar* 8 μm

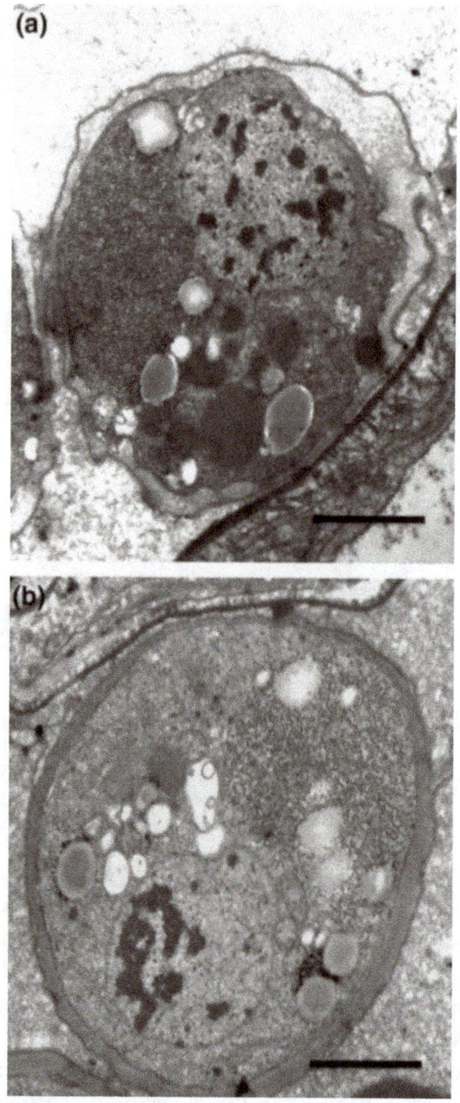

Fig. 9.9 Sporoblast development. Ultrastructural aspects by TEM. **a** Early sporoblast showing a single nucleus and a thin sporoblast cover. **b** Late sporoblast showing a thicker cover. *Scale bars* **a**, **b** 30 μm

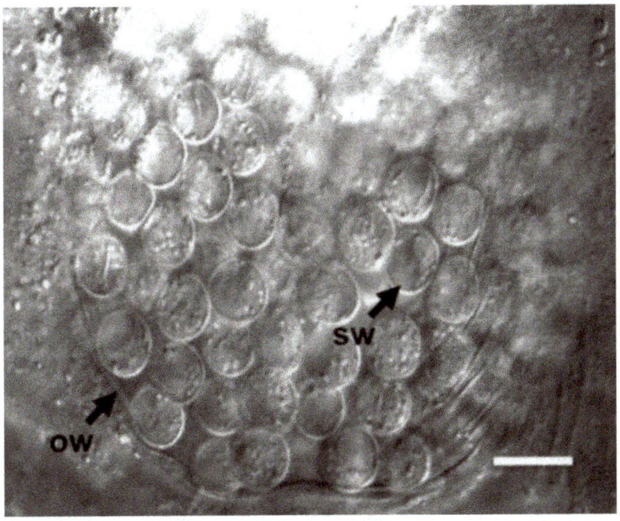

Fig. 9.10 Phase contrast microscopy photography of *A. octopiana* oocyst showing inside the sporocysts containing sporozoites. Note the sporocyst (sw) and oocyst wall (ow). *Scale bar* 30 μm

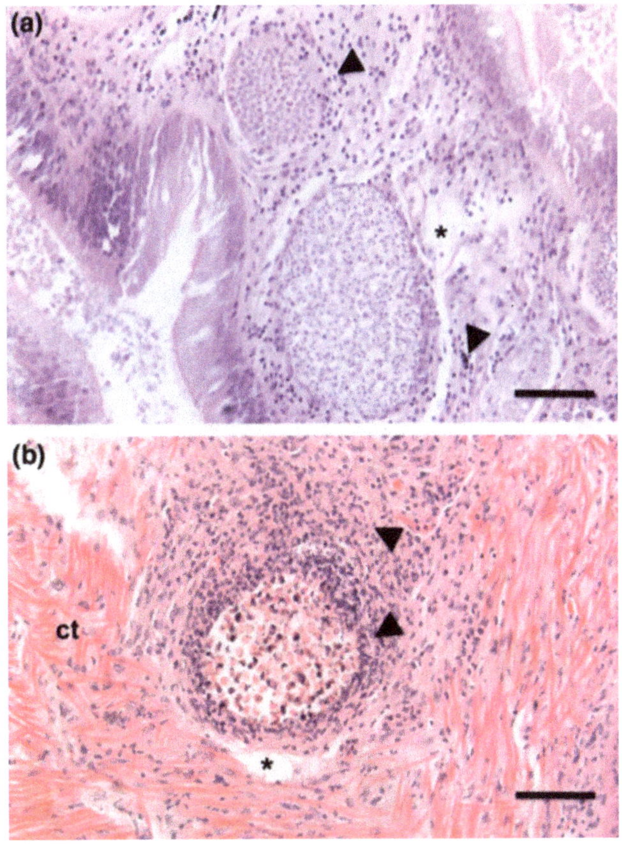

Fig. 9.11 Hemocytic infiltration in the cecum epithelium of *O. vulgaris*. **a** Oocysts surrounded by numerous hemocytes (arrowhead) accompanied by distention (asterisk) of the tissue. **b** Pericyst reaction against oocyst triggered by hemocytes (arrowhead) which formed a barrier around the cysts, connective tissue (ct), distention (asterisk) of the tissue. *Scale bars* **a**, **b** 200 μm

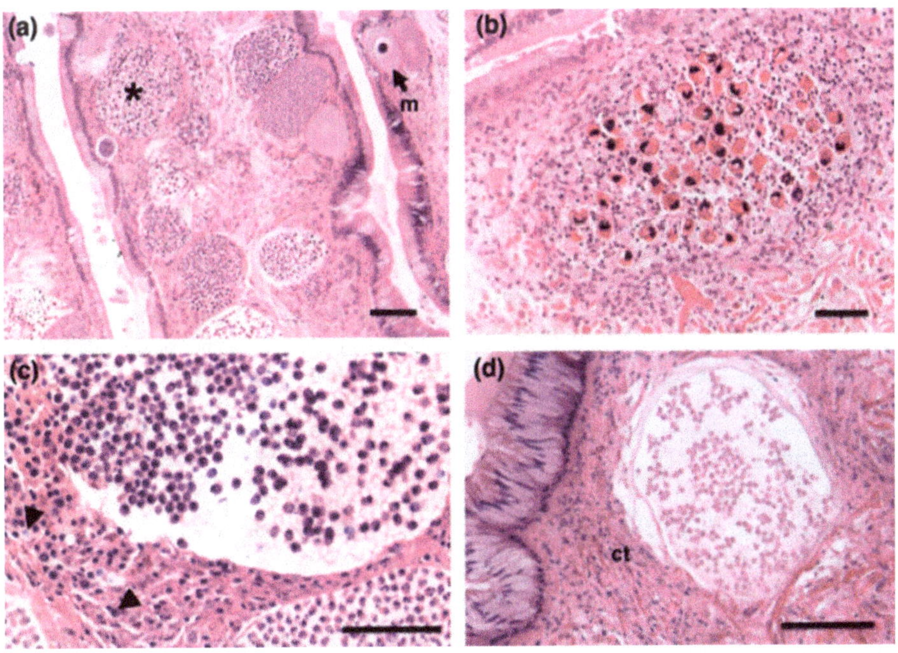

Fig. 9.12 Cecum of *O. vulgaris* infected by *A. octopiana* and host immune response. **a** Longitudinal folds of cecum showing the tissue totally replaced by coccidia at different stages of development; m: macrogamete, asterisk: oocyst. **b** Oocyst of *A. eberthi* phagocytosed by hemocytes. Note the lack of oocyst border and hemocytes dispersed among sporocyst **c** Mature oocyst of *A. eberthi* partially emptied and encapsulated by hemocytes. Note sporocyst (arrowhead) outside the oocyst and attacked by hemocytes. **d** Oocyst encysted by fibrous layer of connective tissue (ct) as a result of pericyst reaction against the parasite. *Scale bars* **a** 0.4 mm; **b** 60 μm; **c**, **d** 100 μm

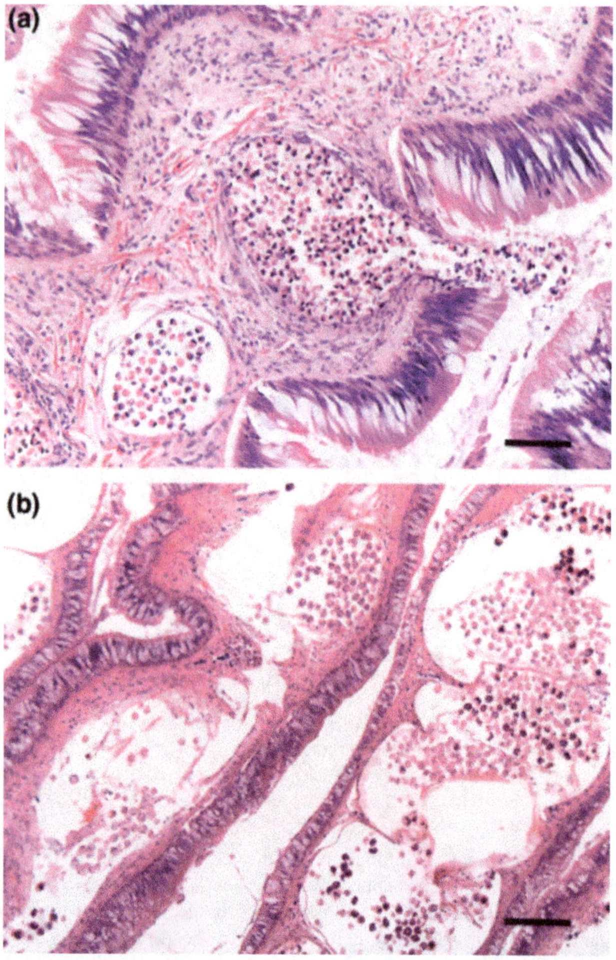

Fig. 9.13 Damage caused to the cecum host tissue after parasite release. **a** Release of *A. octopiana* sporocyst to the lumen of the host digestive tract. Note the rupture of the epithelial cells in order to release the sporocysts. **b** Ulcerated cecum mucosal folds in a host severely infected and after parasite release. *Scale bars* **a**, **b** 200 μm

animals alive (Gestal et al. 2002a; Sykes and Gestal 2014; Sykes et al. 2017). However, while this approach is reached, the positive detection of developmental stages of *Aggregata* spp. is still performed by standard histological procedure of the digestive tissue tract of dead hosts. Further stain with hematoxylin–eosin is enough to clarify the presence of parasitic stages and assess tissue damage.

9.5 Concluding Remarks

Coccidiosis is a common, chronic disease in cephalopods that destroy the cecum and intestinal mucosa of host, although extraintestinal infection can also affect mantle, arms, and gills connective tissue. From the 10 *Aggregata* species described, all of them are pathogenic and causative of coccidiosis in cephalopods that can be hard to detect. However, malabsorption syndrome, decrease in the number of hemocytes, plasmatic protein, and iron in hemolymph, as well as up-regulation of immune genes, are among the notable signs of disease and may be accompanied by discharge of small pieces of tissue lumen. The age of cephalopods when they are infected by *Aggregata* spp. for the first time has not been determined; however, specimens as small as 5 mm mantle length have been found infected in the Ria of Vigo (NW Atlantic). Any risk group based on age or length has been determined and studied for differences in severity effects of the infection. However, clear differential effects have been noted regarding the number of sporocyst infecting the digestive tract of hosts. The cephalopod rearing is still depending on wild specimens; therefore, detection of coccidian species has become an important task to prevent fattening of severely infected hosts. Preventive strategies of coccidiosis are difficult to apply in cephalopods, and no coccidiostats are available to date. Currently, avoiding the intake of infected food is the best strategy to prevent coccidia infection or reinfection, particularly, to those specimens reared in the wild.

References

Castellanos-Martínez S, Arteta D, Catarino S, Gestal C (2014a) *De Novo* transcriptome sequencing of the *Octopus vulgaris* hemocytes using Illumina RNASeq Technology: response to the infection by the gastrointestinal parasite *Aggregata octopiana*. PLoS ONE 9(10): e107873. https://doi.org/10.1371/journal.pone.0107873

Castellanos-Martínez S, Diz AP, Álvarez-Chaver P, Gestal C (2014b) Proteomic characterization of the hemolymph of *Octopus vulgaris* infected by the protozoan parasite *Aggregata octopiana*. J Proteomics 13(105):151–163. https://doi.org/10.1016/j.jprot.2013.12.008

Castellanos-Martínez S, Gestal C (2013) Pathogens and immune response of cephalopods. J Exp Mar Biol Ecol 447:14–22

Castellanos-Martínez S, Pérez-Losada M, Gestal C (2013) Molecular phylogenetic analysis of the coccidian cephalopod parasites *Aggregata octopiana* and *Aggregata eberthi* (Apicomplexa: Aggregatidae) from the NE Atlantic coast using 18S rRNA sequences. Eur J Protistol 49:373–380

Dobell CC (1925) The life-history and chromosome cycle of *Aggregata eberthi* (Protozoa: Sporozoa: Coccidia). Parasitol 17:1–136

Garri RG, Lauria de Cidre L (2013) Microanatomy of the digestive system of *Enteroctopus megalocyathus* (Cephalopoda: Octopoda) of the southwest Atlantic. Bol Invest Mar Cost 42:255–274

Gestal C (2000) Epidemiología y patología de las coccidiosis en cefalópodos. Ph. D. Thesis. University of Vigo, p 157

Gestal C, Abollo E, Pascual S (2002a) Observations on associated histopathology with *Aggregata octopiana* infection (Protista: Apicomplexa) in *Octopus vulgaris*. Dis Aquat Org 50:45–49

Gestal C, Guerra A, Abollo E, Pascual S (2000) *Aggregata sagittata* n. sp. (Apicomplexa: Aggregatidae), a coccidian parasite from the European flying squid *Todarodes sagittatus* (Mollusca: Cephalopoda). Syst Parasitol 47:203–206

Gestal C, Guerra A, Pascual S (2007) *Aggregata octopiana* (Protista: Apicomplexa): a dangerous pathogen during commercial *Octopus vulgaris* ongrowing. ICES J Mar Sci 64:1743–1748

Gestal C, Nigmatullin ChM, Hochberg FG, Guerra A, Pascual S (2005) *Aggregata andresi* n. sp. (Apicomplexa: Aggregatidae) from the ommastrephid squid *Martialia hyadesi* in the SW Atlantic Ocean and some general remarks on *Aggregata* spp. in cephalopod hosts. Syst Parasitol 60:65–73

Gestal C, Páez de la Cadena M, Pascual S (2002b) Malabsorption syndrome observed in the common octopus *Octopus vulgaris* infected with *Aggregata octopiana* (Protista: Apicomplexa). Dis Aquat Org 51:61–65

Gestal C, Pascual S, Corral L, Azevedo C (1999) Ultrastructural aspects of the sporogony of *Aggregata octopiana* (Apicomplexa, Aggregatidae), a coccidian parasite of *Octopus vulgaris* (Mollusca, Cephalopoda) from NE Atlantic Coast Eur J Protistol 35:417–425

Gestal C, Pascual S, Hochberg FG (2010) *Aggregata bathytherma* sp. nov. (Apicomplexa: Aggregatidae), a new coccidian parasite associated with a deep-sea hydrothermal ventoctopus. Dis Aquat Organ 91:237–242

Hochberg FG (1983) The parasites of cephalopods: a review. Mem Nat Mus Vict 44:109–145

Hochberg FG (1990) Diseases of Mollusca: Cephalopoda. Diseases caused by protistans and metazoans. In: Kinne O (ed) Diseases of marine animals, vol III. Cephalopoda to Urochordata. BiolŮogische Anstalt Helgoland, Hamburg, pp 47–227

Kopečná J, Jirků M, Oborník M, Tokarev YS, Lukeš J, Modrý D (2006) Phylogenetic analysis of coccidian parasites from invertebrates: search for missing links. Protist 157:173–183

Labbé A (1895) Sur le noyau et la division nucléaire chez les Benedenia. C R Acad Sci Paris, CXX, p 381

Mayo-Hernández E, Barcala E, Berriatura E, García-Ayala A, Muñoz P (2013) *Aggregata* (Protozoa: Apicomplexa) infection in the common octopus *Octopus vulgaris* from the West Mediterranean Sea: The infection rates and possible effect of faunistic, environmental and ecological factors. J Sea Res 83:195–201

Mladineo I, Bočina I (2007) Extraintestinal gamogony of *Aggregata octopiana* in the reared common octopus (*Octopus vulgaris*) (Cephalopoda: Octopodidae). J Invertebr Pathol 96:261–264

Mladineo I, Jozić M (2005) *Aggregata* infection in the common octopus, *Octopus vulgaris* (Linnaeus 1758), Cephalopoda: Octopodidae, reared in a flow-through system. Acta Adriat 46:193–199

Narasimhamurti CC (1979) The eimeriid *Aggregata kudoi* n. sp. from *Sepia eliptica*. Angew Parasitol 20:154–158

Pascual S, Gestal C, Estevez JM, Rodriguez H, Soto M, Abollo E, Arias C (1996) Parasites in commercially-exploited cephalopods (Mollusca, Cephalopoda) in Spain: an updated perspective. Aquacul 142:1–10

Pascual S, González AF, Guerra A (2006) Unusual sites of *Aggregata octopiana* infection in octopus cultured in floating cages. Aquacul 254:21–23

Poynton S, Reimschuesse R, Stoskopf MK (1992) *Aggregata dobelli* n. sp. and *Aggregata millerorum* n.sp. (Apicomplexa: Aggregatidae) from two species of octopus (Mollusca: Octopodidae) from the Eastern North Pacific Ocean. J Protozool 39:248–256

Sardella NH, Ré ME, Timi JT (2000) Two new *Aggregata* species (Apicomplexa: Aggregatidae) infecting *Octopus tehuelchus* and *Enteroctopus megalocyathus* (Mollusca: Octopodidae) in Patagonia. Argentina. J Parasitol 86:1107–1113

Sykes AV, Almansa E, Cooke GM, Ponte G, Andrews PLR (2017) The digestive tract of cephalopods: a neglected topic of relevance to animal welfare in the laboratory and aquaculture. Front Physiol 8:492. https://doi.org/10.3389/fphys.2017.00492

Sykes AV, Gestal C (2014) Welfare and diseases under culture conditions. In: Iglesias J, Fuentes L, Villanueva R (eds) Cephalopod culture. Springer, Dordrecht, pp 97–112

Tedesco P, Gestal C, Begić K, Mladineo I, Castellanos-Martínez S, Catanese G, Terlizzi A, Fiorito G (2017) Morphological and molecular characterization of *Aggregata* spp. Frenzel 1885 (Apicomplexa: Aggregatidae) in *Octopus vulgaris* Cuvier 1797 (Mollusca: Cephalopoda) from Central Mediterranean. Protist 168:636–648

10 Protist (Ciliates) and Related Diseases

Dhikra Souidenne and Hidetaka Furuya

Abstract

Ciliates are one of the most common protistan parasites in cephalopods. In this chapter, we have undertaken to describe the biology and diversity of parasitic ciliates in European cephalopods and give diagnosis elements to identify the known species. We briefly summarize available data on the ciliates parasitizing the gills and skin of European cephalodops (Ancistrocomidae) and the endoparasitic forms observed in the digestive tract and renal appendages (Opalinopsidae). Ancistrocomidae ectoparasites have been observed in *Octopus vulgaris*. Opalinosidae family harbours two parasitic genera: *Opalinopsis* and *Chromidina*. Species diversity of these two genera seems to be underestimated in Europe.

Keywords

Parasitic ciliates • Opalinopsidae • *Opalinopsis* • *Chromidina* • Ancistrocomidae

10.1 Introduction

Ciliates are one of the most frequently encountered protistan parasites in cephalopods. In addition to the endoparasitic forms observed in the digestive tract, ciliates have been described as ectoparasites parasitizing the gills and skin of different cephalopods.

D. Souidenne (✉)
Muséum National d'Histoire Naturelle de Paris, Biologie Des Organismes et Ecosystèmes Aquatiques (BOREA), Research Group: Reproduction and Development, Evolution, Adaptation, Regulation, CNRS 7208, Sorbonne Université, UCN, IRD 207, 43 rue Cuvier, Paris, France
e-mail: dhikra.souidenne@mnhn.fr

H. Furuya
Department of Biology, Graduate School of Science, Osaka University, Toyonaka, Osaka 560-0043, Japan
e-mail: hfuruya@bio.sci.osaka-u.ac.jp

10.2 Ancistrocomidae (Chatton and Lwoff 1931)

Ancistrocomidae ciliates have been described parasitizing skin and gills of *Octopus bimaculoides* (Forsythee and Hanlon 1991). In European cephalopods they have been identified in *Octopus vulgaris* parasitizing gills (Fig. 10.1) with a high prevalence, and in some occasions the skin. However, no Ancistrocomidae parasites have been observed in *Sepia officinalis*.

Free living and attached forms can be observed, measuring 17–25 µm in length and showing oval or pyriform shaped, with a large centrally located nucleus and a food vacuole in the distal end of the body. Fresh preparations show that the ciliation pattern typically surrounds all the body. Histologically submucosal inflammatory infiltrates producing bronchitis were observed in heavily parasitizied octopus.

C. Gestal et al. (eds.), *Handbook of Pathogens and Diseases in Cephalopods*,
https://doi.org/10.1007/978-3-030-11330-8_10

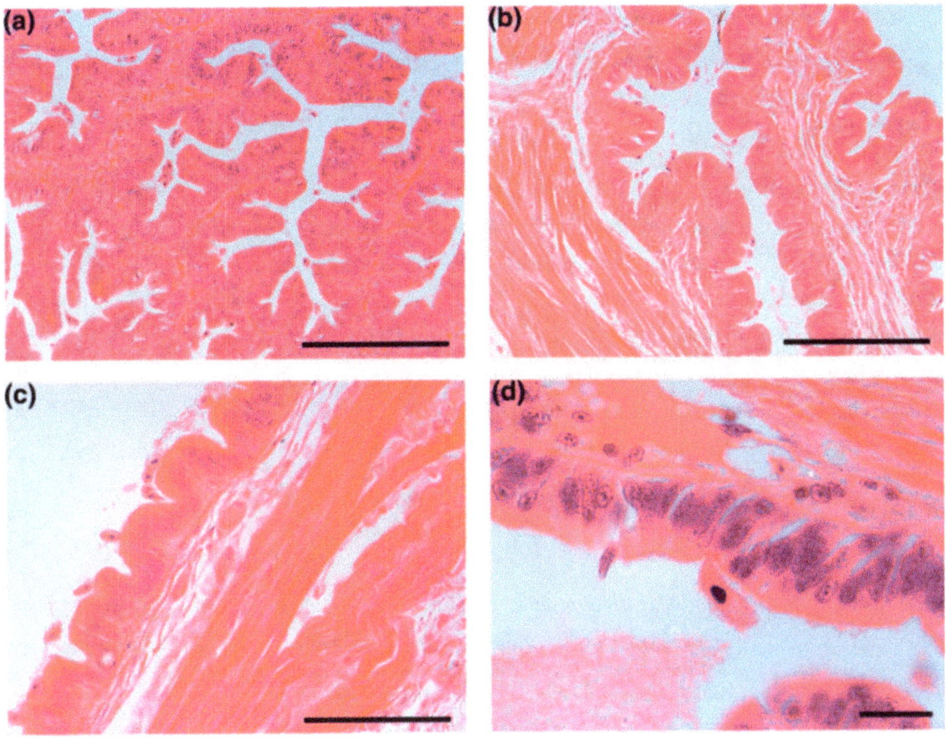

Fig. 10.1 Ancistrocomidae ciliates parasitizing the gills of *O. vulgaris*. **a–b** General aspect of gills infected by the ciliates showing free living and anchored forms. **c–d** Detail of the gill epithelium where anchored ciliates with pyriform shape and large centrally located nucleus are observed. **a–d**: H&E. *Scale bars* **a** 200 μm; **b** 200 μm; **c**100 μm; **d** 20 μm (pictures courtesy of Dr. C. Gestal)

10.3 Opalinopsidae Hartog (1906) (Synonyms: Chromidinida, Chromidinidae)

Although cephalopods and fishes share a wide range of parasite groups that can infest both of them, only one family of parasites, Opalinopsidae Hartog (1906) (synonyms to Chromidinida, Chromidinidae), is restricted to cephalopods and can never infect fishes.

Opalinopsidae are, after the dicyemids, the most common parasites in cephalopods. Their classification is mainly based on their morphology. Gonder (1905) and Dobell (1908) initially described the Apostomes Opalinopsidae as holotrichious protistan parasites of cephalopods.

The macronucleus of Opalinopsidae is a complex, continuous network distributed in parasite body. Regarding a mode of reproduction, there are two ways of interpretation: Foettinger (1881) believed budding is a multiplication mode in Opalinopsidae, while Dobell (1908) regarded it as a segmentation. In most of Opalinopsidae, developmental stages are very labile and sensitive to seawater. Their reproduction mode and complete life cycle remains to be determined. In addition, molecular data still needed to confirm the monophyly of the Opalinopsidae family.

Foettinger (1881) and Dobell (1908) distinguished two genera

- parasites of the renal appendages of cephalopods: *Chromidina* Gonder (1905)
- parasite of the liver and intestine of cephalopods: *Opalinopsis* Foettinger (1881).

Main differences between the two genera are summarized in the table below (Table 10.1):

10.3.1 *Opalinopsis*, Parasites of the Liver of Cephalopods, in Europe

Parasites of the genus *Opalinopsis* are restricted to the digestive tract of cephalopods. The only study to avoid repetition of *Opalinopsis* in Europe was reported by Foettinger (1881), who gave detailed description for these parasites. Later, Chatton and Lwoff (1931, 1935) studied *Opalinopsis* by analogy to *Chromidina* in order to evaluate their distinctive criteria. To date, only two species of *Opalinopsis* were described and named by Foettinger (1881). The following descriptions are bibliographical synthesis between Foettinger (1881), Dobell (1909), Chatton

Table 10.1 Characteristic differences of *Opalinopsis* and *Chromidina*

	Opalinopsis	*Chromidina*
Number of morpho-species described	2	6
Common characteristics		
Ciliature	Holotrichious, helicoidal ciliature, very dense	
Nucleus	Fragmented nucleus, highly crosslinked, dissociated in uniform masses, spherical or vesiculous	
Distinctive characteristics		
Shape	Ovoid	Vermiform
Microhabitat	Liver and intestine of cephalopods	Renal organs of cephalopods
Host habitat	Benthic, mesopelagic cephalopods	Pelagic and mesopelagic cephalopods
Mouth	No mouth observed	Oral blank for tomite stages but no buccal cavity
Nutrition	Diffusion	Eat renal cells when attached to the renal appendages or feed by diffusion when free in the urine
Host (genus)	*Alloteuthis, Heteroteuthis, Histioteuthis, Sepia, Sepietta, Sepiola, Octopus*	Widely in cephalopod genera
Mobility	Free in the liver or fixed massively to the epithelium of the hepatic channels and the intestine by their anterior widened end characterized by distinguishable papillum, kinetie ciliature and infraciliature	Attached their anterior end to the renal epithelium, but detached individuals can swim in the urine.
Kinetie	With gaps	Without gaps
Vacuole	Presence of a contractile vacuole in the posterior end	Present only for the tomite stage
Macronucleus	Macronucleus organized as a network in the medulla zone	Macronucleus organized as a network throughout the cell
Micronucleus	Unique micronucleus with ellipsoidal shape	Unique micronucleus streamlined shape
Number of kineties	30 kineties never reaching neither the anterior end nor the posterior end (both ends are bare)	12–14 kineties
Trichocyst	Absent	Present
Multiplication	Equatorial split	Division of the distal region in several segments. Each segment develops into the adult stage
Physiology	Survives for a long time in sea water	Die in the presence of sea water

and Lwoff (1931, 1935), Hochberg (1971, 1982, 1983, 1990) and Souidenne et al. (2016) descriptions and author's observations on the liver of freshly fished cephalopods.

10.3.1.1 *Opalinopsis sepiolae* (Foettinger 1881)

O. sepiolae is a parasite of the liver of *Sepiola rondeletti* in the gulf of Naples. Foettinger reported the infection 17% of examined hosts and, if present, these ciliates are very dense.

Bodies are ovoid, covered with short vibrative cilia, and have a pointed or round big anterior extremity. The size ranges 60–120 μm length and 30–62 μm width near the anterior end, and 30–44 μm at the posterior end (from the smallest specimens to the biggest specimens). Mobile specimens always have their anterior end in their swimming direction. The trophotomont is attached to its microhabitat (liver/intestine) by a rostrum (Hochberg 1971). Cytostome, rosette or oral cilia are lacked (Foettinger 1881; Gonder 1905; Dobell 1909; Hochberg 1971).

Kineties are oblique and forming a curved radiation, widely spaced, starting from the central part of the body and have gaps at some parts (Foettinger 1881; Chatton and Lwoff 1935).

A fragmented nucleus is observed in a few live specimens. This type of nucleus is dissociated in small fragments, which can be relinked together in a single nucleus afterward.

Generally, the nucleus has network shape; small nuclei linked in a spread, spherical aspect or in sticks shape.

Multiplication of *O. sepiolae* is mainly by transversal segmentation of the body. The division plane results that posterior half is shorter that the anterior half. However, Foettinger (1881) observed just once, two individuals conjugation marked by the fusion of the two bodies followed a traversal division. The survivals in sea water probably can leave the host and swim in the water to infect a new host. However, the complete life cycle and the transmission of the infection mode are still unkown.

10.3.1.2 *Opalinopsis octopi* (Foettinger 1881)

Foettinger (1881) has observed *O. octopi* for the first time when he examined *Octopus tetracirrhus* (Delle Chiaje 1830) and later it was found in *Octopus macropus* by Hochberg (1971).

O. octopi has been obtained from *O. tetracirrhus* (Foettinger 1881; Gonder 1905; Hochberg 1971) in Naples (Italy) and Banyuls (France) (Foettinger 1881; Hochberg 1990).

Today, there is no solid proof that *O. octopi* differs from *O. sepiolae*. The only difference is the host species (Foettinger 1881). It needs to be confirmed that *Opalinopsis* has host specificity.

10.3.2 *Chromidina* in Europe

Apostome ciliates, *Chromidina* Gonder (1905), inhabit in the renal sacs of pelagic cephalopods, while the dicyemids infect mainly the benthic cephalopods (Furuya et al. 2004). They are specific to this microhabitat because they feed from cephalopod tissues and fluids (Hochberg 1971; Souidenne et al. 2016). They have a characteristic nuclear system 'a chromidial system'. *Chromidina* species were reported in 25 cephalopod species. Today, only six species of *Chromidina* have been described (Souidenne et al. 2016).

- *Life cycle*

A hypothetical life cycle was deduced from the different development stages observed and the existence of a crustacean intermediate host was suggested by analogy to other apostomes. The adult stage, unlike the other apostomes, is vermiforme and called trophotomont. It can reach 2 mm length. When the trophotomont is extended posteriorly with only one long bud, the budding process is called monotomy. Later, this bud will develop into a vermiform adult identical to the founder trophotomont. When the trophotomont is extended posteriorly with a chain of small ciliated buds or tomite, the budding process is called palintomy. Tomite stage is probably in charge of the transmission of the infection from a host to another (Landers 2010; Souidenne et al. 2016).

- *Diversity in Europe*

Only two species of *Chromidina* have been reported in Europe.

10.3.2.1 *Chromidina elegans* Foettinger (1881) (Synonym: *Benedenia elegans*)

C. elegans have been first described in Naples by Foettinger (1881) from the renal appendages of *Sepia elegans* d'Orbigny, 1825. Chatton and Lwoff (1935) redescribed this species from cuttlefishes from Banyuls-sur-Mer, France. *C. elegans* can also infect *Sepia orbignyana* Ferussac, 1826, *Illex coindetti* Vérany, 1837; *Todarodes sagittatus* Lamarck, 1798 and *Octopus salutii* Vérany, 1839 in France and England (Hochberg 1971, 1982, 1983). There is no available information about the prevalence of this *Chromidina* species.

C. elegans is considered to be a typical species of the genus *Chromidina* and this is reason why it was redescribed by Chatton and Lwoff (1935) and Souidenne et al. (2016).

The trophotomont is vermiform, that reaches 1.4 mm length. It is easily distinguishable from other *Chromidina* by its club-like apex and 14 Kineties (Collin 1915; Chatton and Lwoff 1935; Souidenne et al. 2016).

Occasionally, some trophotomonts of *C. elegans* grow rapidly and extend up to 5 mm length and they become hypertrophonts.

10.3.2.2 *Chromidina coronata*

C. coronata was described from *O. vulgaris* by Foettinger (1881), then, from *Eledone cirrhosa* by Gonder (1905), and from *Illex coindetii* by Dobell (1909). Foettinger (1881) did not mention the prevalence or mean intensity, but described the dense condition in the renal appendages when parasites were present. *C. coronata* is very similar to *C. elegans* in body length, body shape, nuclear aspect. However, *C. coronate* is easily distinguishable from *C. elegans* and the other *Chromidina* species by the claviform apex and the crown of long cilia surrounding the anterior end.

10.4 Concluding Remarks

Chromidina ciliates are host-specific to the pelagic squids and octopus. However, they are found occasionally in benthic or epibenthic cephalopods when these hosts have a pelagic development stage: like *E. cirrhosa, O. salutii, Scaeurgus unicirrhus* ... implying that they can encounter *Chromidina* (typically present in the water column, avoiding competition with dicyemids present near the seabed and infecting the benthic cephalopods).

The monophyly of *Chromidina* is supported among Oligohymenophorea, Apostomatia, Astomatophorida (Souidenne et al. 2006). However, molecular information of *Opalinopsis* is not available, thus, its phylogenetic position is unclear. The molecular data are essential to clear the relationship between *Opalinopsis* and *Chromidina* and to support the monopholy of the Opalinopsidae family.

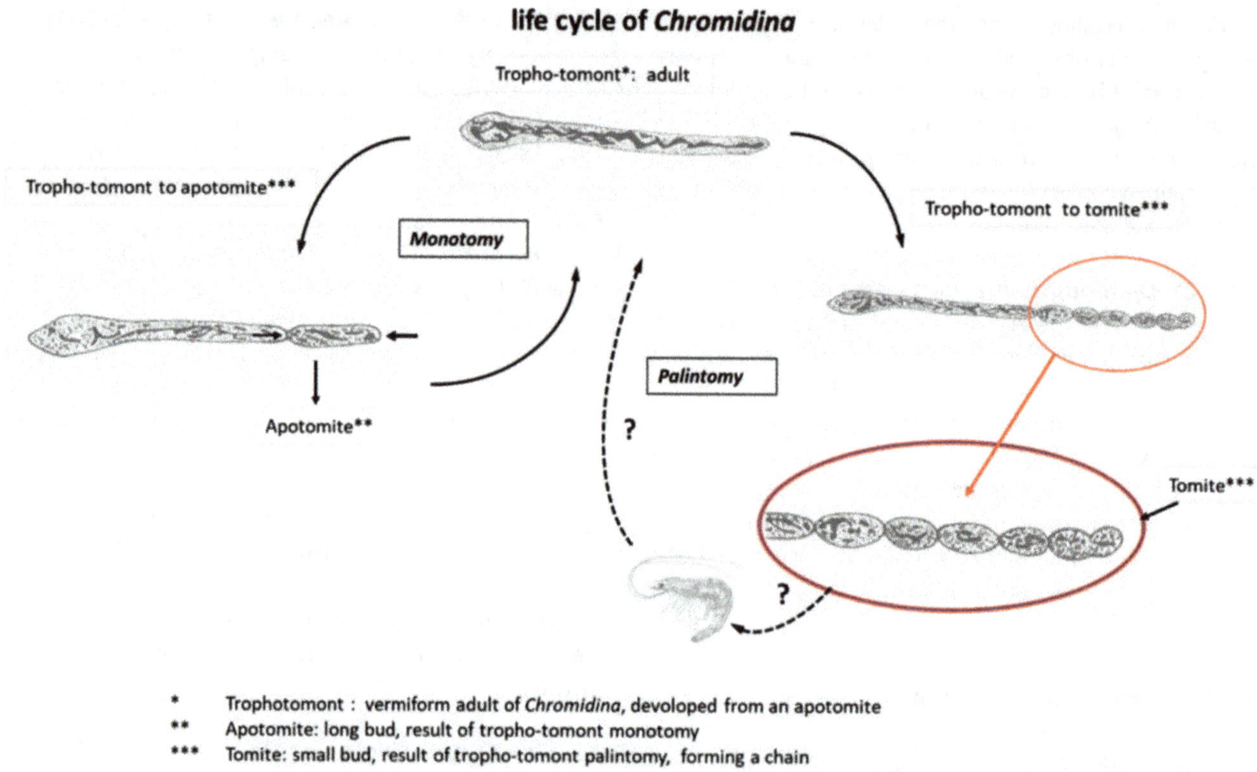

Fig. 10.2 Life cycle of the *Chromidina* (modified from Furuya et al. 2004; on *C. elegans*, modified from Foettinger 1881)

Table 10.2 Summary of Opalinopsidae parasites of European cephalopods

Ciliate parasite of cephalopods	Microhabitat of the parasite	Host species	Locality	Author(s)
O. sepiolae	Liver	*Rossia macrosoma*	Norway (Atlantic Ocean)	Hochberg (1971)
		Sepietta oweniana	France (Mediterranean)	
		Sepiola atlantica	England (English channel)	
		Sepiola rondeletii	Italy, Monaco, France	Foettinger (1881); Gonder (1905); Dobell (1909); Collin (1915); Chatton and Lwoff (1935)
O. octopi	Liver	*O. macropus*	Italy (Mediterranean)	Hochberg (1971)
		O. tetracirrhus	Italy (Mediterranean)	Foettinger (1881); Gonder (1905); Hochberg (1971)
C. elegans	*Renal appendages*	*S. elegans, S. orbignyana, I. coindetti, T. sagittatus, O. salutii*	Italy, France (Mediterranean Sea, Banyuls-sur-Mer), England (English Channel)	Foettinger (1881); Gonder (1905); Dobell (1909); Collin (1915); Chatton and Lwoff (1935); Hochberg (1971); Souidenne et al. (2016)
C. coronata		*O. vulgaris, E. cirrhosa, Sepiola rondeleti, S. unicirrhus, Illex coindetti*	Italy, France (Mediterranean Sea, Banyuls-sur-Mer), England (English Channel)	Foettinger (1881); Dobell (1909); Chatton and Lwoff (1935); Hochberg (1971); Souidenne et al. (2016)

To date, only eight species of Opalinopsidae have been described, and only four have been reported in Europe. This suggests that the diversity of Opalinopsiadae is underestimated.

Their impacts on their host individuals are still unknown. Some authors suggest that they may be a symbiont (Hochberg 1990; Furuya et al. 2004; Souidenne et al. 2006). Further studies on these enigmatic ciliates are needed to understand the host–parasite relationship (Fig. 10.2 and Table 10.2).

References

Chatton E, Lwoff A (1928) Sur la structure, l'évolution et les affinités des Opalinopsides (Ciliés) des Céphalopodes. C R Hebd Acad Sci, Paris 186:1382–1384

Chatton E, Lwoff A (1931) La conception des Ciliés Apostomes (Foettingériidés+Opalinopsidés). Preuve de sa valdité. C R Hebd Acad Sci, Paris 193:1483–1485

Chatton E, Lwoff A (1935) Les ciliés apostomes 1. Aperçu historique et général; étude monographique des genres et des espèces. Arch Zool Exp Gen. 77:1–453

Collin B (1915) A propos de *Chromidina elegans* (Foettinger). C R Hebd Acad Sci 160:406–408

Dobell CC (1908) The structure and life-history of Copromonas subtilis n. g., n. so.: a contribution to our knowledge of the Flagellata. Quart J Micr Sci 52:75–120

Dobell CC (1909) Some observations on the infusoria parasitic in Cephalopoda. Q il microsc Sci 53:183–199

Foettinger A (1881) Recherches sur quelques Infusoires nouveaux parasites des Céphalopodes. Arch Biol 2:345–378

Furuya H, Ota M, Kimura R, Tsuneki K (2004) Renal organs of cephalopods: a habitat for dicyemids and chromidinids. J Morphol 262(2):629–643

Gonder R (1905) Beiträge zur Kenntnis der Kernverhältnisse bei den in Cephalopoden schmarotzenden Infusorien. Arch Protis 5:240–262

Hartog M (1906) Protozoa. In: Harmer SF, Shipley AE (eds) The Cambridge natural history, vol 1. pp 1–162

Hochberg FG (1971) Some aspects of the biology of cephalopod kidney parasites. Ph.D. dissertation, University of California, Santa Barbara

Hochberg FG (1982) The 'kidneys' of cephalopods: a unique habitat for parasites. Malacologia 23:121–134

Hochberg FG (1983) The parasite of cephalopods: a review. Mem Nat Mus Vict, Melbourne 44:109–145

Hochberg FG (1990) Diseases caused by protistans and mesozoans. In: Kinne O (ed) Diseases of marine animals, vol III, Biologische Anstalt Helgoland: Hamburg, Germany, pp 47–227

Landers SC (2010) The fine structure of the tropho-tomont of the parasitic apostome Chromidina (Ciliophora, Apostomatida). Protistol 6(4):271–279

Souidenne D, Florent I, Dellinger M, Justine JL, Romdhane MS, Furuya H, Grellier P (2016) Diversity of apostome ciliates, *Chromidina* spp. (Oligohymenophorea, Opalinopsidae), parasites of cephalopods of the Mediterranean Sea. Parasite 23:33

11 Dicyemids

Hidetaka Furuya and Dhikra Souidenne

Abstract

Dicyemids are the most common and characteristic endosymbionts found in the renal sac of benthic cephalopods. In this chapter, we introduce biology and diversity of dicyemids of European typical cephalopods, *Octopus vulgaris* and *Sepia officinalis*. The diphasic life cycle of dicyemids consists of vermiform stages formed asexually and an infusoriform stage developed sexually. Their morphology varies depending on the development stage. Recent molecular studies suggested that dicyemids belong to lophotrochozoans. In Europe, 16 dicyemid species were described from 17 cephalopod species.

Keywords

Dicyemids • Mesozoa • Vermiform • Infusoriform • Renal sac

11.1 Introduction

The renal organs of cephalopods are the renal complex (renal and pancreatic appendages) and the branchial heart complex (branchial heart and pericardial appendage). Prior to release, urine is collected in a renal sac, the fluid-filled coelom of which is a unique environment providing living space for a diversity of endosymbionts (Hochberg 1982; Furuya et al. 2004b). There are phylogenetically distant parasitic organisms, trematodes, dicyemids, and chromidinids, in the kidney of cephalopods (Nouvel 1945; Hochberg and Short 1983; Hochberg 1990; Furuya et al. 2004a). Dicyemids (Phylum Dicyemida) are the commonest and most characteristic endosymbionts that are found in the renal sac of benthic cephalopod molluscs. The body length of dicyemid species ranges from 0.1 to 10 mm. Typically, two or three dicyemid species are found in individuals of each cephalopod species and most are host specific (Furuya 1999). Currently, about 140 dicyemid species have been recorded from cephalopod hosts distributed in a variety of geographical localities: the Okhotsk Sea, Japan Sea, western and eastern North Pacific Ocean, waters around New Zealand, North Indian Ocean, Mediterranean, western North and eastern Atlantic Ocean, Gulf of Mexico, and Antarctic Ocean (Catalano 2013; Castellanos-Martinez et al. 2016; Furuya 1999; Furuya and Tsuneki 2003; Hochberg 1990; McConnaughey 1951; Nouvel 1947; Short 1991). The dicyemids are heavily infecting the renal organs in their host cephalopods (Fig. 11.1). However, this is somewhat surprising; no damage has ever been observed in the tissues. This means that dicyemids are not pathogens to their cephalopod hosts. There must be interaction between dicyemids and their host renal organs; it is possible that dicyemids are beneficial for their hosts.

In this chapter, we introduce biology of dicyemids and dicyemid species of European typical cephalopods, *O. vulgaris* and *S. officinalis*.

H. Furuya (✉)
Department of Biology, Graduate School of Science, Osaka University, Toyonaka, Osaka, 560-0043, Japan
e-mail: hfuruya@bio.sci.osaka-u.ac.jp

D. Souidenne
National Museum of Natural History of Paris, Biologie des Organismes et Ecosystèmes Aquatiques (BOREA), Research Team: Reproduction and Development, Evolution Adaptation, Regulation CNRS 7208, Sorbonne Université, UCN, IRD 207, UA 55 rue Buffon, Paris, France
e-mail: dhikra.souidenne@mnhn.fr

C. Gestal et al. (eds.), *Handbook of Pathogens and Diseases in Cephalopods*,
https://doi.org/10.1007/978-3-030-11330-8_11

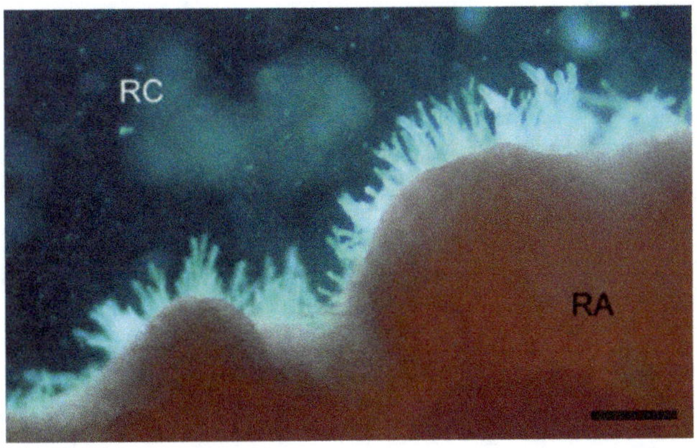

Fig. 11.1 Dicyemids on the renal appendage of *Amphioctopus fangsiao*. The dicyemids attach on the surface areas of renal appendages. Scale bar: 1000 μm. *Abbreviations* RA, renal appendage; RC, renal coelom

11.2 Life Cycle

The diphasic life cycle of dicyemids, with a characteristic asexual phase, likely evolved as an adaptation to parasitism (Fig. 11.2), presumably to enable them to adapt to the cephalopod renal organs. The life cycle of dicyemids consists of two phases of different body organizations (Fig. 11.2). The first phase is the vermiform stages, in which the dicyemid exists as a vermiform embryo formed asexually, and as a final form, the nematogen, or rhombogen. The second phase is the infusoriform embryo that develops from a fertilized egg. The shift from an asexual mode to a sexual mode of reproduction may be caused by a high population density in the cephalopod kidney (Lapan and Morowitz 1975). Vermiform stages are restricted to the renal sac of cephalopods, whereas the infusoriform embryos escape from the host into the sea to search for a new host. However, it is not clear how infusoriform larvae develop into vermiform stages in the new host.

11.3 General Morphology

Vermiform stages, vermiform embryos, nematogens, and rhombogens are similar in shape (Fig. 11.2). The body surface of dicyemids has numerous cilia and the folded structure, which is considered to contribute to absorb nutrients more efficiently from urine (Bresciani and Fenchel 1965; Ridley 1968; Furuya et al. 1997). The number of peripheral cells is species specific and constant. At the anterior region, 4–10 peripheral cells form the calotte, of which cilia are shorter and denser than in more posterior peripheral cells (Fig. 11.2). The calotte shape varies, depending on the species, and adapts to attach to the various regions of renal tissues in the host kidneys (Furuya et al. 2003a) (Figs. 11.3 and 11.4). There is a central cylindrical cell called the axial cell, which extends to 100 mm in length in the largest dicyemid.

Regarding the number of somatic cells, the dicyemid is a multicellular animal that is composed of the fewest in number of cells in metazoans except for aberrant myxozoans. This organization does not correspond to metazoan two-layered construction of endoderm and ectoderm, and dicyemids have neither body cavities nor differentiated organs.

Infusoriform embryos are ovoid and have both antero-posterior axis and dorsoventral axis. Embryos mostly consist of 37 or 39 cells (Short 1971; Furuya 1999), which are more differentiated than those of vermiform stages (Matsubara and Dudley 1976; Furuya et al. 2004b). Internally, there are four large cells called urn cells, each containing a germinal cell that probably gives rise to the next generation (Fig. 11.2). At the anterior region of embryo, there is a pair of unique cell called the apical cell (Fig. 11.5), each containing a refringent body composed of magnesium inositol hexaphosphate (Lapan 1975a). The external cells are mostly ciliated. Infusoriform embryos swim while spinning the body.

The bodies of vermiform stages might be simplified as a reflection of their specialization in their parasitic habitat composed of renal tubules (Nouvel 1947). By contrast, infusoriform embryos seem to represent the true level of organization due to free-swimming organisms (Furuya et al. 1997). However, the body organization of infusoriform embryos cannot be regarded as achieving the grade of tissue level.

11.4 Relationship with Cephalopods

Dicyemids are usually found to be heavily infecting the renal organs in their host cephalopods (Fig. 11.1). No damage has ever been observed in the infected renal tissue, so dicyemids apparently do no harm to their cephalopod hosts. Lapan (1975b) has even suggested that dicyemids facilitate host excretion of ammonia by contributing to acidification of the urine. In addition to the normal muscular contraction of the renal appendages, the ciliary activity of dicyemids present in the kidneys maintains a constant flow of urine, and as a result dicyemids assist in removal of urine. Thus, dicyemids are symbiotic, rather than parasitic, in their relationship with cephalopods.

The majority of the dicyemid species studied were found to be host specific (Furuya 1999). Typically, two or more species of dicyemids are present in each host species or each host individual. There is a certain relationship between the calotte configuration of vermiform stages and the co-occurrence pattern in hosts (Fig. 11.6). Vermiform individuals live specifically within the renal sac. Their anterior region, termed a "calotte", is critical in adapting to their habitats in the renal sac. They insert the distinct anterior region into renal tubules or crypts of the renal appendages of

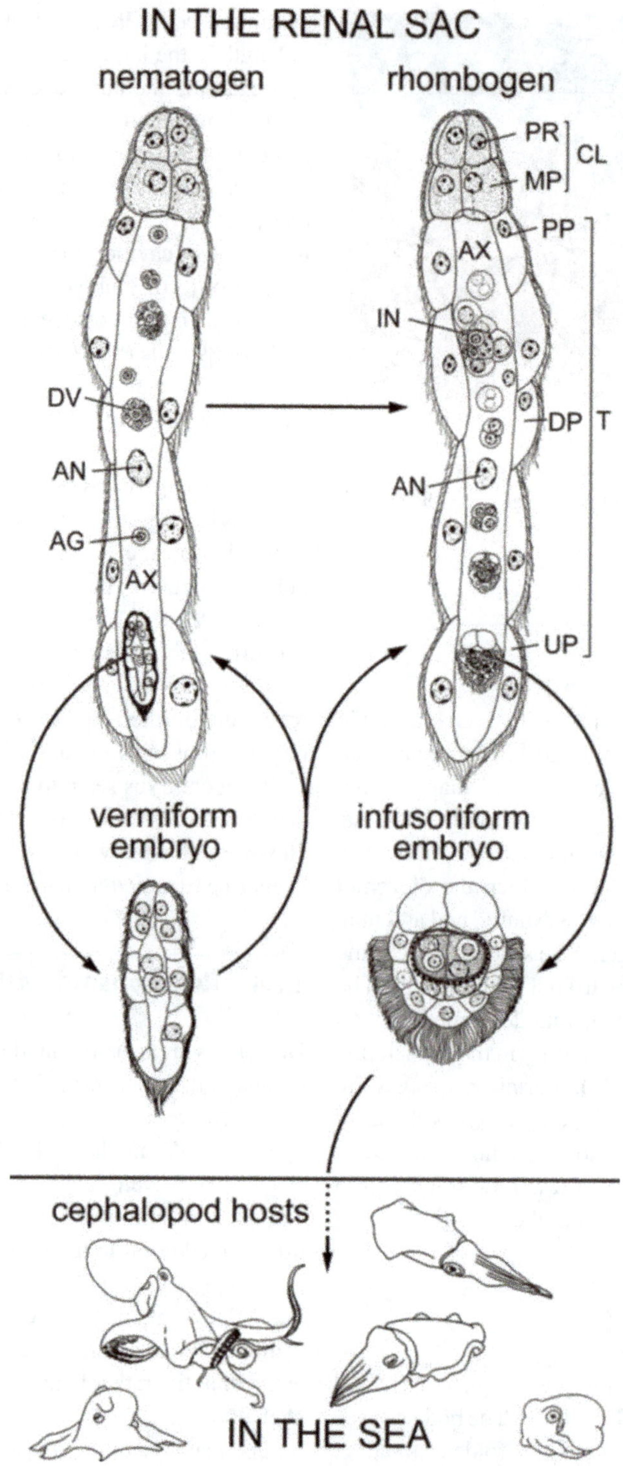

Fig. 11.2 Dicyemid life cycle (modified from Furuya 2016). The dashed line indicates an unknown process involved in the infection of a new cephalopod and development into adult forms. In vermiform stages (nematogen, rhombogen, and vermiform embryo), a large cylindrical axial cell is surrounded by peripheral cells. A calotte is formed by four to ten anterior peripheral cells (propolars and metapolars). The other peripheral cells are diapolars and two of those posterior cells are somewhat specialized as uropolars. The development of hermaphroditic gonads (infusorigens), gametegenesis around the gonads and development of two types of embryos all proceed within the cytoplasm of the axial cell. *Abbreviations* AG, agamete; AN, axial cell nucleus; AX, axial cell; CL, calotte; DP, diapolar cell; DV, developing vermiform embryo; IN, infusorigen; MP, metapolar cell; PP, parapolar cell; PR, propolar cell; T, trunk; UP, uropolar cell

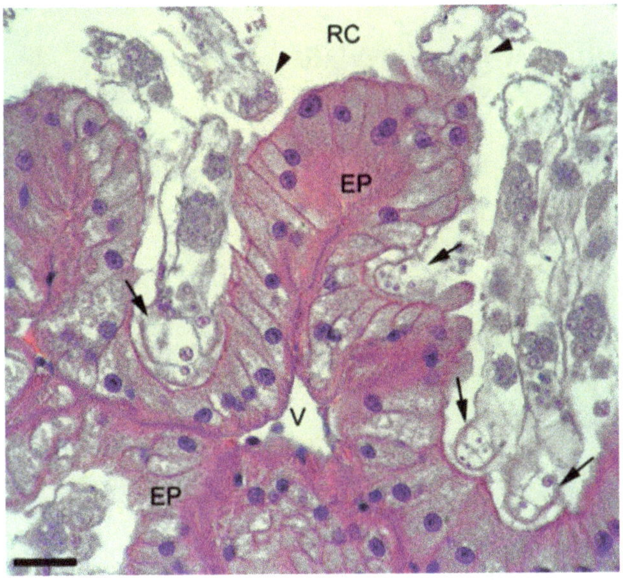

Fig. 11.3 Light micrographs of stained sections through the renal organ of *A. fangsiao*. The niche separation occurs between dicyemid species inhabiting in the renal appendages. *Dicyema akashiense* (arrowhead) lives in the fold of renal appendages, while *D. helocephalum* (arrow) attached on the surface of renal appendages. Scale bar: 20 μm. *Abbreviations* EP, epithelial cell of renal appendage; RC, renal coelom; V, vein

the host (Ridley 1968; Furuya et al. 1997) or attach to surfaces of the renal appendages with a flat anterior region (Furuya et al. 2003a; Furuya 2005, 2006) (Fig. 11.3).

11.5 Systematic Position

Van Beneden (1876) regarded the dicyemids as intermediate in the body plan between Protozoa and Metazoa, and thus gave them the name Mesozoa. This phylum included other several microscopical enigmatic organisms, *Trichoplax*, *Haplozoon*, *Neresheimeria*, *Salinella*, and orthonectids, which were not assignable to any of phyla. Most of these organisms were subsequently belonged to the other phyla (Hyman 1940). Only dicyemids and orthonectids were often united into a single phylum Mesozoa. Later, Hochberg (1990) and Kozloff (1990) treated them independently as a separate phylum, Dicyemida and Orthonectida, in each review. However, they were still treated as the Mesozoa in the many zoological textbooks, because of their unclear relationships among animals. Several zoologists regard the simple organization of dicyemids to be the result of specialization for parasitism (Nouvel 1947; Stunkard 1954; Ginetsinskaya 1988). However, Hyman (1956), Lapan and Morowitz (1975), and Ohama et al. (1984) concurred that dicyemids are primitive multicellular organisms. Since dicyemids have several protozoan-like features, an affinity to the protozoans has been pointed out (Czaker 2006; Noto and Endoh 2004). Current analyses of molecular sequences have revealed that, rather than truly primitive animals that deserve the name "mesozoan", they probably belong to the lophotrochozoans (Katayama et al. 1995; Kobayashi et al. 1999; Aruga et al. 2007; Suzuki et al.

Fig. 11.4 European dicyemid species. **a** *C. polymorpha*; **b** *M. vespa*; **c** *D. typus*; **d** *Dicyema moschatum*; **e** *Dicyemennea eledones*; **f** *P. truncatum*

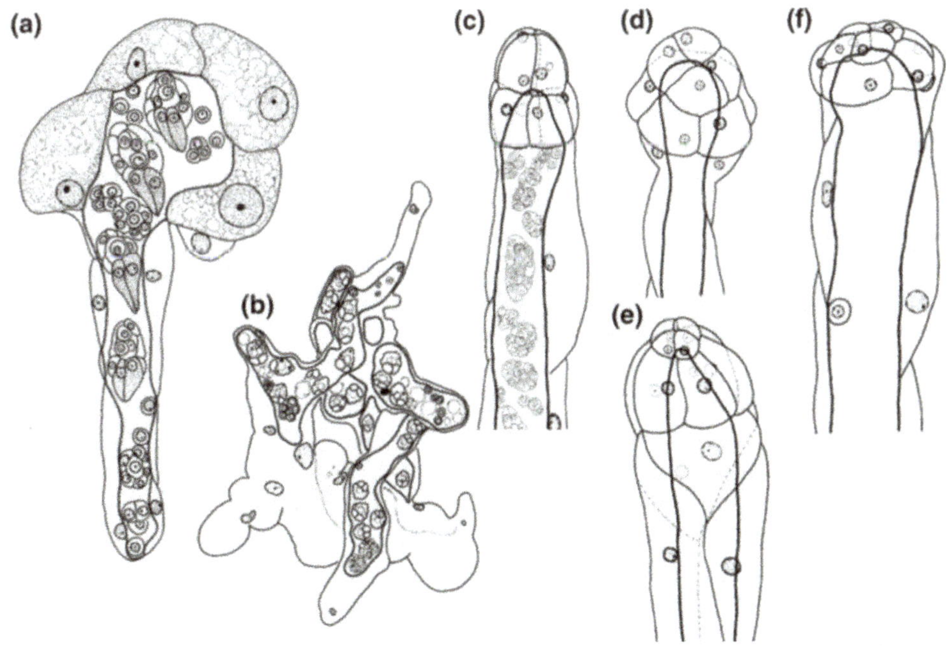

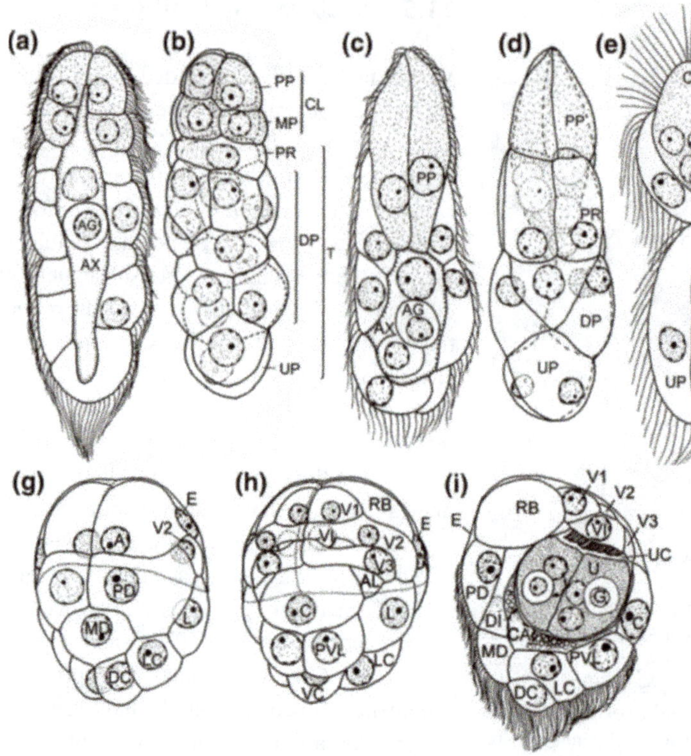

Fig. 11.5 Schematic drawings of vermiform larvae with 22 peripheral cells (**a**, **b**), vermiform larvae of *C. polymorpha* (**c**, **d**), vermiform larvae of *M. vespa* (**e**, **f**), infusoriform larvae with 39 cells (**g–i**) (modified from Furuya and Tsuneki 2003; Furuya 2016). **a**, **f**, lateral view; **b**, **c**, sagittal section; **d**, ventral view; **e**, dorsal view. *Abbreviations* A, apical cell; AG, agamete; AX, axial cell; C, couvercle cell; CA, capsule cell; CL, calotte; DC, dorsal caudal cell; DI, dorsal internal cell; DP, diapolar cell; E, enveloping cell; G, germinal cell; L, lateral cell; LC, lateral caudal cell; MD, median dorsal cell; MP, metapolar cell; PD, paired dorsal cell; PP, parapolar cell; PR, propolar cell; PVL, posteroventral lateral cell; RB, refringent body; SC, short cilia; T, trunk; U, urn cell; UC urn cavity; UP, uropolar cell; VC, ventral caudal cell; VI, ventral internal cell; V1, first ventral cell; V2, second ventral cell; V3, third ventral cell

2010; Mikhailov et al. 2016; Lu et al. 2017). Despite their extremely reduced body plan, dicyemids still appear to exhibit some degree of cell differentiation (Ogino et al. 2011). In this reason, the name Mesozoa is not suited for their phylogenetic place; the Dicyemida, which is the first name of dicyemids by Khrone (1839), has been used as the phylum name of dicyemids in 1999 (Furuya 1999).

11.6 Diversity of Dicyemids in Europe

Cephalopods are commercially important in European countries. Many species of cephalopods have been examined for parasites in European waters. Sixteen species of dicyemids were described from 17 species of cephalopods, so far (Table 11.1). From one to four dicyemid species have been recorded in a single species of cephalopods. Most dicyemid species are host specific. However, 18 dicyemid species are known to have a relatively wide host range (Furuya 1999). In European dicyemids, for instance, *Dicyema macrocephalum* van Beneden (1876) appears to infect five cephalopod species belonging to three genera. The other species with a wide host range have been described mostly without using characters of the infusoriform embryos, so it will be necessary to examine the cellular composition of the infusoriform embryos of these other species to confirm their occurrence in more than one species.

O. vulgaris, the common octopus, is the commercially most important species in the European cephalopods. Therefore, this species has been well studied for the parasite. Four species of dicyemids, *Conocyema polymorpha*, *Dicyema paradoxum*, *Dicyema typus*, and *Dicyemennea lameerei*, have been described from *O. vulgaris* in the Mediterranean Sea, the English Channel, and the Eastern North Atlantic Ocean (Table 11.1). Typically, two or three species of dicyemids are present in each host species or each

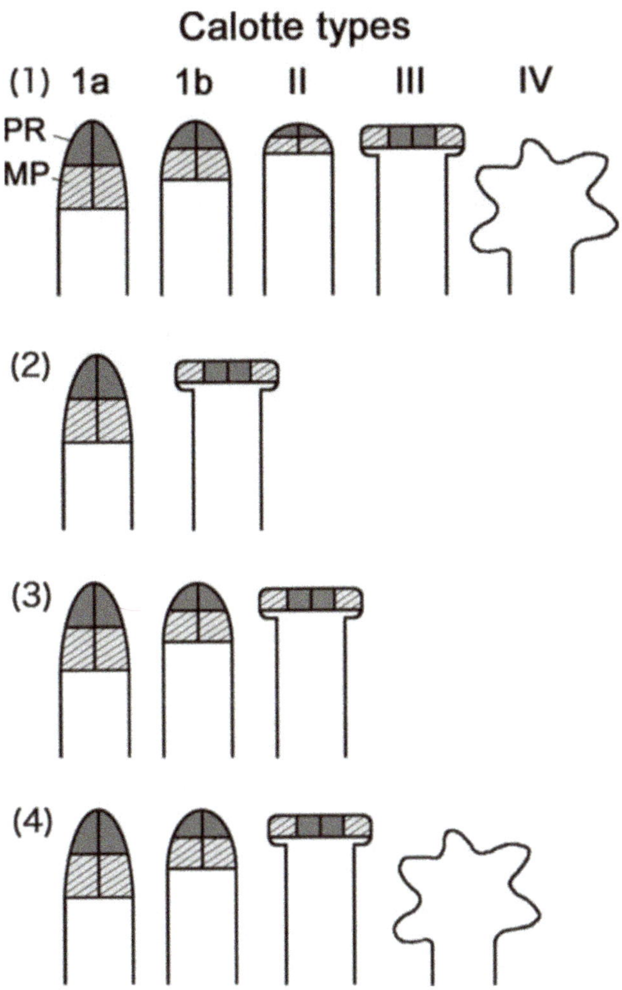

Fig. 11.6 Co-occurrence pattern of calotte shapes usually detected within host individual. (1) Stylized drawings of the main three types of regular calotte configurations and a type of irregular configuration found in vermiform stages. Type I, conical-shaped, is divided into two types (Type Ia and Ib); Type II, cap-shaped; Type III, discoidal; Type IV, an irregular configuration. Shaded and striped areas indicate propolar cells and metapolar cells, respectively. (2) When two species of dicyemids are present, two distinct calotte shapes, conical and discoidal, are usually observed. (3) When three species of dicyemids are present, three types of calotte configurations are usually observed, conical (two grades) and discoidal. (4) When more than four species of dicyemids are present, at least one species is characterized by its rare irregular shaped calotte that spreads, connects with other individuals, and forms a syncytium

host individual, all four species were never simultaneously present in a single-host individual (Furuya et al. 2003b). *Dicyema* and *Dicyemennea* are common, and the largest number of species is placed in these genera. Several other genera are monotypic or contain only a small number of species. *C. polymorpha* is the unusual dicyemid, which is irregular in shape and lacking external cilia (Fig. 11.7). It has relatively small-sized species with 12 peripheral cells. The vermiform larvae are cuneiform and have distinct calottes, which consist of only single tier of four propolar cells. In this species, four parapolar cells are located in the posterior part of propolar cells instead of metapolar cells (Fig. 11.5).

S. officinalis is also commercial species in Europe countries; it is a common inhabitant of the English Channel and Mediterranean Sea. Four species of dicyemids are also recorded from this host cephalopod, namely, *Dicyemennea gracile*, *Pseudicyema truncatum*, *Dicyema whitmani*, and *Microcyema vespa* (Table 11.1). *M. vespa* is unusual in that the body forms a syncytium and the calotte is irregular (Fig. 11.7). In *M. vespa*, the calotte region can only be recognized in the larval stage (Fig. 11.5) (Furuya et al. 2001). *P. truncatum* is the most common species observed with the highest prevalence, nearly 80%. In contrast, *D. whitmani* is a very rare species that has been found in only one cuttlefish host individual collected off Naples, Italy (Furuya and Hochberg 1998).

The dicyemid fauna in the coastal areas of the United States and Japan has been well studied (Furuya 2016), as well as in European waters. The cephalopod fauna in European waters is similar to the Japanese waters, not to the United States, because no cuttlefish (*Sepia*) lives in the coastal areas of the United States. From the ecological viewpoint, *O. vulgaris* and *S. officinalis* are comparable to the Japanese species, *Octopus sinensis* and *Sepia esculenta*, respectively. *O. sinensis* has been regarded as the same species as *O. vulgaris* (Gleadall 2016). *S. esculenta* is a common cuttlefish in Japanese waters. However, *Conocyema* and *Microcyema* species have never been found in these host species and the other Japanese cephalopods. The presence of various genera may be characteristic of the dicyemid fauna in Europe.

Table 11.1 Dicyemids from cephalopod species in European waters

Cephalopods	Dicyemids	Locality	References
Octopoda			
Bathypolypus sponsalis	*Dicyemodeca delamarei*	Mediterranean (Spain)	Nouvel (1961)
Eledone cirrhosa	*D. eledones*	Eastern North Atlantic Ocean (Sweden, Norway), English Channel (France), Mediterranean (Italy, France)	Wagener (1857); Whitmann (1883); Hartmann (1906); Nouvel (1947); Dhikra et al. (2016)
	D. lameerei	English Channel (France)	Nouvel (1947)
Eledone moschata	*D. moschatum*	Mediterranean (Italy, France)	van Beneden (1876); Whitmann (1883); Hartmann (1906); Nouvel (1947)
	D. eledones	Mediterranean (Italy, France)	Wagener (1857); Whitmann (1883); Nouvel (1947)
Octopus defilippi	*Dicyema microcephalum*	Mediterranean (Italy, France)	Whitmann (1883); Nouvel (1947)
Octopus macropus	*D. paradoxum*	Mediterranean (Italy, Monaco, France)	van Beneden (1876); Whitmann (1883), Nouvel (1947)
Octopus salutii	*Dicyema banyulensis*	Mediterranean (Italy, France)	Furuya and Hochberg (1998)
	Dicyema benedeni	Mediterranean (Italy, France)	Furuya and Hochberg (1998)
	D. eledones	Mediterranean (Italy, France)	Wagener (1857); Whitmann (1883); Hartmann (1906); Nouvel (1947)
O. vulgaris	*C. polymorpha*	Mediterranean (Italy, Monaco, France)	Whitmann (1883); Hartmann (1939); Nouvel (1947)
	D. paradoxum	English Channel (France), Mediterranean (Italy, France)	von Kolliker (1849); van Beneden (1876); Whitmann (1883); Nouvel (1947)
	D. typus	English Channel (France, England), Eastern North Atlantic Ocean (France), Mediterranean (Italy, Monaco, France)	van Beneden (1876); Nouvel (1947)
	D. lameerei	English Channel (France), Eastern North Atlantic Ocean (France), Mediterranean (Italy, Monaco, France)	Nouvel (1947)
Sepioidea			
Sepia elegans	*D. macrocephalum*	Mediterranean (Italy, Monaco, France)	van Beneden (1876); Whitmann (1883); Hartmann (1906); Nouvel (1947)
	Dicyema schulzianum	Mediterranean (Italy, Monaco, France)	van Beneden (1876); Nouvel (1947)
S. officinalis	*D. whitmani*	Mediterranean (Italy, France)	Furuya and Hochberg (1998)
	D. gracile	English Channel (France), Mediterranean (Italy, Monaco, France)	Wagener (1857); Whitmann (1883); Nouvel (1947)
	M. vespa	English Channel (France), Mediterranean (Italy, Monaco, France)	van Beneden (1882); Nouvel (1947)
	P. truncatum	English Channel (France), Eastern North Atlantic Ocean (France), Mediterranean (Italy, France, Spain)	Whitmann (1883); Nouvel (1947)
Sepia orbignyana	*D. gracile*	Mediterranean (France, Spain)	Wagener (1857); Whitmann (1883); Nouvel (1947)
	P. truncatum	Mediterranean (Italy, Monaco, France)	Whitmann (1883); Nouvel (1947)
Sepiolioidea			
Rondeletia minor	*Dicyema rondeletia*	Mediterranean (Italy, Monaco, France)	Nouvel (1944)
	D. schulzianum	Mediterranean (Italy, Monaco, France)	van Beneden (1876); Whitmann (1883); Nouvel (1947)

(continued)

Table 11.1 (continued)

Cephalopods	Dicyemids	Locality	References
Rossia macrosoma	*P. truncatum*	Mediterranean (Italy, Monaco, France)	Whitmann (1883); Nouvel (1947)
Sepetta neglecta	*D. rondeletiolae*	Mediterranean (Italy, Monaco, France)	Nouvel (1944)
Sepietta obscura	*D. macrocephalum*	Mediterranean (Italy, Monaco, France)	van Beneden (1876); Whitmann (1883); Nouvel (1947)
Sepietta oweniana	*D. macrocephalum*	Mediterranean (Italy, Monaco, France)	van Beneden (1876); Whitmann (1883); Nouvel (1947)
	D. rondeletiolae	Mediterranean (Italy, Monaco, France)	Nouvel (1944)
Sepiola rondeleti	*D. moschatum*	Mediterranean (Monaco, France)	Whitmann (1883); Nouvel (1947)
Sepiola steenstrupiana	*D. macrocephalum*	Mediterranean (Italy, Monaco, France)	van Beneden (1876); Whitmann (1883); Nouvel (1947)
	D. microcephalum	Mediterranean (Italy, Monaco, France)	Whitmann (1883); Nouvel (1947)

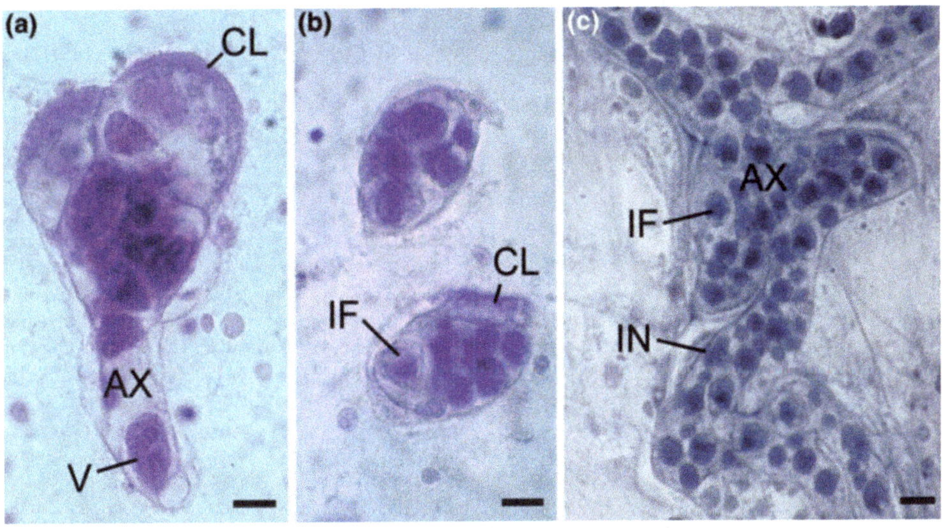

Fig. 11.7 Light micrographs of *C. polymorpha* (**a**, **b**) and *M. vespa* (**c**). Scale bars represent 20 μm. *Abbreviations* AX, axial cell; CL, calotte; IF, infusoriform embryo; IN, infusorigen; V, vermiform embryo

11.7 Concluding Remarks

What I always consider first is when they met cephalopods and where dicyemids come from. The earliest dicyemids must be harmful as well as many other parasites. However, it seems that dicyemids took a new way of life call the "symbiosis". Now dicyemids do no harm to their host cephalopods, rather may give benefits. In this sense, dicyemids are considered to be one of the most advanced parasites.

References

Aruga J, Odaka YS, Kamiya A, Furuya H (2007) Dicyema Pax6 and Zic: tool-kit genes in a highly simplified bilaterian. BMC Evol Biol 7:201

Bresciani J, Fenchel T (1965) Studies on dicyemid Mesozoa. I. The fine structure of the adult (nematogen and rhombogen stage). Vidensk Med Dansk Naturh For 124:367–408

Castellanos-Martinez S, Aguirre-Macedo ML, Furuya H (2016) Two new species of dicyemid mesozoans (Dicyemida: Dicyemidae) from *Octopus maya* Voss and Solis-Ramirez (Octopodidae) off Yucatan, Mexico. Syst Parasitol 93:551–564

Catalano SR (2013) First descriptions of dicyemid mesozoans (Dicyemida: Dicyemidae) from Australian octopus (Octopodidae) and cuttlefish (Sepiidae) species, including a new record of *Dicyemennea* in Australian waters. Folia Parasitol 60:306–320

Czaker R (2006) Serotonin immunoreactivity in a highly enigmatic metazoan phylum, the pre-nervous Dicyemida. Cell Tiss Res 326:843–850

Dhikra S, Florent I, Dellinger M, Justine JL, Romdhane MS, Grellier P, Furuya H (2016) Redescription of *Dicyemennea eledones* (Wagener, 1857) (Phylum Dicyemida) from *Eledone cirrhosa* (Lamark, 1789) (Mollusca: Cephalopoda: Octopoda). Syst Parasitol 93:905–915

Furuya H (1999) Fourteen new species of dicyemid mesozoans from six Japanese cephalopods, with comments on host specificity. Species Diver 4:257–319

Furuya H (2005) Three new species of *Dicyema* (Phylum Dicyemida) from *Amphioctopus kagoshimensis* (Mollusca: Cephalopoda: Octopodidae). Species Diver 10:231–247

Furuya H (2006) Three new species of dicyemid mesozoans (Phylum Dicyemida) from *Amphioctopus fangsiao* (Mollusca: Cephalopoda), with comments on the occurrence patterns of dicyemids. Zool Sci 23:105–119

Furuya H (2016) Diversity and morphological adaptation of dicyemids in Japan. Springer, Anim Diver Gener, pp 401–417

Furuya H, Hochberg FG (1998) Three new species of *Dicyema* (Phylum Dicyemida) from cephalopods in the Western Mediterranean. Vie et Milieu 49:117–128

Furuya H, Tsuneki K (2003) Biology of Dicyemid Mesozoan. Zool Sci 20:519–532

Furuya H, Tsuneki K, Koshida Y (1997) Fine structure of a dicyemid mesozoan, *Dicyema acuticephalum*, with special reference to cell junctions. J Morphol 231:297–305

Furuya H, Hochberg FG, Tsuneki K (2001) Developmental patterns and cell lineages of vermiform embryos in dicyemid mesozoans. Biol Bull 201:405–416

Furuya H, Hochberg FG, Tsuneki K (2003a) Calotte morphology in the phylum Dicyemida: niche separation and convergence. J Zool 259:361–373

Furuya H, Hochberg FG, Tsuneki K (2003b) Reproductive traits of dicyemids. Mar Biol 142:693–706

Furuya H, Hochberg FG, Tsuneki K (2004a) Cell number and cellular composition in infusoriform larvae of Dicyemid Mesozoans (Phylum Dicyemida). Zool Sci 21:877–889

Furuya H, Ota M, Kimura R, Tsuneki K (2004b) The renal organs of cephalopods: a habitat for dicyemids and chromidinids. J Morphol 262:629–643

Ginetsinskaya TA (1988) Trematodes, their life cycles, biology and evolution. (Translation of the original Russian edition, 1968) Amerind Publishing Co. Pvt. Ltd., New Delhi

Gleadall IG (2016) *Octopus sinensis* d'Orbigny, 1841 (Cephalopoda: Octopodidae): valid species name for the commercially valuable East Asian common octopus. Species Diver 21:31–42

Hartmann M (1906) "Untersuchungen ueber den Generationswechsel der Diyemedin" Mem Acad Roy Belgique Serie 2, 17

Hochberg FG (1982) The "kidneys" of cephalopods: a unique habitat for parasites. Malacologia 23:121–134

Hochberg FG, Short RB (1983) *Dicyemennea discocephala* sp. n. (Mesozoa Dicyemidae) in a finned octopod from the Antarctic. J Parasitol 69:963–966

Hochberg FG (1990) Diseases caused by protistans and mesozoans. In: Kinne O (ed) Diseases of marine animals, vol III. Biologische Anstalt Helgoland, Hamburg, pp 47–202

Hyman LH (1940) The invertebrates. Protozoa through Ctenophora, vol I. McGraw Hill, New York, pp 233–247

Hyman LH (1956) The invertebrates. Smaller coelomate groups, vol V. McGraw Hill, New York, pp 713–715

Katayama T, Wada H, Furuya H, Sato N, Yamamoto M (1995) Phylogenetic position of the dicyemid Mesozoa inferred from 18S rDNA sequences. Biol Bull 189:81–90

Kobayashi M, Furuya H, Holland WH (1999) Dicyemids are higher animals. Nature 401:762

Kozloff EN (1990) Phyla Placozoa, Dicyemida, and Orthonectida. In: Invertebrates. Saunders College Publishing, Philadelphia, pp 210–220

Lapan EA (1975a) Studies on the chemistry of the octopus renal system and an observation on the symbiotic relationship of the dicyemid Mesozoa. Comp Biochem Physiol 52:651–657

Lapan EA (1975b) Inositol polyphosphate deposits in the dense bodies of mesozoan dispersal larvae. Exp Cell Res 83:143–151

Lapan EA, Morowitz HJ (1975) The dicyemid Mesozoa as an integrated system for morphogenetic studies. 1. Description, isolation and maintenance. J Exp Zool 193:147–160

Lu T-M, Kanda M, Satoh N, Furuya H (2017) The phylogenetic position of dicyemid mesozoans offers insights into spiralian evolution. Zool Letters 3:6

Matsubara JA, Dudley PL (1976) Fine structural studies of the dicyemid mesozoan, *Dicyemennea californica* McConnaughey, II. The young vermiform stage and the infusoriform larva. J Parasitol 62:390–409

McConnaughey BH (1951) The life cycle of the dicyemid Mesozoa. University of California Press, Berkeley and Los Ángeles 55:295–336

Mikhailov KV, Slyusarev GS, Nikitin MA, Logacheva MD, Penin AA, Aleoshin VV (2016) The genome of *Intoshia linei* affirms orthonectids as highly simplified spiralians. Curr Biol 26:1–7

Noto T, Endoh H (2004) A "chimera" theory on the origin of dicyemid mesozoans: evolution driven by frequent lateral gene transfer from host to parasite. Biosystem 73:73–83

Nouvel H (1944) Les Dicyémides des Sepiolidae des côtes françaises. Bull Inst Océanogr Monaco 869:1–12

Nouvel H (1945) Les Dicyémides de quelque Céphalopodes côtes françaises avec indication de la presence de Chromidinides. Bull Inst Océanog Monaco 887:1–8

Nouvel H (1947) Les Dicyémides. 1re partie: systématique, générations, vermiformes, infusorigène et sexualité. Arch Biol, Paris 58:59–220

Nouvel H (1961) Un Dicyémide nouveau, *Pleodicyema delamarei* n. g., n. sp., parasite du Céphalopode *Bathypolypus sponsalis*, remarques sur la validité des genres *Dicyemodeca* Wheeler, *Pseudicyema* Nouvel et *Microcyema* v. Bened. Vie Milieu 12:565–574

Ogino K, Tsuneki K, Furuya H (2011) Distinction of cell types in *Dicyema japonicum* (Phylum Dicyemida) by expression patterns of 16 genes. J Parasitol 97: 596–601

Ohama T, Kumazaki T, Hori T, Osawa S (1984) Evolution of multicellular animals as deduced from 5Sribosomal RNA sequences: a possible early emergence of the Mesozoa. Nucleic Acids Res 12:5101–5108

Ridley RK (1968) Electron microscopic studies on dicyemid mesozoa. I. Vermiform stages. J Parasitol 54:975–998

Short RB (1971) Three new species of *Dicyema* (Mesozoa: Dicyemidae) from New Zealand. Antarc Res Ser (Biology of the Antarctic Seas 4) 17:231–249

Short RB (1991) Marine Flora and Fauna of the Eastern United States, Dicyemida. NOAA Tech Rep NMFS 100

Stunkard HW (1954) The life history and systematic relations of the Mesozoa. Q Rev Biol 29:230–244

Suzuki GT, Ogino K, Tsuneki K, Furuya H (2010) Phylogenetic analysis of dicyemid mesozoans (Phylum Dicyemida) from innexin

amino acid sequences: dicyemids are not related to Platyhelminthes. J Parasitol 96:614–625
van Beneden É (1876) Recherches sur les Dicyémides, survivants actuels d'un embranchement des Mésozoaires. Bull Acad Roy Belg 42:3–111
van Beneden É (1882) Contribution à l'histoire des Dicyémides. Arch Biol Paris 3:195–228
von Kölliker A (1849) Über *Dicyema paradoxum*, den Schmarotzer der Venenanhänge der Cephalopoden. Ber König Zootom Anst Würzburg 2:53–58
Wagener GR (1857) Über *Dicyema* Kölliker. Arch Patholo Anat Physiol 1857:354–364
Whitmann CO (1883) A contribution to the embryology, life history, and classification of the dicyemids. Mitt Zoolo Station Neapel 4:1–89

Metazoa and Related Diseases

12

Santiago Pascual, Elvira Abollo, Ivona Mladineo, and Camino Gestal

Abstract

Cephalopods and their metazoan parasites have coevolved in wild fisheries for many years. In fact, helminth larvae and parasitic copepods have been recorded in cephalopods worldwide. This is not surprising considering the important role cephalopods play in the transfer of energy and contaminants in marine food webs. Nerito-oceanic ommastrephid squids are by far the most noticeable trophic bridge for helminth parasites in the marine realm, coastal octopus, and cuttlefish serving as primary host for crustaceans. Although it is highly likely that parasitic infections occurred, relatively little is known about the pathogenic potential of metazoan parasites in naturally infected cephalopods. It is stated that heavy parasitic infections may probably cause host morbidity or poor condition but signs of disease are singularly rare with very few specimens exhibiting disease conditions. Unfortunately, neither robust scientific evidence nor available material is available to support this statement. It is more likely that metazoans may deplete energy stores of infected cephalopods, which are directed toward tissue repair and the host's defense mechanisms. Parasitic infection may thus be considered an environmental stressor and as such a source of uncertainty in the evaluation of the potential productivity of cephalopod populations.

Keywords

Metazoan parasites • Pathogens • Trematodes • Cestodes • Nematodes • Crustaceans • Seafood security

S. Pascual (✉)
Ecology and Biodiversity Department, Institute of Marine Research, Spanish National Research Council (CSIC), 36208 Vigo, Pontevedra, Spain
e-mail: spascual@iim.csic.es

E. Abollo
Centro Tecnológico del Mar, Fundación CETMAR, 36208 Vigo, Pontevedra, Spain
e-mail: eabollo@cetmar.org

I. Mladineo
Institute of Oceanography and Fisheries, 21000 Split, Croatia
e-mail: mladineo@izor.hr

C. Gestal
Aquatic Molecular Pathobiology Group, Institute of Marine Research, Spanish National Research Council (CSIC), 36208 Vigo, Pontevedra, Spain
e-mail: cgestal@iim.csic.es

12.1 Introduction

Metazoan parasites comprise a polyphyletic group made up of six parasitic taxa: flatworms (Platyhelminthes), tapeworms (cestodes), trematodes (flukes), roundworms (nematodes), acanthocephalans, and crustaceans. They exhibit complex life cycles and reproductive strategies, with a remarkable high diversity and prevalence in marine ecosystems. Ecto- and endoparasitic metazoans including monoxenous/heteroxenous and specialist/generalist species have been largely recorded in the different components (zooplankton, fish, large fish, marine mammals, and seabirds) of the trophic cascades characteristically defined in the marine realm (Rohde 2002).

C. Gestal et al. (eds.), *Handbook of Pathogens and Diseases in Cephalopods*,
https://doi.org/10.1007/978-3-030-11330-8_12

Recently, spatially explicit modeling revealed that European cephalopod distributions match contrasting trophic pathways (Puerta et al. 2015), and therefore it is expected that cephalopods are common hosts for metazoan parasites. Such statement is not surprising considering that cephalopods are key element in the food web, its foraging behavior and diet facilitates endoparasite transmission. Furthermore, cephalopods inhabit in a wide array of biotopes (shallow to deeper waters)/ecosystems (benthic to pelagic), and its varied social structure and behavior capabilities (solitary, scholar) may also enable an ectoparasitic recruitment into major cephalopod stocks. The above both arguments provide us a broad perspective to understand the great availability of ubiquitous microhabitats offered by cephalopods to colonization by metazoan parasites. In fact, the reported species composition of the metazoan fauna-infecting cephalopods being characterized by a relatively uniform and limited composition remains far from saturated, with empty microniches to be colonized.

The general qualitative character of the metazoan fauna of European Atlantic populations of octopus/cuttlefish/squid (coastal-slope species) and short-finned squid (slope-shelf and nerito-oceanic species) is almost the same as that of Mediterranean populations; only a few differences in species composition were observed, which clearly reflects that infection by metazoans (mostly at larval stage) are nonspecific. Overall, the community structure of parasitic metazoans of European cephalopods is similar among ecologically and taxonomically close species. On the basis of 2000 individuals comprising 10 cephalopod species collected at a microgeographic area (Galician waters, NW Spain), González et al. (2003) found some associations between parasite relative species diversity and cephalopod life cycle characteristics. Results showed that those species with similar risk of becoming infected with a given parasite fauna belong to one of three ecological groupings (coastal, intermediate, or nerito-oceanic). It was suggested that the ecological niche of a cephalopod species is more important in determining its risk of parasitic infection than is phylogeny.

Mostly, the narrow range of metazoan parasites found in European cephalopod populations is thus characterized by wide host specificity. In the life cycles of the reported parasitic helminths, cephalopods may be considered second intermediate or transport/paratenic hosts serving as trophic bridges for parasite flow to top predators (final hosts) (Pascual et al. 1996a; Abollo et al. 1998).

Moreover, the composition of the parasitocoenoses of European cephalopods seems to remain stable over time. Another issue is the marked differences noted in the infection rate. The demographic infection parameters of a given cephalopod species within a particular ecological group may vary among ecoregions and even province of a particular European marine realm. As a rule, infections by metazoan parasites are significantly higher in northern European seas and Lusitanian provinces than in the Mediterranean basin. Furthermore, the size/weight/sexual maturity structure of a given cephalopod grouping is recognized as the key categorical predictor of parasite epidemiological values determining the intra- and interspecific variability of the metazoan fauna of European cephalopod stocks. Generally, no significant differences in the infection rate of males and females are observed, but as the size/weight/maturity increase the infection values substantially raise. Additionally, parasite recruitment may vary depending on the definitive host distribution (Kuhn et al. 2016) but especially, at the mesoscale, the recruitment in the mesozooplankton and hyperbenthos are affected by the oceanographic regime (Pascual and González 2007; Gregori et al. 2015). The latter authors gave evidence that at in upwelling systems parasite faunas are impoverished, whereas downwelling relaxing conditions propitiate optimal conditions to successful. Similarly, ontogenetic shifts in cephalopod diet from planktonic invertebrates and small fish planktophages on one side to largest fish preys on the other may contribute to age-related variations in the helminthofauna (from trematodes to cestodes/nematodes). These shifts may also enhance the accumulation process of parasites which largely favors the typical skewed binomial distribution of metazoans in cephalopod populations.

Fragmentary information on the metazoan fauna of European cephalopods based on opportunistic sampling plans within commercial fisheries or market surveys has been produced in 20 papers published in the last 30 years accounting from the latter revision provided by Hochberg (1990). This knowledge progress made on the biodiversity, pathology, and ecological relationships of metazoan parasites affecting cephalopods reflects a poor coverage for species/geographical areas. There can be no doubt of the lack of sufficient critical mass of European scientists in this field, but in a comparative analysis with other commercially important taxa, a historical negligible financial support for research on cephalopod diseases animal group was noted (Pascual and Guerra 2003). The rate of knowledge progress on cephalopod diseases becomes, therefore, a vexing, unbalanced question in fisheries research.

There is, nevertheless, some current regional and national surveillance plans for zoonotic parasites implicated in human allergy (following the scientific opinion on parasite risk in fishery products published by the European Food Safety Authority; EFSA 2010) which may serve as a promising platform for future biodiversity studies on metazoan parasites of cephalopods. The use of already certified biobanking tools in fish parasite research (González et al. 2018) can also aid to establish network opportunities for sampling and collection of traceable metazoan cephalopod parasites.

Against the overall background, the strategy defined in this chapter is not to make a comprehensive literature review of host–parasite systems, but illustrate the role of the most prevalent and relevant metazoan parasites as pathogens and diseases-related agents in European cephalopods. Thereafter, scientific focus for the different taxa which is discussed under the new challenge perspectives.

12.2 Metazoan Parasites as Pathogens

12.2.1 Trematodes

Several monogeneans have been described from European cephalopods (Hochberg 1990), but some forms were considered *incertae sedis* and the type material (holotype, paratype, and syntype) is not largely available. The single extent of evidence came by Llewellyn (1984), who reported gyrodactylids as epidermal browsers in the mantle cavity and on the gills of *Alloteuthis* squids from the North Sea and the English Channel off France and England. These monogeneans are thought to be recruited to the squids through direct contact of adults at the time of mating.

Cephalopods are also parasitized by digenean trematodes, at larval stages (metacercaria) or adults, acting as second intermediate, paratenic, or final host, but never as first intermediate host (Hochberg 1990). Metacercariae of didymozoid are the most important group of digeneans which infects oceanic squids, and some of them have been described in Illex coindetii (Fig. 12.1a) or *Todaropsis eblanae* in European waters (Hochberg 1990). Other groups of digenean trematodes were reported in 10 species of squids, cuttlefish, and octopus from the French and Italian coasts (Mediterranean) and from the English Channel off France and England (Hochberg 1990). Again, the several morphs recognized present taxonomic uncertainty. *Derogenes varicus* were reported in *Sepia officinalis* in the coast of Plymouth, England, where more than 80% of the specimens over 10 cm mantle length appeared to be infected. *Lecithochirium* sp. was reported in *Octopus vulgaris* in the North East Atlantic, NW Spain (Fig. 12.1b–d). This hemiurid shows a fusiform body, with a sub-terminal oral sucker, a small pharynx, big acetabulum, or ventral sucker, with conspicuous acetabular cleft, and excretory vesicle with a characteristic Y-shape.

With some exceptions, most reports of trematodes in cephalopods show a low prevalence of infection, acting as paratenic hosts. Metacercaria and adult digeneans infected the digestive system (especially, the stomach and caecum) and despite they can form oval cysts with thin, transparent envelopes no significant host tissue reaction was noted.

12.2.2 Cestodes

Larval and post-larval stages of cestodes repeatedly have been described from European cephalopods (Hochberg 1990). The prevalence and intensity of infection are high in theuthoid squids, showing a wide range of sizes and shapes in relation to the squid host (Fig. 12.2a, b). Plerocercoid larvae belonging to the orders Tetraphyllidea and Trypanorhynchidea dominate among cestodes (Pascual et al. 1996b), which become sexually mature in the digestive tracts of elasmobranch fishes, sharks, and rays. The scolex of Tetraphyllidean larvae has characteristically four large

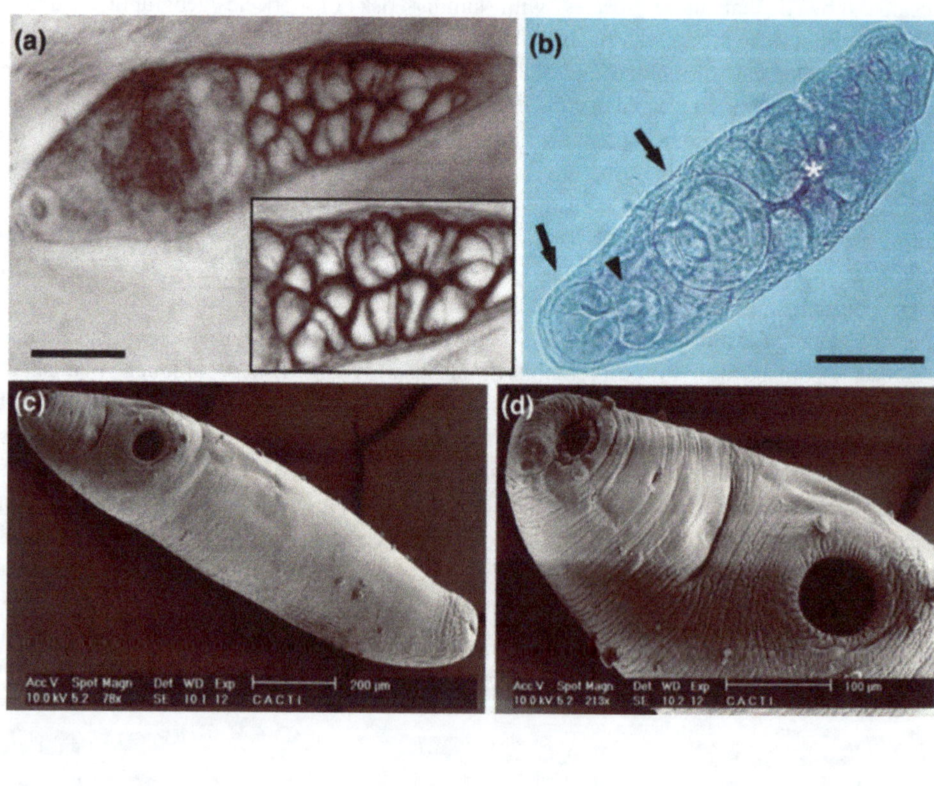

Fig. 12.1 Digenean trematodes from European cephalopods. Whole specimens (ventral view) of didymozoid from from *Illex coindetii* (**a**), and adult *Lecitochirium* sp. (**b**, **c**, **c**) from *Octopus vulgaris* showing oral and ventral sucker, pharynx, acetabular cleft, and excretory vesicle. View at light microscopy (**a**, **b**), and (**c**, **d**) scanning electron microscopy (SEM). Scale bars: A: 200 µm; B: 200 µm; C. 200 µm; D 100 µm

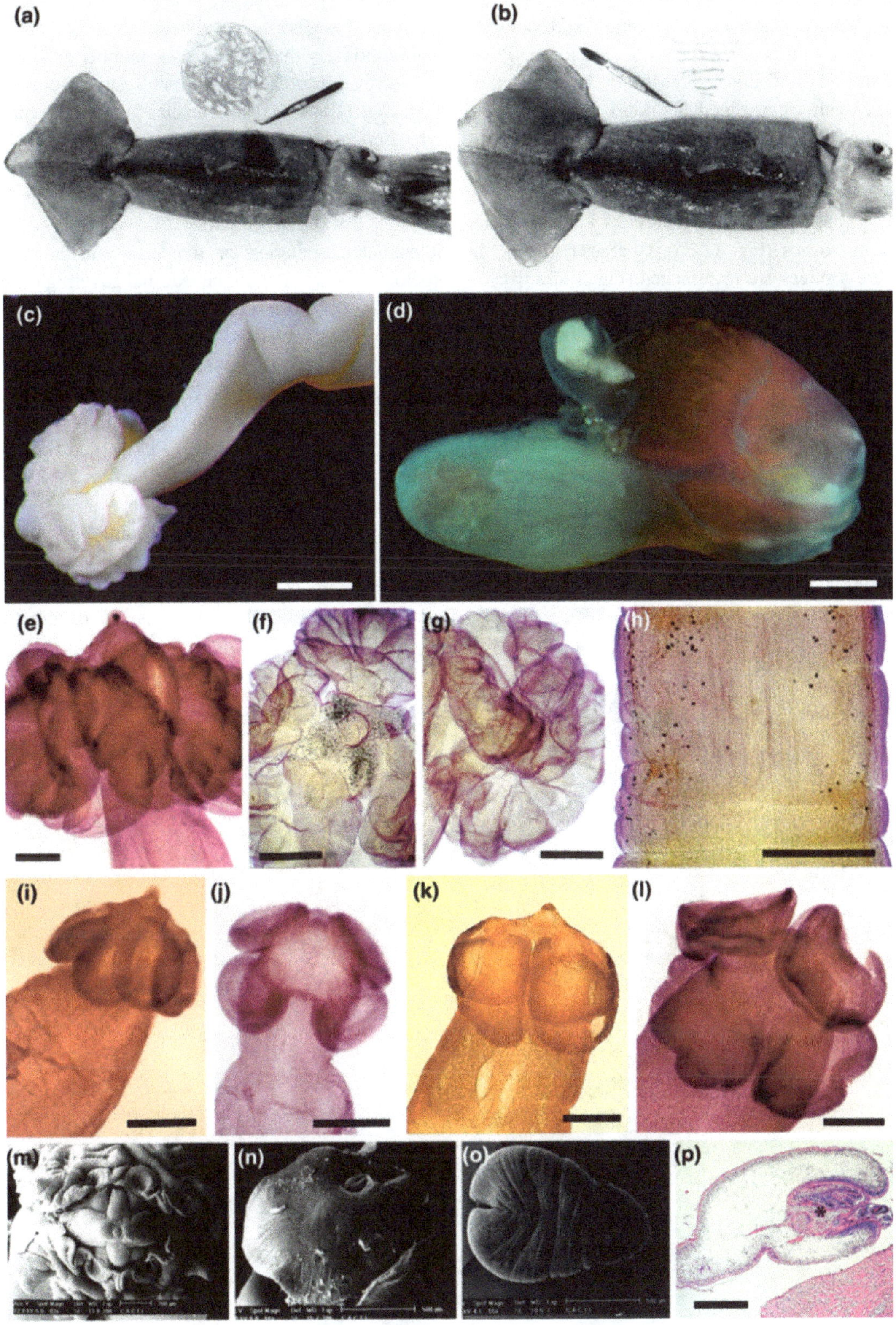

Fig. 12.2 Larval cestodes tetraphyllidean taken from a variety of cephalopod species of Europe. Note the biomass of plerocercoids (**a**) and the range of sizes and shapes (**b**) in relation to the squid host. Light microscopy of two typical body architecture of tetraphyllideans (**c**, **d**), showing the phenotypic plasticity of their scolices: with wavy-edged bothridia (**e–g**), smooth-oval bothridia (**i–k**), and scalloped-edged bothridia (**l**). Tegument (**h**) and apical and bothridial sucker in apical (**m**, **n**) view of scolex. Characteristically, in some cases, the scolices are invaginated as seen in scanning electron microscopy (**o**) and histological section (**p**). (**e–h**) Alcoholic Gill's Haematoxylin. (**p**) H&E. Scale bars: C: 1 mm; D: 5 mm; E: 100 μm; F: 100 μm; G: 100 μm; H: 500 μm; I: 200 μm; J: 100 μm; K: 100 μm; L: 100 μm; M: 200 μm; N: 500 μm; O: 500 μm; P: 250 μm

leaf-like bothridia. The genus *Phyllobothrium* is the most common and widely dispersed in decapod and octopod cephalopods from European waters (Fig. 12.2c, d). Phyllobothriid larvae are divided into three groups by the form of their bothridia: with wavy-edged bothridia (Fig. 12.2e, g), smooth-oval bothridia (Fig. 12.2i, k), and scalloped-edged bothridia (Fig. 12.2l). An apical sucker is also observed (M, N). They show one accessory sucker by bothridia and one apical sucker. The tegument of the body is covered by microvilli or microtrics (Fig. 12.2h). Characteristically, in some cases, the scolices are invaginated (Fig. 12.2o, p).

Plerocercoids are mainly lying free in the lumen or attached to the organs of the digestive tract (stomach, caecum, and rectum) (Fig. 12.2p), although sometimes found free in the liver, mantle cavity, and even leaving the host. Plerocercoids move freely between these organs, especially when changes in temperature and other physico-chemical factors occurred in postmortem condition. This movement of large forms has been suggested to impair the marketability of the infected specimens considerably due to the unaesthetic appearance of the fish product.

Other Tetraphyllidean larvae have been reported from European cephalopods within the *Scolex spp.* species complex. Despite the yet unresolved uncertainty of their taxonomic affinities, these forms are well recognized by their smaller sizes and bothridia with a characteristic number of suckers.

Larval Tetrarhynchidean metacestodes characteristically with four hook-armed tentacles are well represented by *Nybelinia* plercocerci in European cephalopods. *Nybelinia* is commonly encountered found in a variety of cephalopods in the NE Atlantic and Mediterranean cephalopods (Pascual et al. 1996a). *N. lingualis* (Cuvier 1817) localizes in intestinal mesenteries, on the ovary, on the linings of the coelomic cavity, and on the external covering of the stomach (Fig. 12.3a). The scolex is composed of four sessile bothridia showing four tentacles or proboscids armed by small helicoidally placed hooks (Fig. 12.3b). They can be observed evaginated (Fig. 12.3a, b, d), or invaginated into the body (Fig. 12.3c). Despite the intensity of infection can be significantly high in larger squids and the tentacles are used to anchor the host's tissues, no noticeable report on the pathological effect of these cestodes was found in the literature, with the exception of specific light infiltration of hemocytes in the infected area (Fig. 12.3e).

Most reports of cestodes in European cephalopods simply document the presence of cestodes, site of infection, sample

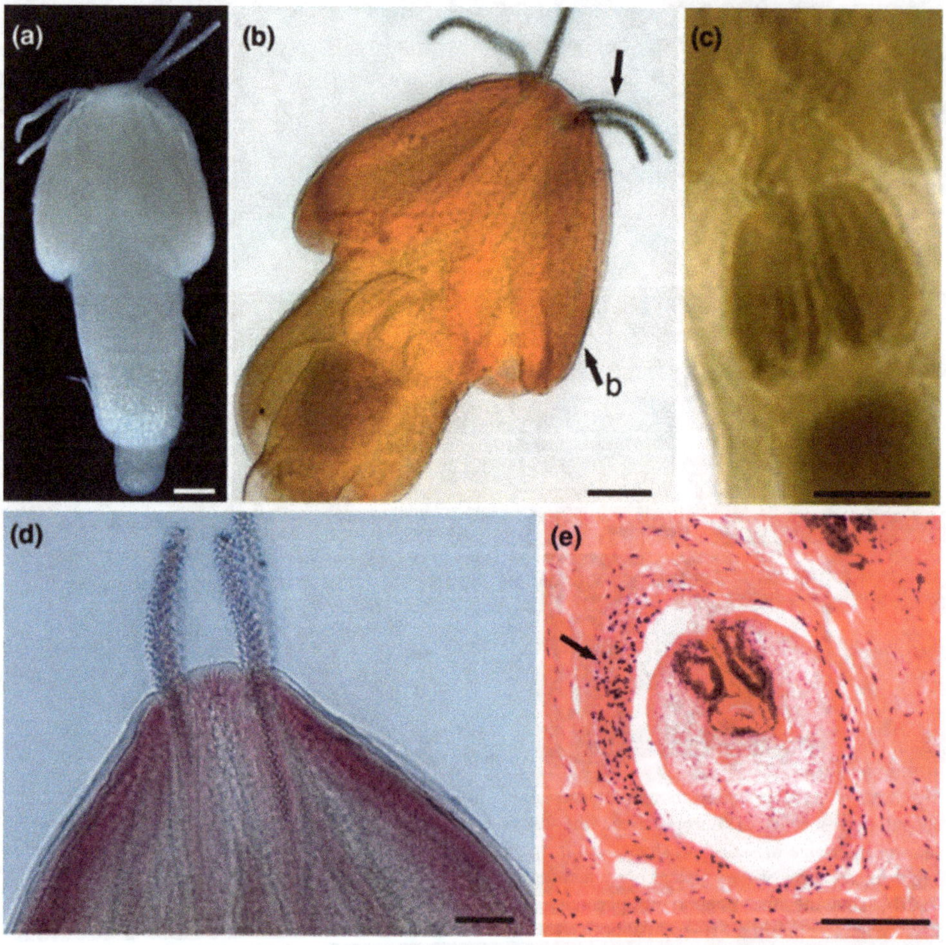

Fig. 12.3 Larval tetrarhynchidean of *Nybelinia lingualis* from a variety of hosts. Stereomicroscopy (**a**) and light microscopy (**b**) image of the typical body architecture of tetrarhynchideans, showing four sessile bothridia with four tentacles armed with hooks in spirals. Detail of the hooks observed invaginated into the body (**c**) or evaginated (**d**). Histological section showing specific light infiltration of hemocytes surrounding the infected area (**e**) H&E stain. Scale bars: A: 250 μm; B: 250 μm; C: 250 μm; D:250 μm; E: 100 μm

locality, and some demographic infection parameter. Despite singular effort has been concentrated on the ecological relationships of cephalopod–cestode systems (e.g., Gaevskaya and Nigmatulli 1978; Pascual et al. 1996b) as a whole neither pathological nor disease symptoms have been mentioned or figured associated to the cestode infections.

12.2.3 Nematodes

In the last years, larval ascaridoid nematodes are by far the most commonly reported parasitic agent in European cephalopods. Survey of anisakids with zoonotic and human allergic potential in cephalopod food products has been a target of some national surveillance plans. In fact, despite in the older literature specific identification for nematode larval types in cephalopods has been suggested as a main taxonomic concern, from the Hochberg's revision (1990) molecular methods have been largely applied to specifically identify the anisakids and their distribution in the organs and tissues of the host (Abollo et al. 2001; Melani et al. 2014; Serracca et al. 2013; Pico-Duran et al. 2016; Cost et al. 2016). Larval stages of *Anisakis simplex* sensu stricto and *A. pegreffii* have been identified parasitizing *Octopus vulgaris*, *Eledone cirrhosa*, *Sepia officinalis*, and other sepiidae species, and with higher prevalence have been identified in loliginids and ommastrephids in European waters (Abollo et al. 1998, 2001). As a rule, anisakids are found covering the outer and inner membranes of internal organs, especially the gonads (ovary and testes), nidamental glands and on the wall of stomach. Sometimes they were found on the coelomic membrane of the mantle wall (Fig. 12.4a, b). In cephalopods at fresh postmortem condition, the viable anisakid larvae can be also found actively moving within the mantle cavity. This provokes commercial rejection by consumers due to the unaesthetic appearance of squid products.

General morphological diagnostic characteristics of larval stages of Anisakis, such as anterior end showing a boring

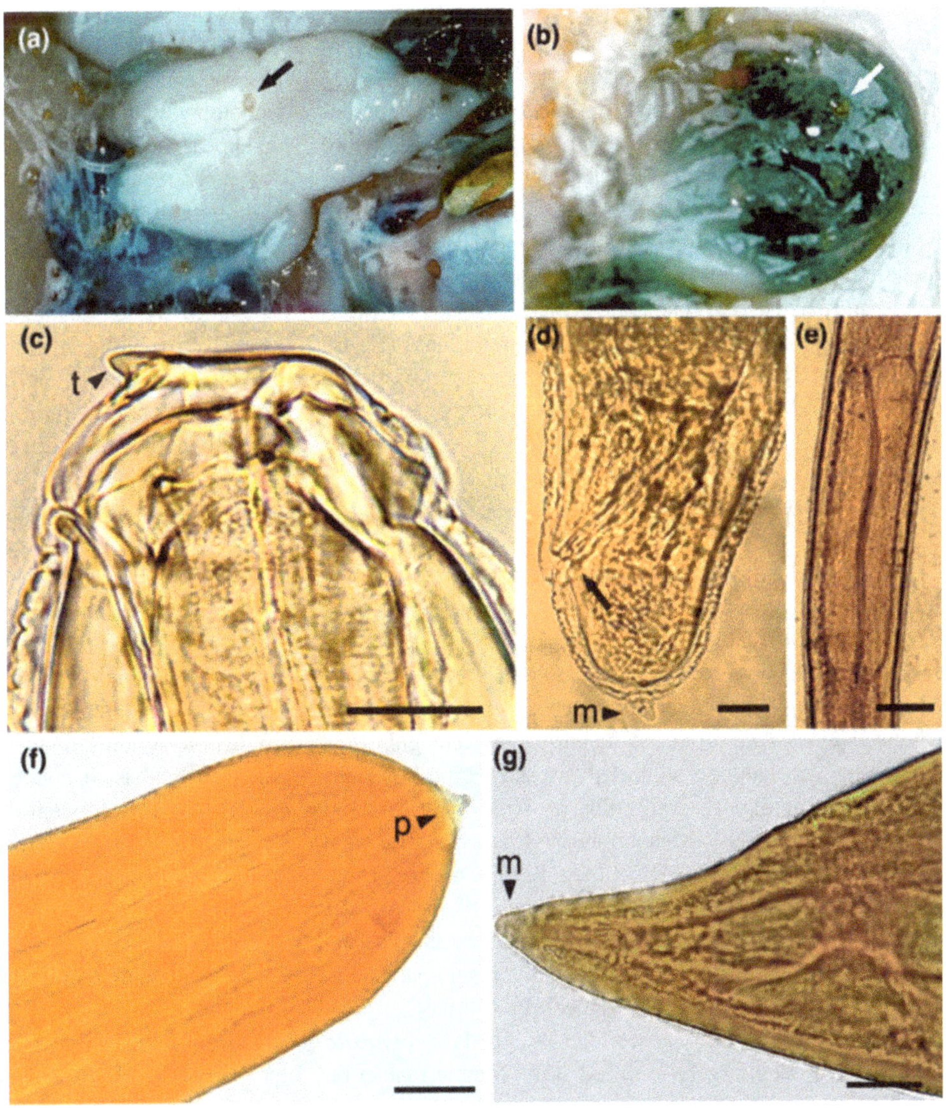

Fig. 12.4 Anisakid nematodes from various cephalopod species in Europe. Third-larval stages are easily recognized macroscopically (**a**, **b**) coiled and encysted in different organs (arrows). Light microscopy images of the anterior (**c**) and posterior (**d**) extremities with the characteristic ventriculus (**e**) of *Anisakis simplex* showing some morphological structures (striated cuticle, boring tooth, excretory pore, lips, esophagus, intestine, anal gland, anus, and mucron) in lateral view. *Cystidicola* sp. nematode from *Octopus vulgaris* (**f**, **g**). Anterior (**f**) and posterior (**g**) extremities showing the characteristic pseudolabia and mucron, respectively. Scale bars: C: 50 µm; D: 30 µm; E: 150 µm; F: 20 µm; G: 20 µm

tooth, mouth, lips with papilla and excretory pore, ventriculous with specific length and shape, and tail end showing the anus and mucron terminal, are shown in Fig. 12.4c, e.

Some nematodes other than ascaridoids occasionally have been observed in European cephalopods. As an example, spirurida larval nematodes of a cystidicolid were found encapsulated in the external and internal walls of the crop, and on the connective tissue sheath surrounding the digestive gland and intestine of the common octopus *O. vulgaris* caught at NW Spain (Gestal et al. 1999a). Larval of Cystidicolidae shows mouth dorsoventrally elongated with a pair of pseudolabia with conical protuberances, two lateral cephalic alae. The esophagus shows an anterior short muscular part and posterior part longer and glandular. Post-anal tail short, with weakly nodulose truncated mucron (Fig. 12.4f, g).

Most recently, some efforts have been made to show the histopathological effect of nematode infections (Pascual et al. 1996b; Gestal et al. 1999a). Early infections consisted of necrotic tissue displaying a light inflammatory reaction followed by haemocyte infiltration. In more advanced case of infection, the response of cephalopod tissues to invading nematodes was a typical cell-mediated immune response (Ford 1992), with parasite encapsulation as an immune strategy to avoid parasite migration and destruction of host tissues (Fig. 12.5a–h). Most infected organs displayed evidence of mechanical compression and displacement of host tissue elements at sites close top or in direct contact with parasitic larvae, with varying degrees of cellular infiltration. The spaces surrounding worms were usually coated with tissue fragments, cell debris, and extensive secretion of mucous. Anisakids were thus postulated as responsible for parasitic castration in those heavily infected mature squids as a consequence of partial destruction and alteration of gonad tissues (Abollo et al. 1998).

12.2.4 Crustaceans

Few published reports dealt with the crustaceans infecting European cephalopods. Branchiurans and cymothoid isopods have been accidentally found on the skin and in the mantle cavity of cuttlefish (*Sepia* and *Sepiola* species). The majority of crustacean reports refer to copepods: harpacticoids of *Cholydia intermedia* from the mantle cavity and gills of a cirroteuthid cephalopod collected in the Faroe-Shetlands Channel; lichomolgids on the gills of *Sepia officinalis* and *T. sagittatus* from NW Mediterranean (Rosas and Banyuls) and the Adriatic (Trieste) (Hochberg 1990; Costanzo et al. 1994), and from the gills of *Illex coindetii* off the Atlantic coast of the Iberian Peninsula (Lopez-González and Pascual 1996); females and males of a cyclopoid copepod parasite in *Octopus vulgaris* from Banyuls (Hochberg 1990).

Larval stages of Lernaeoceridae assigned to *Pennella varians* have been largely recorded at the Mediterranean on the gills of teuthoids (*L. vulgaris, T. eblanae*), cuttlefish (*Sepia officinalis, S. elegans, S. orbignyana, Rossia caroli, Sepietta oweniana*) and octopus (*Octopus vulgaris, E. moschata, Bathypolypus sponsalis*) (Gestal et al. 1999b) (Fig. 12.6a–e).

Heavy infestation by the postembryonic stages of the siphonostomid copepod *Pennella* sp. has also been commonly reported in the gills of several commercially important cephalopod species from temperate waters of the NE Atlantic (Pascual et al. 1996a). The spatiotemporal distribution of this mesoparasitic copepod revealed a marked aggregated and seasonal pattern of parasites that fits well with their mating behavior in the gills of cephalopods (Pascual et al. 2001). Adults of the cyclopoid copepod of the genus Octopicola, *Octopicula superbus* have been identified in European octopuses at the English Channel, Mediterranean, and Atlantic at NW Spain (Fig. 12.6i–l).

Although in the older literature the cephalopod-copepod relationships have been categorized as highly host specific, most of the species were considered commensals. They moved on the skin (of head, arm, or mantle), mantle cavity, and gills, and feed on mucous (Fig. 12.6f–h, m–o), thereby they were considered not true parasites when affecting wild cephalopod populations. In fact, the infected cephalopods did not appear stressed and no damage to the tissues was reported. However, pennellid larvae deserve a special mention. Correlation between heavy gill infections and poorer squid condition at the infrapopulation level has also been demonstrated (Pascual et al. 2005). This work provides strong evidence that mechanical lysing of large areas of functional tissues produced by pennellids contributes to the variability in squid growth, being one of the multiple categorical predictors of size-at-age data in several infested cephalopod species commercially exploited in European waters.

12.3 New Coming Challenges

Modern conception of fisheries management under the Common Fishery Policy and the H2020 Research and Innovation Framework is based on two driven pillars: the ecosystem-based concept and the accommodation of fish production systems to the new seafood system challenge. The final goal is to conquer a better understanding of the natural and anthropogenic impacts on fish resources at the ecosystem level to render productive ecosystems and healthy seafood products.

12.3.1 Seafood Security

Parasitic diseases have been largely recognized as a bottleneck that hampers fish production systems (Shinn et al. 2014).

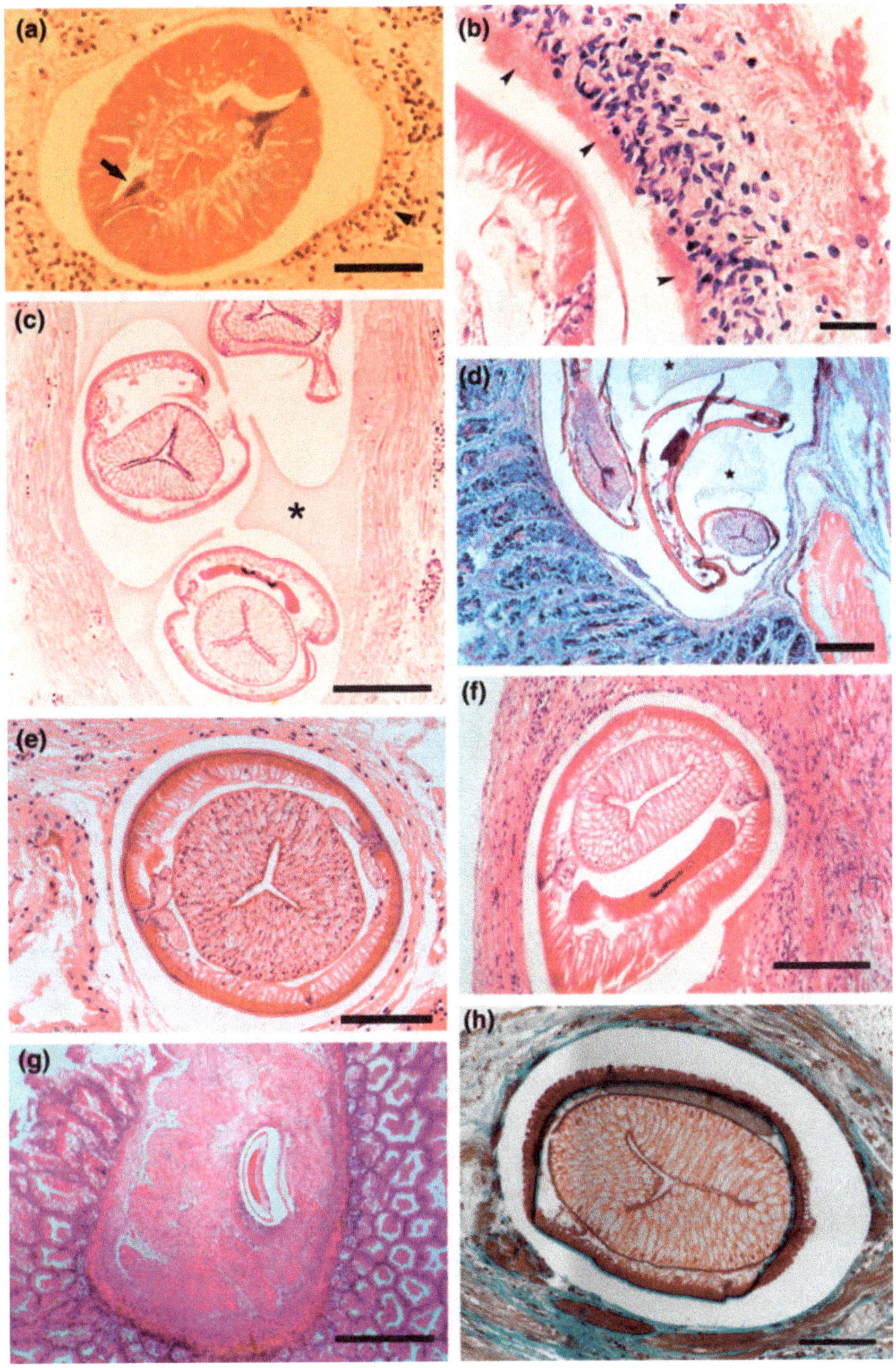

Fig. 12.5 Histopathology caused by larval nematodes in various cephalopod species in Europe. Histological sections showing different aspects of the encapsulation process of nematode larvae in squids (**a**, **b**, **c**, **d**) and octopuses (**e–h**). (**a**) Early infection showing an encapsulated larva of *Anisakis simplex* with the Y-shape lateral chords, and hemocytic infiltration. (**b**) Histological section showing heavy hemocyte infiltration in response to the infection by larval nematodes (arrowheads). (**c**) Later anisakid infection showing extensive secretion of mucous in the spaces surrounding the worms. (**d**) Histological section of connective-muscular tissue of the testis of squid showing mechanical compression and displacement of host tissue elements (*, cell debris). (**e–h**) Later infection in *Octopus vulgaris* showing nematodes larvae encysted in connective tissue capsule with various degrees of hemocyte infiltration. (**g**) Cystidicolid larvae infecting the connective tissue of the digestive gland. (**a**, **b**, **c**, **e**, **f**, **g**) H&E stain. (**d**, **h**) Masson's trichrome stain. Scale bars: A: 100 μm; B: 100 μm; C: 200 μm; D: 250 μm; E: 100 μm; F: 200 μm; G: 20 μm; H: 100 μm

However, as it was summarized in this chapter, apart from histopathological evidences the role of metazoans as etiological agents of pathologies in cephalopod species, stocks, or individuals still remains unexplored. Of particular interest is to estimate the impact of aggregated metazoan infrapopulations on the condition and productivity of cephalopod populations, especially for those species that have fast-growing potential in open-caged systems. Similarly, considering that multiple

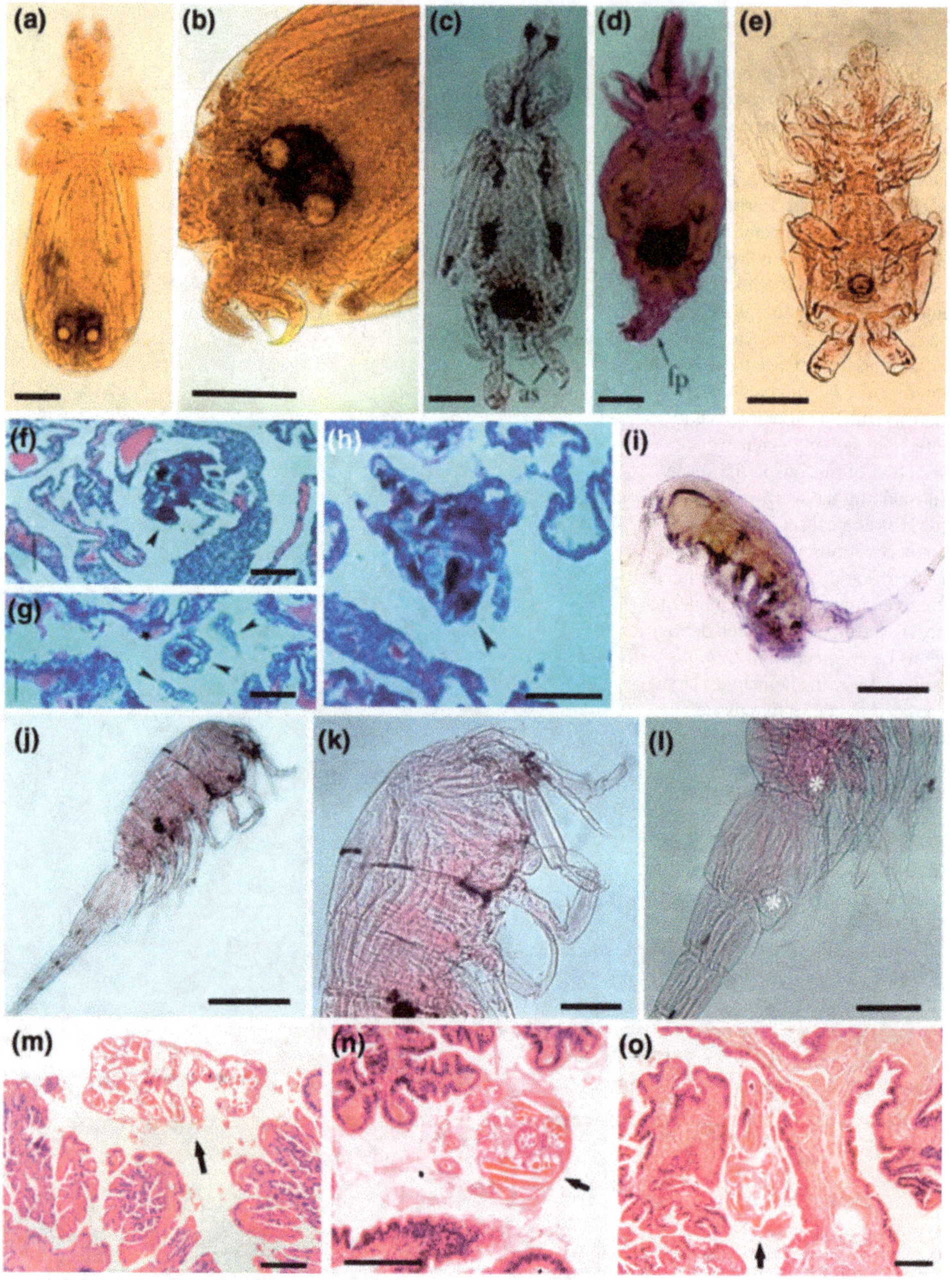

Fig. 12.6 Various ontogenetic stages of the most prevalent copepod (*Pennella* sp.) from the gills of many cephalopod species of Europe. (**a–c**) Copepodid with characteristic second antenna (as); (**d**) chalimus with polar filament (fp); (**e**) free-living adult male. Histological sections of squid gills showing pennellids (arrows) associated to mechanical displacement of host tissues (**f**); secretion of mucous (*) (**g**); mating behavior (arrow) of an adult male and female (**h**). Lichomolgids *Octopicola superbus* (habitus, lateral) from the gills of octopuses (**i–o**). Free-living adults showing the specific morphological characters of the thorax, rostrum, and legs, with specific distribution of spiny and seta (*) (**i–l**). Histological sections of octopus gills showing Lichomolgids free living or anchored to the host tissue (**m–o**). (**f–h**) Masson's trichrome stain. (**m–o**) H&E stain. Scale bars: A: 100 μm; B: 100 μm; C: 100 μm; D: 100 μm; E: 100 μm; F: 200 μm; G: 200 μm; H: 150 μm; I: 300 μm; J: 300 μm; K: 100 μm; L: 50 μm; M: 200 μm; N: 150 μm

infections are common in nature, it would be desirable to analyze the synergistic/antagonistic effect of the different parasitic agents in the well-being of cephalopod populations.

12.3.2 Seafood Safety

Problems in the rational utilization of commercial fisheries include the management of biohazards along fish production value chains. The high pathogenicity for man of the anisakid larvae and their high prevalence and abundance in various commercially exploited fish and cephalopod species draws particular attention to this biohazard (EFSA 2010). Parasites have zoonotic potential (i.e., cause anisakidosis in humans) but also they affect the marketability of seafood products. Exposure to the anisakidosis pathogens at high rate in the mantle cavity of European squids should be properly evaluated as a causative vector in risk analysis of this emerging zoonotic and allergic disease in southern European countries (EFSA 2010).

To achieve the above challenges, systematic study on the biodiversity of the metazoan parasitic fauna of European cephalopods should clearly be a hot spot. Considering the larval stage for most recorded metazoans and in many cases the absence of type specimens, biobanking, and genetic markers are relevant tools to assure the identification of the etiological agent, the characterization of the hazard and the implementation of critical control points.

12.4 Concluding Remarks

Relatively little is known about the pathogenic potential of metazoan parasites in naturally infected cephalopods. It is stated that heavy parasitic infections may probably cause morbidity or poor condition of cephalopods but signs of disease are singularly rare with very few specimens exhibiting disease conditions. Gaevskaya and Nigmatullin (1981) suggested that the greatest injury to the cephalopod *Sthenoteuthis pteropus* may be done by *Tentacularia* larvae, large *Porrocaecum* (which destroy the integrity of the mantle musculature), *Phyllobothrium* (which assimilate part of the nutrients of the squid´s food as they undergo growth and development), and anisakid larvae (which apparently destroy oocytes). Unfortunately, neither robust scientific evidence nor available material is available to support this statement.

As a whole, judging by the magnitude of the extent/intensity of infection, the site of infection, and the fact they can undergo growth, it seems that metazoans may deplete energy stores of infected cephalopods, which are directed toward tissue repair and the host's defense mechanisms. Parasitic infection may thus be considered an environmental stressor and as such a source of uncertainty in the evaluation of the potential productivity of cephalopod populations (Pascual et al. 2007a, b, c).

References

Abollo E, Gestal C, López A, González A, Guerra A, Pascual S (1998) Squid as trophic bridges for parasite flow within marine ecosystems: the case of *Anisakis simplex* (Nematoda: Anisakidae), or when the wrong way can be right. S Afr J Mar Sci 20:223–232

Abollo E, Gestal C, Pascual S (2001) *Anisakis* infestation in marine fish and cephalopods from Galician waters: an updated perspective. Parasitol Res 87:492–499

Cost A, Cammilleri G, Graci S, Buscemi MD et al (2016) Survey on the presence of *A. simplex* s.s. and *A. pegreffii* hybrid forms in Central-Western Mediterranean Sea. Parasitol Inter 65 (6):696–701

Costanzo G, Calafiore N, Crescenti N (1994) Copepodids of *Doridicola longicauda* (Claus, 1860) (Copepoda: Poecilostomatoida: Lichomolgidae) associated with *Sepia officinalis* L. J Crust Biol 14(3):601–608

European Food Safety Agency (2010) Scientific opinion on risk assessment of parasites in fishery products. EFSA 8(4):1543

Ford L (1992) Host defense mechanisms of cephalopods. Annu Rev Fish Disea 1:25–41

Gaevskaya AV, Nigmatullin CM (1978) The helminth fauna ofAtlantic squids of the Family Ommastrephidae (Cephalopoda: Oegopsida). Malcol Rev 11:134–135

Gaevskaya AV, Nigmatullin CM (1981) Several ecological aspects of the parasitic relationships of the flying squid (*Sthenoteuthis pteropus*, Steenstrup, 1855). (In Russian). Biol. Nauki (Mosk.) 1:52–57. (Translation available from F.G. Hochberg)

Gestal C, Abollo E, Arias C, Pascual S (1999a) Larval nematodes (Spiruroidea: Cystidicolidae) in *Octopus vulgaris* (Mollusca: Cephalopoda: Octopodidae) from Northeastern Atlantic Ocean. J Parasitol 85(3):508–511

Gestal C, Belcari P, Abollo E, Pascual S. (1999b) Parasites of cephalopods in the northern Thyrrenian Sea (Western Mediterranean): new host records and host specificity. Sci Mar 63 (1):39–43

González AF, Pascual S, Gestal C, Abollo E, Guerra A (2003) What makes a cephalopod a suitable host for parasites? The case of Galician waters. Fish Res 60(1):177–183

González AF, Rodríguez H, Outeiriño L, Vello C, Larsson C, Pascual S (2018) A biobanking platform for fish-borne zoonotic parasites: a traceable system to preserve samples, data and money. Fish Res 202:29–37

Gregori M, Roura A, Abollo E, González AF, Pascual S (2015) *Anisakis simplex* complex (Nematoda: Anisakidae) in zooplankton communities from temperate NE Atlantic waters. J Nat Hist 49(13–14):755–773

Hochberg FG (1990) Diseases of Mollusca: Cephalopoda (Diseases caused by protistans and metazoans). In: Kinne O (ed), pp 47–200. Diseases of Marine Animals. Biologische Anstalt Helgoland, Germany

Kuhn T, Cunze S, Kochmann J, Klimpel S (2016) Environmental variables and definitive host distribution: a habitat suitability modelling for endohelminth parasites in the marine realm. Sci Rep 6:30246

Llewellyn J (1984) The biology of *Isancistrum subulatae* n. sp. a monogenean parasitic on the squid, *Alloteuthis subulata*, at Plymouth. J Mar Biol Ass UK 64:285–302

López-González J, Pascual S (1996) A new species of *Stellicola* Kossmann, 1877 (Copepoda, Lichomolgidae) associated with the squid *Illex coindetii* (Cephalopoda, Ommastrephidae) in the Atlantic Ocean. Hydrobiol 336:1–6

Meloni M, Ángelucci G, Merella P, Siddi R, Deiana C, Orru G, Salati F (2014) Molecular characterization of *Anisakis* larvae from fish cuaght off Sardinia. J Parasitol 97(5):908–914

Pascual S, González AF (2007) Parasite recruitment and oceanographic regime: evidence suggesting a relationship on a global scale. Biol Rev Camb Philo Soc 82(2):257–63

Pascual S, Guerra A (2003) Vexing question on fisheries research: the study of cephalopods and their parasites. Iberus 19(2):87–95

Pascual S, González AF, Arias C, Guerra A (1996a) Biotic relationships of *Illex coindetii* and *Todaropsis eblanae* (Cephalopoda, Ommastrephidae) in the Northeastern Atlantic: evidence from parasites. Sarsia 81:265–274

Pascual S, Gestal C, Estévez JM, Rodríguez H, Soto M, Abollo Arias C (1996b) Parasites in commercially-exploited Cephalopods (Mollusca, Cephalopoda) in Spain: an updated perspective. Aquacul 142:1–10

Pascual S, González AF, Gestal C, Abollo E, Guerra A (2001) Epidemiology of *Pennella* sp. (Crustacea: Copepoda) in exploited *Illex coindetii* stock in the NE Atlantic. Sci Mar 65 (4):307–312

Pascual S, González AF, Guerra A (2005) The recruitment of gill-infecting *Pennella* (Crustacea, Copepoda) as a categorical predictor of size-at-age data in squid populations. ICES J Mar Sci 62:629–633

Pascual S, Gestal C, Abollo E, Arias C (2007a) 9 Effect of *Pennella* sp. (Copepoda, Pennellidae) on the condition of *Illex coindetii* and *Todaropsis eblanae* (Cephalopoda, Ommastrephidae). Bull Europ Assoc Fish Pathol 17 (3/4):91–95

Pascual S, González AF, Guerra A (2007b) Parasites and cephalopod fisheries uncertainty: towards a waterfall understanding. Rev Fish Biol Fish 17:139–144

Pascual S, González AF, Guerra A (2007c) Parasite Recruitment and Oceanographic Regime: a working hypothesis on a global. Biol Rev 82:257–263

Pico-Duran G, Pulleiro-Potel L, Abollo E, Pascual S, Muñoz P (2016) Molecular identification of *Anisakis* and *Hysterothylacium* larvae in commercial cephalopods from the Spanish Mediterranean Coast. Vet Parasitol 220:47–53

Puerta P, Hunsicker ME, Quetglas A, Álvarez-Berastegui D, Esteban A, González M, Hidalgo M (2015) Spatially explicit modelling reveals cephalopod distributions match contrasting trophic pathways in the Western Mediterranean Sea. PLoS ONE 10(7):e013343

Rohde K (2002) Ecology and biogeography of marine parasites. Adv Mar Biol 43:1–86

Serracca L, Cencetti E, Battistini R, Rossini I et al. (2013) Survey on the presence of Anisalis and Hysterothylacium larvae in fishes and quids caught in Ligurian Sea. Vet Parasitol 196(83–4):547–51

Shinn AP, Pratoomyot J, Bron JE, Paladini G, Brooker EE, Brooker AJ (2014) Economic costs of protistan and metazoan parasites to global mariculture. Parasitol 142:196–270. https://doi.org/10.1017/S0031182014001437

Aquarium Maintenance Related Diseases 13

Antonio V. Sykes, Kerry Perkins, Panos Grigoriou, and Eduardo Almansa

Abstract

This chapter reviews the mechanical (physical) and chemical (water quality) related pathologies that have been reported since cephalopods are maintained, reared or cultured in captivity. For the first time, it builds up on the existing knowledge from researchers and aquarists (which are represented as authors of the chapter) in order to provide the most updated and inclusive revision on this theme. It is organized in terms of pathologies that are reported and eventual described for one or more species, which are commonly kept for research and display purposes, and exemplified with photos when possible. It includes pathologies of the mantle, arms, eyes, shell; egg infections, malformations of the shell and eggs; and causes of disease or mortality related with water quality focusing on pH and trace elements.

Keywords

Cephalopoda • Chemical related pathologies • Egg infections • Malformations • Shell fracture • Skin wounds

13.1 Introduction

Since 2013, cephalopods used in experimentation are protected in the European Union through the application of Directive 2010/63/EU (EU 2010). The application of this law generated an impact in research and aquaculture (Sykes et al. 2012; Ponte et al. 2013; Smith et al. 2013; Fiorito et al. 2014; Di Cristina et al. 2015). Unfortunately, at time of publication (2010) and until the end of 2017, the Directive omitted important information regarding the housing and husbandry conditions of this class. This has prompted the cephalopod community to join and write the first set of guidelines for the use of this class in the laboratory (Fiorito et al. 2015). Under this framework and that of COST Action Cephs*In*Action (FA1301—http://www.cephsinaction.org/), the community has suggested the definition of *mandate minima* [minimal requirements in Annex III (Care and Accommodation) and Annex IV (Humane killing)] for cephalopod to be included in the update of Directive 2010/63/EU. Through a consensus approach on published data, the community has established the species-specific requirements for the care and accommodation of cephalopods.

The health and welfare of cephalopods are directly related to how these animals are housed and treated. 'Pathologies registered under captive conditions derive most of the times from bad welfare practice' (Sykes and Gestal 2014). Interestingly, despite this cephalopods have been used as laboratory animals

A. V. Sykes (✉)
Centro de Ciências Do Mar, Universidade Do Algarve|CCMAR, Campus de Gambelas, Faro, Portugal
e-mail: asykes@ualg.pt

K. Perkins
Sea Life Brighton—Merlin Entertainments, Marine Parade, Brighton, BN2 1TB, UK
e-mail: Kerry.Perkins@merlinentertainments.biz

P. Grigoriou
HCMR, Gournes Pediados, P.O. Box 2214 71003 Irakleion, Crete, Greece
e-mail: pgrigoriou@her.hcmr.gr

E. Almansa
Instituto Español de Oceanografía, Centro Oceanográfico de Canarias, Santa Cruz de Tenerife, Canary Islands, Spain
e-mail: eduardo.almansa@ieo.es

C. Gestal et al. (eds.), *Handbook of Pathogens and Diseases in Cephalopods*,
https://doi.org/10.1007/978-3-030-11330-8_13

for more than a century (Dröscher 2016), most of the existing literature regarding pathologies observed in cephalopods in captivity was published at the end of the 1980s and beginning of 1990s, resulting from the booming interest on culturing individuals of this class (Sykes et al. 2014b).

Pathologies in cephalopods are related to the method of capture, transportation (from the type of container used, to biting or cannibalism, when animals are transported in group), handling (from rough materials used in nets to slipping from the hand of the operator), housing (seawater systems not meeting the minimal requirements of seawater quality, space, illumination, etc.) and husbandry (live prey may become predators and try to eat the cephalopod) conditions (Forsythe et al. 1987; Hanlon 1990; Boyle 1991; Oestmann et al. 1997; Fiorito et al. 2015). Good (positive) or bad (negative) welfare practice in research, maintenance, rearing or culture conditions will determine the existence of pathologies in cephalopods in any of these. The cause of pathologies in cephalopods may be divided in viral, bacterial, fungi, parasite, chemical and mechanical (Sykes and Gestal 2014). This chapter focuses on mechanical (physical) and chemical (water quality) related pathologies, which will be presented according to the pathologies observed in one or more situations identified above for all.

13.2 Mechanical (Physical) Damage Related Pathologies

13.2.1 Skin Wounds

Apart from being the outer barrier of the muscle tissue beneath, the skin of coleoid cephalopods is used to express behaviour through the dynamic patterns of the chromatophores (How et al. 2017), communication and camouflage (Hanlon and Messenger 1996). The skin also has cells with the ability to sense light (Kingston et al. 2015) and, eventually, smell (Campinho et al. 2017). This integumentary system is composed by (from top to bottom): (a) a mono-stratified epidermis consisting of columnar epithelial cells with a microvillous border (Smith et al. 2011), which is intermingled with mucus-secreting cells (Hanlon et al. 1984); and (b) a deeper dermis (thicker than the previous), composed of connecting tissue (with numerous blood vessels and nerves and some amoebocytes), and containing chromatophores, iridophores, and leucophores (Andouche and Bassaglia 2016).

Because of the delicate nature of the skin, the handling, transportation and housing of cephalopods should be made with utmost care to prevent tears or other trauma to the skin tissue. Any skin wound is an open door for opportunistic secondary infections (particularly bacterial), which can be fatal if untreated (Fiorito et al. 2015). Hanlon et al. (1984) and Hanlon and Forsythe (1990a) characterized four stages of ulceration: (a) Stage 1—The epidermis is destroyed mostly or completely, chromatophores become nonfunctional, with oblong or elliptical shape or they disintegrate (originating a slight grey colour in the skin). The dermis becomes thicker with collagen, but the layers of muscle cells are disrupted, and the tissue display an increased number of amoebocytes and blood vascular vessels; (b) Stage 2—Total destruction of the epidermis, and total destruction of the chromatophores with ulcerated zones increasing in size over the mantle surface. Amoebocytes are present in the superficial layers of the dermis. Bacteria populate and embed exposed surface and tissue; (c) Stage 3—Full penetration of the skin and muscle layers (deep wounds). Fast progression of ulcers and bacteria spread to the ventral part of the mantle; Stage 4—Spreading of lesions to the head and arms. Wounds in Stages 3 and 4 are fatal. All cephalopods are known to be susceptible to the infection of the skin by bacteria (Forsythe et al. 1987; Hanlon et al. 1988). The most common secondary bacterial infections associated with skin wounds were reported by Sherrill et al. (2000), Hanlon et al. (1984), and Ford et al. (1986) for cuttlefish, octopus and squid species, respectively. Nonetheless, cephalopods are known to have the ability to fully recover from arm injuries or amputation through regeneration (Feral 1978, 1979, 1988; Rohrbach and Schmidtberg 2006; Tressler et al. 2014; Shaw et al. 2016).

13.2.1.1 Mantle and Arms

Mantle tip damage, resulting from hitting the tank walls, is known to occur in octopus, squid and cuttlefish (Forsythe et al. 1987; Hanlon et al. 1988; Scimeca and Oestmann 1995; Hanley et al. 1998; Scimeca 2011). It is characterized by extensive, deep ulcerative dermatitis and cellulitis (Fig. 13.1a, b), with exposure of the cuttlebone tip in cuttlefish (Fig. 13.1e, f, g). One way of mitigating such damage is to apply the soft-sided tanks technology (Hanley et al. 1999). Another way is lowering density or increasing the sex ratio of females (Sykes et al. unpublished results). Ford et al. (1986) reported a skin lesion that led to the split of the mantle and exposure of the gladius in *Lolliguncula brevis*.

In octopus and cuttlefish, the mere contact of the suckers of one individual to another is sufficient to cause skin damage (Forsythe et al. 1987; Hanlon et al. 1988; Hanley et al. 1998). Cuttlefish copulate on a head-to-head position, where the arms of both are tangled and males exert some strength to keep the female in the position. Males also fight for the opportunity of copula (either with a female or another smaller male, if the latter is showing signs that may lead to sexual misleading; Brown et al. 2012) and this will result in multiple skin wounds (Fig. 13.1d, g). Either cuttlefish or octopus can show extended biting wounds (Fig. 13.1c) resulting from the latter, with eventual internal organ exposure [Fig. 6.3 in Sykes and Gestal (2014)].

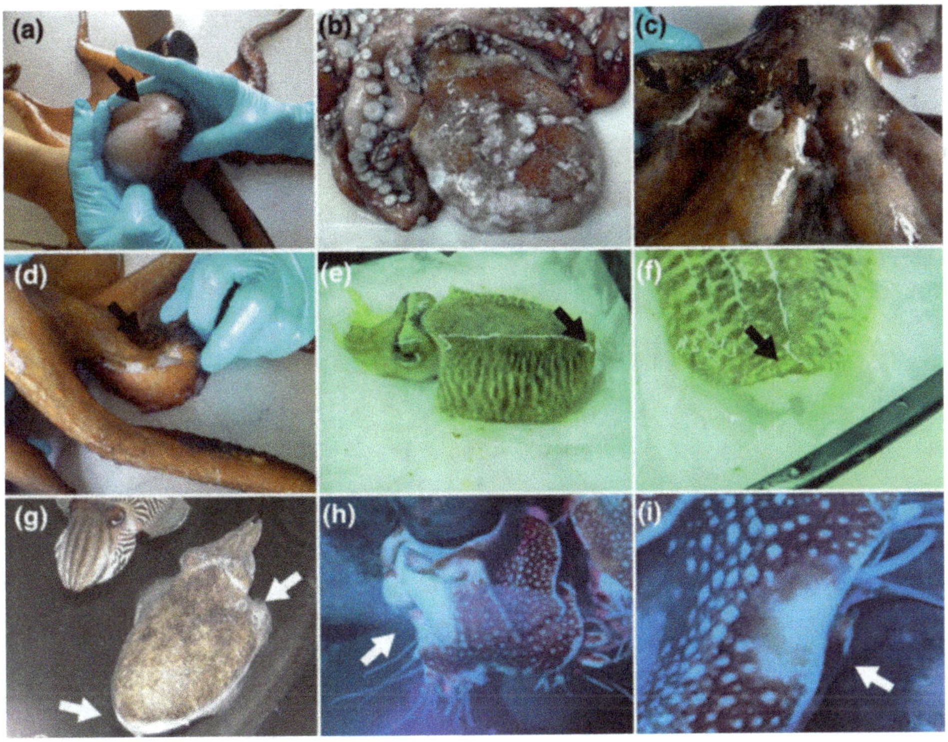

Fig. 13.1 Mechanical damage of cephalopod skin: **a** Skin abrasion (ulcerative dermatitis of the mantle apex) in the head of juvenile *Octopus vulgaris* (probably derived from hitting the tank wall); **b** Generalized skin wound with probable bacterial sepsis in a senescent *O. vulgaris* female; **c** Extended biting marks in the connection of the arms with the head in an *O. vulgaris* juvenile caused by male fighting; **d** Minor biting marks in the arm of an *O. vulgaris* juvenile; **e** Ulcerative dermatitis of the mantle apex in *Sepia officinalis*, due to hitting the tank wall; **f** Detail image of wound described in E, where the lack of skin and the appearance of the distal tip of the cuttlebone is now visible; **g** Mantle skin wounds in female *S. officinalis* (arrow on the left shows a similar ulcerative dermatitis of the mantle apex as in E and F, while the arrow on the right shows multifocal ulcerative dermatitis provoked by male cuttlefish suckers during the act of copulation); **h** Skin wound near the mantle cavity in *Nautilus pompilius*; **i** Skin wound in the tissue right above the eye in *N. pompilius*

There are reports (Reimschuessel and Stoskopf 1990; Budelmann 1998, 2010) regarding autophagy or automutilation syndrome (OAS) to occur in at least four species of octopus (*Octopus dolfleini*, *O. vulgaris*, *O. bimaculoides* and *O. maya*). This syndrome is reported to affect both mantle and arms. There is no consensus on if it caused by a substance (released by the octopus) or eventually by a virus or bacteria.

In squid, skin lesions related to tank wall contact often result in internal infections (apart from the skin itself), which are chronic and develop slowly, requiring weeks or months to be fatal (Forsythe et al. 1987). According to the same authors, the most common of these infections is a localized necrosis of mantle tissue that surrounds the wound, spreading from the mantle apex towards the head and looking like 'an opaque dagger-shaped abscess in the lateral mantle tissue'.

In Nautilus, Scimeca (2011) reported skin abrasion, associated with a deep infection originated by a fungus, which generate pigment loss (Fig. 13.1h, i). There have also been several anecdotal reports of hood discolouration, with fast spreading growth, being these patches often colonised by other pathogens (Barord 2014).

13.2.1.2 Eyes

Pathologies of the eyes in cephalopods have been reported to occur in octopus, squid and cuttlefish (Forsythe et al. 1987; Hanlon 1990; Sykes and Gestal 2014).

Forsythe et al. (1987) reported that the eye ball of octopuses may sometimes swell and rupture, being fatal within 2 days. According to these same authors, Hanlon et al. (1989b) and Hanlon and Forsythe (1990a), a similar condition may also occur in squid. However, in the latter the cause is the incrustation of bacterial colonies due to tissue abrasion, which turns the lens and the corneal covering of the eye opaque and the eye larger than normal. This condition may also be found in octopus and cuttlefish (Fig. 13.2a and b, respectively).

Idiopathic bulbus protusions of one or two eyes have been registered during reproduction in cuttlefish (Sykes and Gestal 2014) and affect both male and female (Fig. 13.2b, c). According to Hanley et al. (1998), this condition also affects juveniles and may eventually lead to the eye pathology previously described above. There are no reports of alike idiopathic bulbus protusions of the eye in nautilus. However, a similar skin abrasion, associated with a deep infection

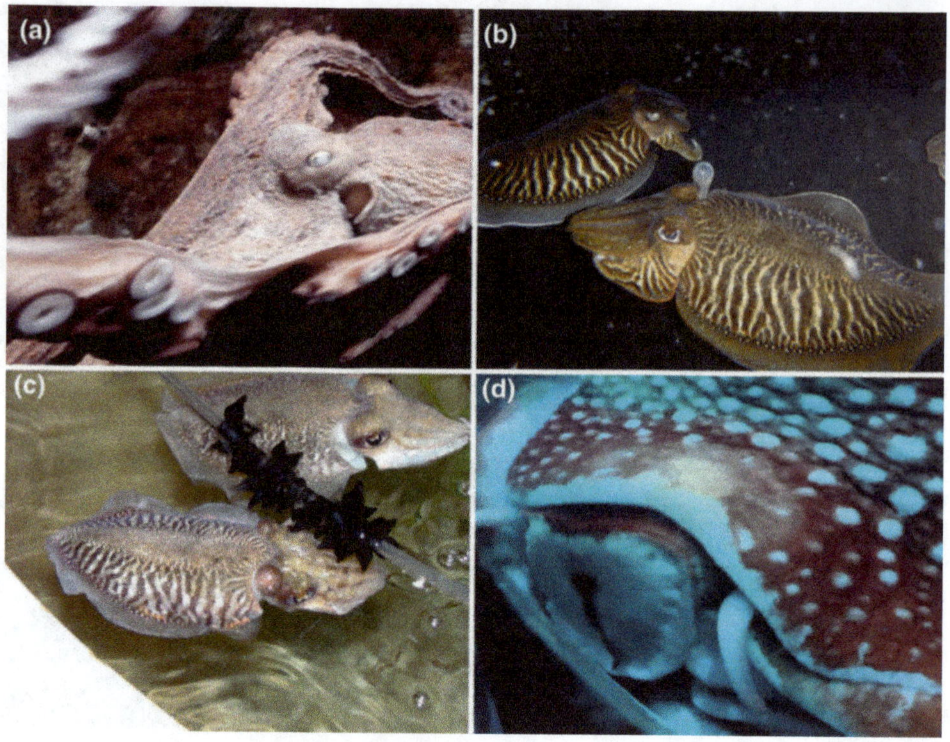

Fig. 13.2 Mechanical damage of cephalopod skin 2: **a** Opaque lens in *O. vulgaris*; **b** Opaque lens and idiopathic bulbous protrusions of the eye in *S. officinalis* males (on the left and right individuals, respectively); **c** Idiopathic bulbous protrusions of both eyes in a *S. officinalis* female; **d** Skin wound in the tissue right above the eye in *Nautilus pompilius*

originated by a fungus, which will generate pigment loss has been seen in captive individuals (Fig. 13.2d) and previously reported by Scimeca (2011). The inexistence of idiopathic bulbus protusions in nautilus is most likely due to the anatomy of the eye, which is more primitive than that of other cephalopods. However, excessive mucus production around the eyes can suggest a more serious condition or infection and further diagnostics would be required to determine that it is not a potentially fatal mucodegenerative disease (Barord 2014).

13.2.2 Shell Wounds/Fracture

Cuttlefish have an internal shell, commonly known as the cuttlebone or *sepion*, which corresponds to approximately 9% of the animal volume, acts as a rigid buoyancy device, and is made of a matrix of calcium carbonate (Denton 1961; Denton and Gilpin-Brown 1961, 1973; Birchall and Thomas 1983; Jacobs 1996), in its aragonite polymorph with a mixture of β-chitin and other protein complexes (Florek et al. 2009; North et al. 2017). This structure is made of a dorsal shield that covers the lamellar matrix below. The latter is arranged as over a hundred superposed narrow chambers and organic membranes. The chambers have a complex internal arrangement of calcified pillars (made from 0.01 mm thick septa supported by intracameral walls) that allow resisting external pressures greater than 1 MPa (Hewitt 1975; Birchall and Thomas 1983; Checa et al. 2015; North et al. 2017). The buoyancy and movement in the water column of cuttlefish is attained through the cuttlebone by: (a) varying the volume of gas space in these chambers and, therefore, of the overall cuttlebone density by moving liquid into or out of those via an osmotic process (Denton et al. 1961; Denton and Gilpin-Brown 1973) and (b) being highly porous (93%) and having a low specific gravity (Checa et al. 2015). The gas inside the cuttlebone has traces of CO_2, 2–3% of O_2 and the remaining is N_2 (Denton and Taylor 1964).

Despite having a low occurrence (Sherrill et al. 2000), the fracture of the cuttlebone is one the most common pathologies reported to occur when holding cuttlefishes in captivity. We believe that the higher the occurrence, the lower the welfare the overall rearing conditions, which might be related to available space, tank colour, light conditions or even sex ratios (Sykes and Gestal 2014). It is commonly seen in mature animals due to fighting or banging against the tank walls (Hanlon and Forsythe 1990b; Hanley et al. 1999).

Cuttlebone pathologies in captivity can be categorized into fractures that are (a) partial, in the distal (striated siphuncular zone) and proximal tips (Fig. 13.3a and b, respectively); (b) full transversal (Fig. 13.3c and e); and (c) full longitudinal (Fig. 13.3i and l). Any of these may or may not include the rupture of the tissues that separate the cuttlebone from the viscera (Fig. 13.3h) and the possible consequent exposure to seawater (Fig. 13.3f, g and k). When the latter happens the individual will die in a few days.

There is an additional pathology related to the cuttlebone. This is characterized by the disruption of the mantle tissue of

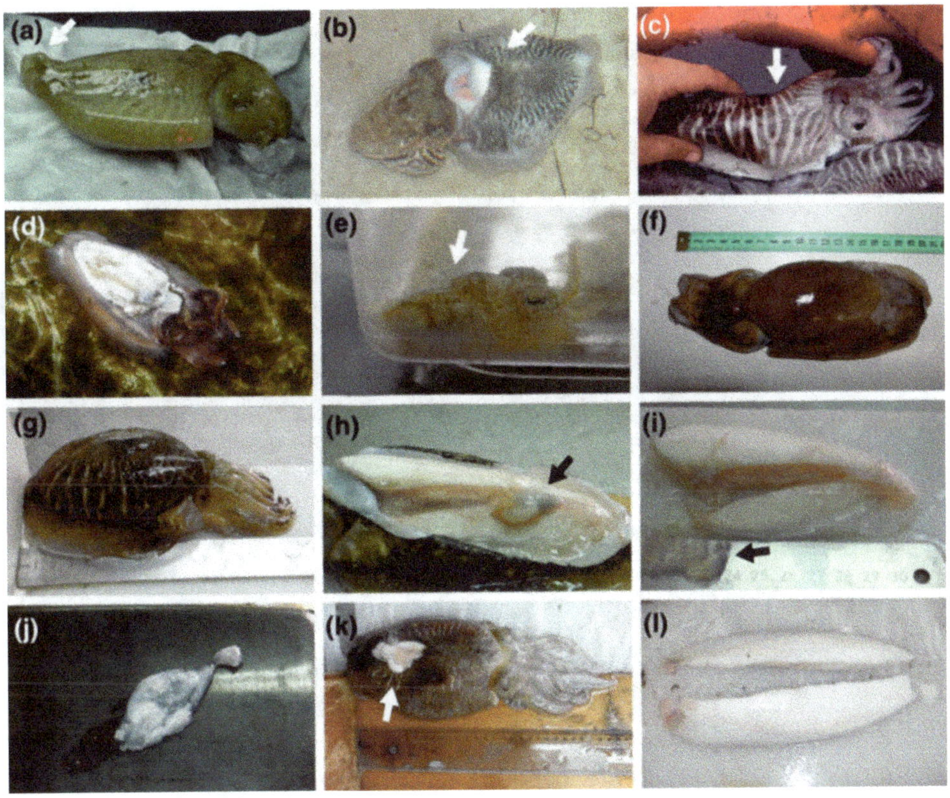

Fig. 13.3 Shell fracture in *S. officinalis*: **a** fracture at the distal tip of the cuttlebone; **b** fracture at the proximal tip of the cuttlebone; **c** fracture in the middle of the cuttlebone; **d** live female where the cuttlebone is not present; **e** fracture in the middle of the cuttlebone with increased production of the shell; **f** and **g** shell fracture in a female and a male (respectively), where the animal is trying to re-unite the shell by massively producing a solution of calcium carbonate; **h** detail of shell fracture of animal in (**g**), where part of the digestive system (stomach and caecum) has passed between the shell parts; **i** detail of the broken shell and tissue regeneration; **j** detail of tissue regeneration of shell; **k** male exhibiting a shell fracture and exposure of digestive system organs (stomach, caecum and digestive gland duct appendages) through the skin; **l** detail of shell fracture of animal in (**k**)

the shell sac due to senescence and the natural displacement of the cuttlebone from its normal site due to its floating capacity (Fig. 13.3d). The animals that show this condition die a few days later after the loss of the cuttlebone (Sykes, unpublished results).

It is not however clear if in these two conditions cause of death is directly related to the fracture/loss of the cuttlebone or to wounds that are generated. Table 6 of Fiorito et al. (2015) resumes the most common bacteria found in wounds of several cephalopod species. None of the bacteria in that table were reported to be linked to wounds of such nature.

Cuttlebone fracture also occurs in nature as studied by Boletzky and Overath (1991). The full longitudinal fracture in *S. officinalis* was reported to occur during rearing by these authors, Hanlon and Forsythe (1990a) and Scimeca (2011).

When exposed to a fracture, the cuttlebone will be 're-generated' by a similar process to the construction described by Boletzky and Overath (1991) and Čadež et al. (2017) with the secretion of a chitin-protein complex (Figs. 13.3f, g, i and j) (Checa et al. 2015) and up to 100 mL of slightly milky fluid that accumulates between the dermis and the cuttlebone (Hanley et al. 1998).

Feeding conditions (malnutrition) will also affect the proper development of the cuttlebone, generating aberrant forms in juveniles and adults (Boletzky 1974). Black lines in the striated siphuncular zone [Fig. 13.4b; (Keupp 2012)] are usually seen in underfed or starving animals.

Black lines have also been recorded in nautilus and are often found with new shell growth in captivity. However, they are not considered to be detrimental to the health or welfare of the nautilus or linked to nutritional deficit (Barord 2014). Further analysis of nautilus shells under scanning electron microscope (SEM) suggests that the individuals kept in aquaria display a shell made of disorderly crystalline structures when compared to those living in the wild (Moini et al. 2014). It is hypothesised that these differences are due to lower Ca and Mg concentrations in the shell; and the resulting brittleness or shell deformities are due to the lack of equilibrium in the biomineralisation process.

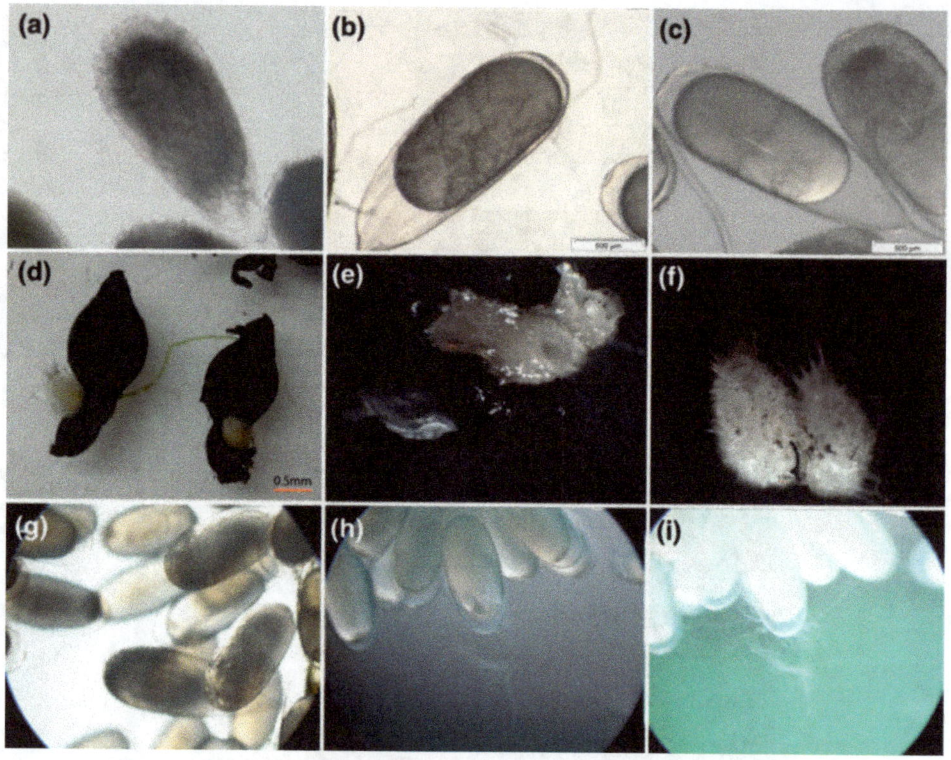

Fig. 13.4 Fungus or parasites in cephalopods eggs: **a–c** fungi infestation in *Octopus insularis* eggs (photos courtesy of Érica Vidal); **d–f** sponges attached to *S. officinalis* eggs; **g–f** fungi infestation in *O. vulgaris* eggs

13.3 Egg Infections and Cephalopods Malformations

One of the major issues when keeping eggs of cephalopods through embryogenesis is the eventual spread of fungus (Sykes et al. 2006). However, reports of such occurrence are very scarce. In cuttlefish, fungal activity may be prevented by using the methods described in Sykes et al. (2014a).

Fungal infections in cephalopods were reported to be very limited and are mostly relate to eggs and embryos (Sykes and Gestal 2014; Fiorito et al. 2015). They are reviewed in detail in Chap. 4, but, in here, we report the existence of fungus and possible parasites in cephalopod eggs kept in a captive environment. Both eggs of *Octopus insularis* (Fig. 13.4a–c) and *Octopus vulgaris* (Fig. 13.4g–f) displayed mycelia covering the chorion at early stages of embryonic development in Érica Vidal laboratory (Center for Marine Studies, Universidade Federal do Paraná, Brasil) and Eduardo Almansa laboratory (Instituto Español de Oceanografia, Centro Oceanográfico de Canarias, Spain), respectively. In September 2013, at the Sykes laboratory (CCMAR, Universidade do Algarve, Portugal), *Sepia officinalis* eggs obtained in captivity aborted their development due to an infestation by siliceous sponges that penetrated the chorion (Fig. 13.4d–f). The causes for such infestations are surely due to the seawater quality in the systems, which most probably did not have any sterilization or any appropriate filter prior to the application of the disinfection agent (being the latter either physical or chemical). Fungal activity may be prevented in cuttlefish by individualizing the eggs and using a special tank setup that promotes their gentle movement and proper oxygenation (Sykes et al. 2006, 2014a). This setup has been replicated for rearing other cephalopod eggs through embryogenesis under captivity.

Despite cuttlefish *S. officinalis* non-viable eggs (Fig. 13.5) were classified and described by Sykes et al. (2014a), similar reports are lacking for other cephalopods. As regards *S. officinalis*, the most typical non-viable eggs are those described as orange (Fig. 13.5a), grey and white (Fig. 13.5b), and malformations (Fig. 13.5c). It is known that non-viable eggs also occur in nature but, until now, there is not a trend that might explain the high variability of their occurrence in captivity (Sykes et al. 2013, 2017).

Overall, malformations are even less reported than existing pathologies in cephalopods. Malformations of the cuttlebone have been reported in literature for *S. officinalis* (Ruggiero 1980; Battiato 1983) and other cuttlefish (Keupp 2012). A cuttlebone with a full transversal fracture might regenerate (Fig. 13.3j) with an excess of calcified material in the dorsal shield (Fig. 13.6a). While repairing the cuttlebone, cuttlefish uses a similar process of lamellar deposition to the normal construction being self-organized layer-by-layer as seen with CT-Scan (X-ray computed tomography; Fig. 13.6c and d). The same cuttlebone shows signs of possible decay of the last lamella and black lines in

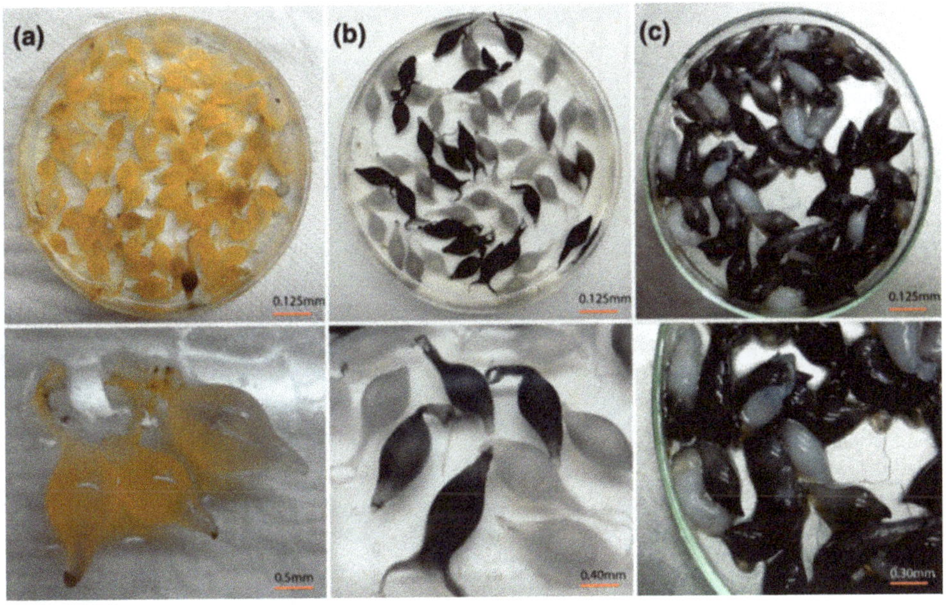

Fig. 13.5 Non-viable eggs of *S. officinalis*, according to the nomenclature given in Table 11.2 of Sykes et al. (2014): **a** Orange eggs; **b** Grey and White eggs; **c** Malformation eggs

the striated siphuncular zone (Fig. 13.6b). The use of x-ray-computed tomography will allow a better knowledge on the process of cuttlebone repair (Tiseanu et al. 2005) or eventually in nautilus (Hoffmann et al. 2018), even in living organisms.

Other types of malformations exist and are related to the eye (Fig. 13.7a, b), fin (Fig. 13.7a, c), arms (Fig. 13.7e, f) and mantle to arm tissue (Fig. 13.7g) development in cuttlefish and octopus. This was previously reported by Hanlon and Forsythe (1990b). Neoplasia (Fig. 13.7d) is not common in cephalopods (Scimeca 2011) but will result in massive death of animals. Hanlon and Forsythe (1990b) reported that at least two authors have verified the existence of 'tumours' in cuttlefish and wild octopus, but the description of such is related to something completely different to what is seen in Fig. 13.7d. Interestingly, malformations (in this case, the split of an arm into 3 new arms) might develop due to regeneration of an arm after a wound by biting (Fig. 13.7h, i). Arm regeneration is described in literature for cuttlefish (Tressler et al. 2014) and octopus (Shaw et al. 2016). There are no causes reported for these malformations.

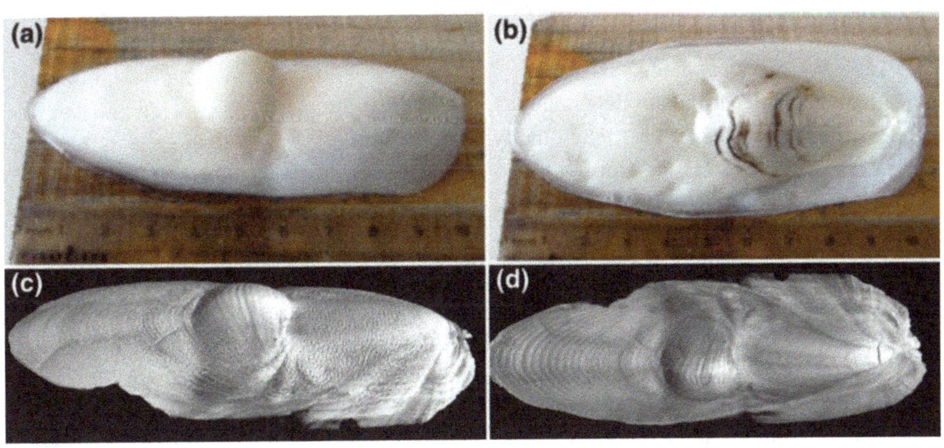

Fig. 13.6 Cuttlebone regeneration in *S. officinalis*: **a** and **b** anterior and posterior image of cuttlebone that suffered a transversal shell fracture in the middle and regenerated with an increased amount of shell in the upper part; **c** and **d** CT-Scan of the same cuttlebone from the side and from above respectively, where the growth rings are perfectly visible (images courtesy of René Hoffmann)

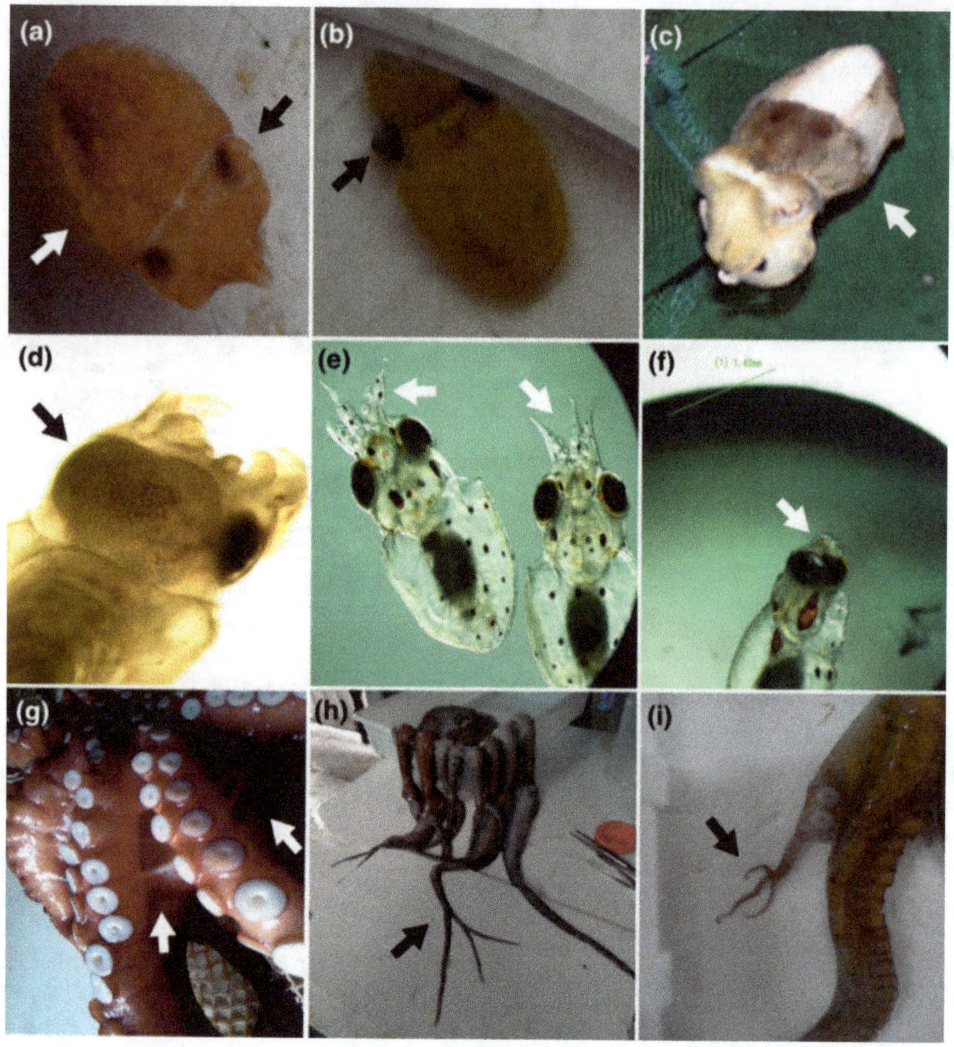

Fig. 13.7 Malformations in development of specific organs in cephalopods: **a** malformation in development of the *S. officinalis* fin and eye in a newly hatched hatchling; **b** malformation of the eye in a *S. officinalis* hatchling; **c** malformation of the fin in a *S. officinalis* juvenile; **d** neoplasia in the head of a newly hatched *S. officinalis*; **e** and **f**—malformations of the arms in *O. vulgaris* paralarvae (only 3 arms and absence of arms, respectively); **g** malformation of the connecting muscle of the mantle to the arms in a *O. vulgaris* juvenile; **h** and **i** development of three arms in one arm that was subject to biting in *O. vulgaris* juveniles

13.4 Chemical (Water Quality) Damage Related Pathologies

Cephalopods are marine animals, and as such, they are influenced by the seawater chemical quality, at collection or after being filtered in open, semi-open and closed systems. According to Sykes and Gestal (2014), the impact of diseases/lesions increases with the physicochemical quality and existing stress (which might be generated due to handling or housing conditions), which might promote a suppression of the immune response and proliferation of opportunistic microorganisms. The guidelines for the care and welfare of cephalopods in research (Fiorito et al. 2015) provide a list of water quality criteria for optimum health and welfare of cephalopods in its Appendix 2 and their routine monitoring, while Hanlon (1990) and Smith et al. (2011) described the basic filtering of the seawater systems used for housing cephalopods. Species-specific conditions for every life stage may also be found in Iglesias et al. (2014).

A low seawater pH has an effect on the carriage of oxygen blood pigments but not in all the species, such as *S. officinalis* juveniles which displays an acid–base regulatory ability (Gutowska et al. 2008, 2010a). However, as a response, this species will increase the calcification of its cuttlebone that may affect its buoyancy function (Gutowska et al. 2010b). On the other hand, hypercapnia promoted reduced growth, extended embryogenesis and smaller cuttlebones (with denser cuttlebone laminae) in embryos and hatchlings (Sigwart et al. 2016).

Colmers et al. (1984) reported the absence or malformation of the statolith and the gravity receptor system and also the absence of cupulae of the angular acceleration receptor systems in seven species of coleoid cephalopods (*Octopus joubini*, *O. maya*, *O. bimaculoides*, *S. officinalis*, *Loligo vulgaris*, *L. pealei*, and *L. plei*). This condition was described to affect the control and orientation in cephalopods and was concluded that it was due to the lack of strontium in seawater (Hanlon et al. 1989a).

Still concerning rearing in regards to seawater trace elements, despite the copper role in cephalopod haemocyanins

(Decleir et al. 1978; Thonig et al. 2014), Paulij et al. (1990) verified that copper concentrations of 50–200 ppb Cu^{2+} exerted shorter embryogenesis and premature hatching in *S. officinalis*, while Establier and Pascual (1983) reported that 0.08 ppm of copper will provoke total mortality in freshly laid eggs in the same species. According to Smith et al. (2011) copper is toxic to all cephalopods. There are some reports (Kuba, personal communication) that an excess of copper in seawater might generate a similar orientation problem and death in *S. officinalis*. This is probably due to this metal either triggering or inhibiting the phenoloxidase-like activity, which is implicated in the innate immune system (Lacoue-Labarthe et al. 2009). On the other hand, 6 ppm of copper in seawater (used as a way to increase the availability of this trace element) has been used in *O. vulgaris* paralarvae rearing (Garrido et al. 2014) or even up to 115 ppm in formulated feeds for juveniles of this same species (Sancho et al. 2015) without deleterious effects. The differences found between *S. officinalis* and *O. vulgaris* might be due to the possibility of this trace element being essential for the proper development of the latter, as suggested by Villanueva and Bustamante (2006) and García--García and Cerezo-Valverde (2006).

13.5 Concluding Remarks

Despite cephalopods being kept in captivity for more than 50 years, our knowledge regarding their pathologies are scarcely reported in literature. This chapter focused on the on mechanical (physical) and chemical (water quality) related pathologies. This is a research field in need of more attention in the years to come, not only because of existing EU welfare legislation, and that arising in other non-EU countries, but also because of the intrinsic importance of this subject in cephalopod maintenance/rearing/culture (Sykes and Gestal 2014). From the several pathologies that are already identified in the laboratory, the community has established the basics for healing and antibiotics application [see Forsythe et al. (1990) and Hanlon and Forsythe (1990a)], and changes to culture setups (some examples given in here). However, the overall existing knowledge regarding the exact causes, its effects and posology for healing is poor when compared with what is available in fish. This is a major gap in our knowledge if we want to provide the best welfare conditions to the animals of this class. Therefore, not only further research is needed but its availability as scientific reports is of major importance.

Acknowledgements The authors would like to thank both Dr. Érica Vidal and Dr. René Hoffmann for allowing us to use their photos and images in this chapter. AVS was funded through Fundação para a Ciência e a Tecnologia (FCT) Investigator Grant (IF/00576/2014). FCT (Project SEPIABREED PTDC/MAR/120876/2010 and UID/Multi/04326/2016), PROMAR (Project SEPIATECH 31.03.05.FEP.002) and Mar2020 (Project SEPIACUL MAR-02.01.01-FEAMP-0053) funded this work. EA acknowledges the funding of OCTOMICs (Project AGL2017-89475-C2-2-R) and OCTOWELF (Project AGL2013-49101-C2-1-R) to this chapter. This work benefited from networking activities carried out under the COST ACTION FA1301, and is considered a contribution to the COST (European COoperation on Science and Technology) Action FA1301 'A network for improvement of cephalopod welfare and husbandry in research, aquaculture and fisheries' (http://www.cephsinaction.org/).

References

Andouche A, Bassaglia Y (2016) Coleoid cephalopod color patterns: adult skin structures and their emergence during development in *Sepia Officinalis*. Vie Milieu 66:43–55

Barord GJ (2014) 1—800 Diagnose My Nautilus. Drum and Croaker 24–34

Battiato A (1983) Su un sepiostario aberrante di *Sepia officinalis L.* (Cefalopoda, Sepiidae). Thalassia Salentina 12/13:152–153

Birchall JD, Thomas NL (1983) On the architecture and function of cuttlefish bone. J Mater Sci 18:2081–2086

Boletzky SV (1974) Effects of continuous malnutrition on development of cuttlebone in *Sepia officinalis L.* (Mollusca, Cephalopoda). B Soc Zool Fr 99:667–673

Boletzky SV, Overath H (1991) Shell fracture and repair in the cuttlefish *Sepia officinalis*. In: Boucaud-Camou E (ed) La Seiche—The Cuttlefish, pp 69–78. Centre de Publications de la Université de Caen, France

Boyle PR (1991) The UFAW handbook on the care and management of the cephalopods in the laboratory. UFAW, Herts

Brown C, Garwood MP, Williamson JE (2012) It pays to cheat: tactical deception in a cephalopod social signalling system. Biol Lett 8:729–732

Budelmann BU (1998) Autophagy in octopus. S Afri J Mar Sci 20:101–108

Budelmann BU (2010) Cephalopoda. In: The UFAW Handbook on the care and management of laboratory and other research animals. Wiley-Blackwell, pp 785–817

Čadež V, Škapin SD, Leonardi A et al (2017) Formation and morphogenesis of a cuttlebone's aragonite biomineral structures for the common cuttlefish (*Sepia officinalis*) on the nanoscale: revisited. J Coll Interface Sci 508:95–104

Campinho MA, Oliveira AR, Sykes AV (2017) Olfactory-like neurons are present in the forehead of common cuttlefish, *Sepia officinalis* Linnaeus, 1758 (Cephalopoda: Sepiidae). Zool J Linnean Soc:zlx083

Checa AG, Cartwright JHE, Sanchez-Almazo I et al. (2015) The cuttlefish *Sepia officinalis* (Sepiidae, Cephalopoda) constructs cuttlebone from a liquid-crystal precursor. Sci Rep 5

Colmers WF, Hixon RF, Hanlon RT et al (1984) Spinner cephalopods—defects of statocyst suprastructures in an invertebrate analog of the vestibular apparatus. Cell Tissue Res 236:505–515

Decleir W, Vlaeminck A, Geladi P et al (1978) Determination of protein-bound copper and zinc in some organs of the cuttlefish *Sepia officinalis L.* Comp Biochem Physiol 60B:347–35

Denton EJ (1961) The buoyancy of fish and cephalopods. Progr Biophys Mol Biol 11:177–234

Denton EJ, Gilpin-Brown JB (1961) Buoyancy of cuttlefish, *Sepia officinalis* (L). J Mar Biol Assoc UK 41:319–342

Denton EJ, Gilpin-Brown JB, Howarth JV (1961) The osmotic mechanism of the cuttlebone. J Mar Biol Assoc UK 41:351–364

Denton EJ, Taylor DW (1964) Composition of gas in chambers of cuttlebone of *Sepia officinalis*. J Mar Biol Assoc UK 44:203–207
Denton EJ, Gilpin-Brown JB (1973) Floatation mechanisms in modern and fossil cephalopods. Adv Mar Biol 11:197–268
Di Cristina G, Andrews P, Ponte G et al (2015) The impact of Directive 2010/63/EU on cephalopod research. Invert Neurosci 15:1–7
Dröscher A (2016) Pioneering studies on cephalopod's eye and vision at the Stazione Zoologica Anton Dohrn (1883–1977). Front Physiol 7
Establier R, Pascual E (1983) Effects of cadmium and copper on the development of eggs of *Sepia officinalis* L. Invest Pesq 47:143–150
EU (2010) Directive 2010/63/EU of The European Parliament and of the Council of 22 September 2010 On the protection of animals used for scientific purposes. In: Union E (ed) Official Journal European Union, pp 33–79
Feral JP (1978) Regeneration of arms of cuttlefish *Sepia officinalis L* (Cephalopoda, Sepioidea): 1—Morphological study. Cah Biol Mar 19:355–361
Feral JP (1979) Regeneration of the arms of *Sepia officinalis* L (Cephalopoda, Sepioidea): 2—Histologic and Cytologic Study. Cah Biol Mar 20:29–42
Feral JP (1988) Wound-healing after arm amputation in *Sepia officinalis* (Cephalopoda, Sepioidea). J Invertebr Pathol 52:380–388
Fiorito G, Affuso A, Anderson DB et al (2014) Cephalopods in neuroscience: regulations, research and the 3Rs. Invertebr Neurosci 14:13–36
Fiorito G, Affuso A, Basil J et al (2015) Guidelines for the care and welfare of cephalopods in research—a consensus based on an initiative by CephRes, FELASA and the Boyd Group. Lab Anim 49:1–90
Florek M, Fornal E, Gomez-Romero P et al (2009) Complementary microstructural and chemical analyses of *Sepia officinalis* endoskeleton. Mat Sci Eng C-Bio S 29:1220–1226
Ford LA, Alexander SK, Cooper KM et al (1986) Bacterial populations of normal and ulcerated mantle tissue of the squid, *Lolliguncula brevis*. J Inv Pathol 48:13–26
Forsythe JW, Hanlon RT, Lee PG (1987) A synopsis of cephalopod pathology in captivity. In: Williams TD (ed) 18th annual conference of the international association for aquatic animal medicine. Monterey Bay Aquarium, Monterey, California, pp 130–135
Forsythe JW, Hanlon RT, Lee PG (1990) A formulary for treating cephalopod mollusc diseases. In: Perkins FO, Cheng TC (eds) Third International Colloquium on Pathology in Marine Aquaculture Academic Press Inc., Gloucester Point, Virginia (USA), 2–6 Oct 1988, pp 51–63
García-García B, Cerezo-Valverde J (2006) Optimal proportions of crabs and fish in diet for common octopus (*Octopus vulgaris*) ongrowing. Aquaculture 253:502–511
Garrido D, Rodríguez EM, Felipe B et al (2014) Influence of copper on *Octopus vulgaris* paralarvae rearing. In: Aquaculture Europe 2014—adding value, p 2. Donostia—San Sebastián, Spain
Gutowska MA, Portner HO, Melzner F (2008) Growth and calcification in the cephalopod *Sepia officinalis* under elevated seawater $p\mathrm{CO_2}$. Mar Ecol Progress Ser 373:303–309
Gutowska MA, Melzner F, Langenbuch M et al (2010a) Acid-base regulatory ability of the cephalopod (*Sepia officinalis*) in response to environmental hypercapnia. J Comp Physiol B 180:323–335
Gutowska MA, Melzner F, Portner HO et al (2010b) Cuttlebone calcification increases during exposure to elevated seawater $p\mathrm{CO_2}$ in the cephalopod *Sepia officinalis*. Mar Biol 157:1653–1663
Hanley JS, Shashar N, Smolowitz R et al (1998) Modified laboratory culture techniques for the European cuttlefish *Sepia officinalis*. Biol Bull 195:223–225
Hanley JS, Shashar N, Smolowitz R et al (1999) Soft-sided tanks improve long-term health of cultured cuttlefish. Biol Bull 197:237–238
Hanlon RT, Forsythe JW, Cooper KM et al (1984) Fatal penetrating skin ulcers in laboratory-reared octopuses. J Inv Pathol 44:67–83
Hanlon RT, Forsythe JW, Lee PG (1988) External pathologies of cephalopods in captivity. In: Cheng TC, Perkins FO (eds) Third international colloquium on pathology in marine aquaculture. Academic Press Inc., Gloucester Point, Virginia (USA), pp 17–18
Hanlon RT, Bidwell JP, Tait R (1989a) Strontium is required for statolith development and thus normal swimming behavior of hatchling cephalopods. J Exp Biol 141:187–195
Hanlon RT, Yang WT, Turk PE et al (1989b) Laboratory culture and estimated life span of the Eastern Atlantic squid, *Loligo forbesi* Steenstrup, 1856 (Mollusca: Cephalopoda). Aqua Fish Manage 20:15–34
Hanlon RT (1990) Maintenance, rearing and culture of teuthoid and sepioid squids. In: Adelman WJ Jr, Arnold JM, Guilbert DL (eds) Squid as Experimental Animals. Plenum Press, New York, pp 35–61
Hanlon RT, Forsythe JW (1990a) Diseases caused by microorganisms. In: Kinne O (ed) Diseases of Mollusca: Cephalopoda, pp 23–46. Biologische Anstalt Helgoland, Hamburg
Hanlon RT, Forsythe JW (1990b) Structural abnormalities and neoplasia. In: Kinne O (ed) Diseases of marine animals, pp 203–204. Biologische Anstalt Helgoland, Hamburg
Hanlon RT, Messenger JB (1996) Cephalopod behaviour. Cambridge University Press, New York
Hewitt RA (1975) Analysis of aragonite from cuttlebone of *Sepia officinalis L*. Mar Geol 18:M1–M5
Hoffmann R, Lemanis RE, Falkenberg J et al (2018) Integrating 2D and 3D shell morphology to disentangle the palaeobiology of ammonoids: a virtual approach. Paleontology 61:89–104
How MJ, Norman MD, Finn J et al (2017) Dynamic skin patterns in cephalopods. Front Physiol 8:393
Iglesias J, Fuentes L, Villanueva R (2014) Cephalopod culture. Springer, Netherlands
Jacobs DK (1996) Chambered cephalopod shells, buoyancy, structure and decoupling: history and red herrings. Palaios 11:610–614
Keupp H (2012) Atlas zur paläopathologie der cephalopoden. Berliner Paläobiologische Abhandlungen 12:1–392
Kingston ACN, Kuzirian AM, Hanlon RT et al (2015) Visual phototransduction components in cephalopod chromatophores suggest dermal photoreception. J Exp Biol 218:1596–1602
Lacoue-Labarthe T, Bustamante P, Horlin E et al (2009) Phenoloxidase activation in the embryo of the common cuttlefish *Sepia officinalis* and responses to the Ag and Cu exposure. Fish Shellfish Immun 27:516–521
Moini M, O'halloran A, Peters AM et al (2014) Understanding irregular shell formation of *Nautilus* in aquaria: chemical composition and structural analysis. Zool Biol 33:285–294
North L, Labonte D, Oyen ML et al (2017) Interrelated chemical-microstructural-nanomechanical variations in the structural units of the cuttlebone of *Sepia officinalis*. APL Mater 5:116103
Oestmann DJ, Scimeca JM, Forsythe J et al (1997) Special considerations for keeping cephalopods in laboratory facilities. Cont Topics Lab Animal Sci 36:89–93
Paulij WP, Zurburg W, Denuce JM et al (1990) The effect of copper on the embryonic-development and hatching of *Sepia officinalis L*. Arch Environ Con Tox 19:797–801
Ponte G, Dröscher A, Fiorito G (2013) Fostering cephalopod biology research: past and current trends and topics. Invert Neurosci :1–9
Reimschuessel R, Stoskopf MK (1990) Octopus automutilation syndrome. J Inv Pathol 55:394–400
Rohrbach B, Schmidtberg H (2006) Sepia arms and tentacles: model systems for studying the regeneration of brachial appendages. Vie Milieu 56:175–190

Ruggiero L (1980) Un esemplare aberrante di *Sepia officinalis L.* (Cephalopoda, Sepiidae). Thalassia Salentina 10:131–132
Sancho MDC, Valverde JC, Sironi JS et al (2015) Is copper supplementation required in formulated feeds for octopus vulgaris (Cuvier, 1797)? J Shellfish Res 34:473–480
Scimeca JM, Oestmann DJ (1995) Selected diseases of captive and laboratory reared cephalopods. Proc Int Assoc Aquatic Anim Med 27:26–79
Scimeca JM (2011) Cephalopods. In: Lewbart GA (ed) Invertebrate medicine, pp 113–125. Wiley-Blackwell
Shaw TJ, Osborne M, Ponte G et al (2016) Mechanisms of wound closure following acute arm injury in *Octopus vulgaris*. Zool Lett 2:1–10
Sherrill J, Spelman LH, Reidel CL et al (2000) Common cuttlefish (*Sepia officinalis*) mortality at the National Zoological Park: implications for clinical management. J Zoo Wildlife Med 31:523–531
Sigwart JD, Lyons G, Fink A et al (2016) Elevated *p*CO(2) drives lower growth and yet increased calcification in the early life history of the cuttlefish *Sepia officinalis* (Mollusca: Cephalopoda). ICES J Mar Sci 73:970–980
Smith JA, Andrews PLR, Hawkins P et al (2013) Cephalopod research and EU Directive 2010/63/EU: requirements, impacts and ethical review. J Exp Mar Bio Ecol 447:31–45
Smith SA, Scimeca JM, Mainous ME (2011) Culture and maintenance of selected invertebrates in the laboratory and classroom. ILAR J 52:153–164
Sykes AV, Domingues PM, Correia M et al (2006) Cuttlefish culture—state of the art and future trends. Vie Milieu 56:129–137
Sykes AV, Baptista FD, Gonçalves RA et al (2012) Directive 2010/63/EU on animal welfare: a review on the existing scientific knowledge and implications in cephalopod aquaculture research. Rev Aqua 4:142–162
Sykes AV, Pereira D, Rodríguez C et al (2013) Effects of increased tank bottom areas on cuttlefish (*Sepia officinalis, L.*) reproduction performance. Aqua Res 44:1017–1028
Sykes AV, Domingues P, Andrade JP (2014a) *Sepia officinalis*. In: Iglesias J, Fuentes L, Villanueva R (eds) Cephalopod culture, pp 175–204. Springer, Netherlands
Sykes AV, Gestal C (2014) Welfare and diseases under culture conditions. In: Iglesias J, Fuentes L, Villanueva R (eds) Cephalopod culture, pp 97–112. Springer Netherlands
Sykes AV, Koueta N, Rosas C (2014b) Historical review of cephalopods culture. In: Fuentes L, Villanueva R, Iglesias J (eds) Cephalopod culture. Springer, Netherlands, pp 59–75
Sykes AV, Alves A, Capaz JC et al (2017) Refining tools for studying cuttlefish (*Sepia officinalis*) reproduction in captivity: in vivo sexual determination, tagging and DNA collection. Aquacult 479:13–16
Thonig A, Oellermann M, Lieb B et al (2014) A new haemocyanin in cuttlefish (*Sepia officinalis*) eggs: sequence analysis and relevance during ontogeny. Evodevo 5
Tiseanu I, Craciunescu T, Mandache NB et al (2005) µ-X-ray computer axial tomography application in life sciences. J Optoelectron Adv M 7:1073–1078
Tressler J, Maddox F, Goodwin E et al (2014) Arm regeneration in two species of cuttlefish *Sepia officinalis* and *Sepia pharaonis*. Invert Neurosci 14:37–49
Villanueva R, Bustamante P (2006) Composition in essential and non-essential elements of early stages of cephalopods and dietary effects on the elemental profiles of *Octopus vulgaris* paralarvae. Aquacult 261:225–240

Regeneration and Healing

14

Letizia Zullo and Pamela Imperadore

Abstract

Cephalopods are animals endowed with a high regenerative potential. They can regenerate missing or injured structures such as the cornea, the shell, the arms and tentacles and even peripheral nerves and brain centers. As much as regeneration and healing cannot be considered as pathologies sensu stricto, they are always accompanied by conditions such as inflammation, tissue degeneration and potentially by infection. No treatments are currently available for any of these cases. Although they often get resolved autonomously, the early identification and monitoring of post-traumatic events is fundamental in the context of animal welfare.

Keywords

Tissue damage • Traumatism • Wound healing • Regeneration process

14.1 Introduction

Wild animals often carry on their body signs of pre-experienced traumatic events. Tissues and structures such as skin, fins and arms are reported to be subject to injury in the wild as well as in captivity, mainly due to capture and transport, autotomy, mating and competition (by con-specifics or predators) but also aggression and cannibalism (Budelmann 1998; Bush 2006, 2012; Hanlon et al. 1984).

In order to discriminate among mild to severe body damages, it is important to have a good understanding of the cephalopod physiology. As an example, abnormal body coloration can be due either to a superficial skin damage, which causes chromatophores expansion or skin retraction, or to a more severe damage to internal structures, such as the pallial or optic nerves and tracts, causing deafferentation of targeted organs. That is, alteration of the external appearance is not always the direct consequence of skin lesions but can be the secondary effect of an injury located elsewhere in the body. This aspect is particularly relevant in the context of animal welfare as it allows identifying the primary target to hit to ensure the animal wellness. In response to body damage, most of the cephalopods activate regenerating processes in various organs such as cornea, peripheral nerves, arm and tentacles (Imperadore and Fiorito 2018). Regeneration of the arms is particularly important as when one or more arms are damaged, the impairment of several functions, such as swimming, prey manipulation and posturing can occur (Tressler et al. 2014). This begins with a characteristic process of skin and tissue wound healing consistent within and across species (Fossati et al. 2013, 2015; Lange 1920; Shaw et al. 2016; Tressler et al. 2014).

Cephalopod skin has the vital role of protection against pathogens. The latter function becomes crucial when keeping animals in captivity, as it has been observed that severe ulcers can lead to death if untreated (Hanlon et al. 1984; Mather and Anderson 2007; Polglase 1980). It has also been noticed that undamaged squids adapt better than injured

L. Zullo (✉)
Centre for Synaptic Neuroscience and Technology, Fondazione Istituto Italiano Di Tecnologia, Genoa, Italy
e-mail: Letizia.Zullo@iit.it

P. Imperadore
Association for Cephalopod Research (CephRes), Naples, Italy
e-mail: p_imperadore@cephalopodresearch.org

P. Imperadore
Stazione Zoologica Anton Dohrn, Biology and Evolution of Marine Organisms, Naples, Italy

C. Gestal et al. (eds.), *Handbook of Pathogens and Diseases in Cephalopods*,
https://doi.org/10.1007/978-3-030-11330-8_14

animals to temperature and salinity changes (Hanlon et al. 1983). Skin plays also an important role in cephalopods survival in their natural environment as they use body patterning, obtained through changes in color and shape of the skin, for concealment and communication (Messenger 2001; Packard 1988; Packard and Hochberg 1977). Hence, wounds and lesions have to be carefully monitored in captive animals to ensure a full recovery of their function and appearance and to avoid transferring possible infections to other animals (this can be exacerbated in closed water systems), as also suggested in the Guidelines for the Care and Welfare of Cephalopods in Research (Fiorito et al. 2015).

In this chapter, we will attempt at describing in details the healing and regeneration processes occurring at mantle and arms of *Octopus vulgaris*, a Cephalopods representative.

14.1.1 Skin and Tissue Damage in Wild Animals: From Healing to Regeneration

Traumatic events occurring in wild animals can cause alterations of several aspects of the body appearance. Animals can manifest from simple superficial skin lesions to partial or complete structure loss, as often occurs in the case of arms (Fig. 14.1).

As injured arms normally regenerate, it is not rare to see animals with one or more regenerating arms. Superficial wounds can have various extensions and can be very localized or distributed over the body, although small lesions are more frequently observed. Examples of wounds on mantle and on the eyeballs skin are reported in Fig. 14.1a^{I} and a^{II} where several small scratches are clearly visible. Arms can present unhealed wounds (Fig. 14.1b^{I}) or regenerating arms (Fig. 14.1b^{II} and b^{III}) at various stages of regeneration depending on the time the traumatic event occurred. Lesions can be localized at any point along the arm although they are mostly found at its mid-terminal portion.

14.2 Skin and Tissue Damage After Experimentally Induced Injury

Wound healing in cephalopods has been investigated after experimentally induced mantle injury (Bullock et al. 1987; Polglase et al. 1983) and arm transection during the initial stages of arm regeneration (Féral 1988; Lange 1920; Shaw et al. 2016). In both cases, similar phenomena are observed. Indeed, even though arm regeneration involves recovery and regrowth of several tissues and structures (i.e., nerves, muscles, vessels, skin, etc.) it first requires healing of the wound. Healing starts with muscular contraction and epidermis in-folding (mainly connective tissue of the dermis) soon after injury (30 min). This phenomenon usually lasts for the first 12 h, contributing to reducing the size of the lesion (Fig. 14.2). Here we present an exemplary case where a complete mantle wound closure is established as soon as 4 days after injury (Fig. 14.2a^{I} and a^{II}). Indeed, at 4 days only a thin line (red arrow), due to intense muscular contraction and epidermis in-folding, is still visible around the site of injury.

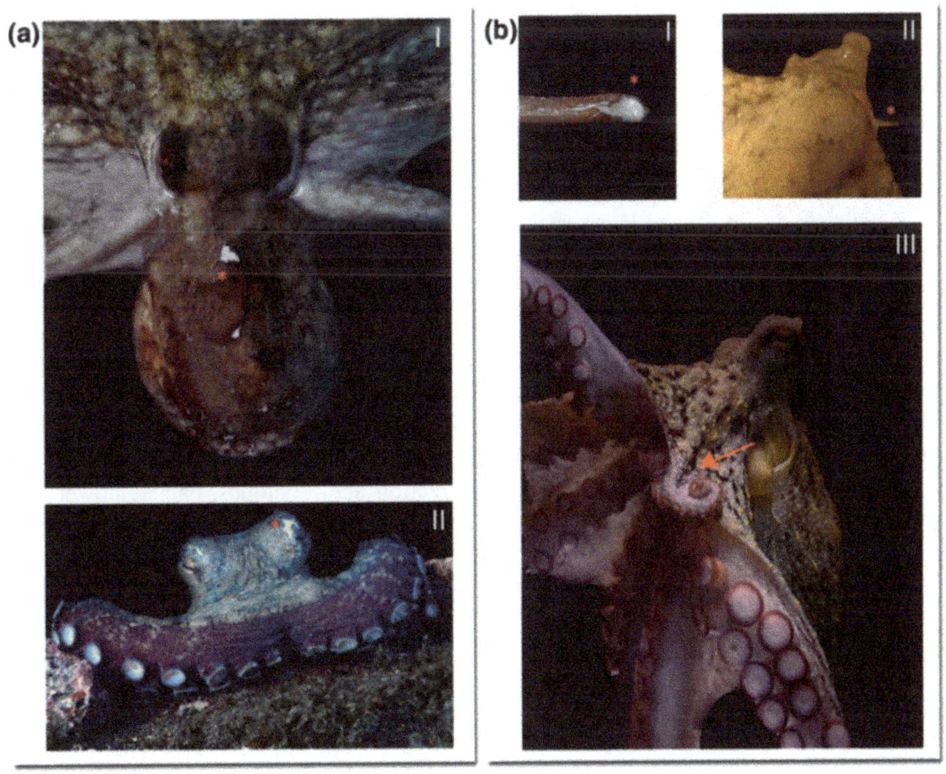

Fig. 14.1 Skin lesions in wild caught animals. **a** Wounds localized at the mantle (I) and around the eyeballs (II) (red asterisks); **b** examples of injured non-regenerating arm tip (I, red asterisk, scale bar 5 mm) and regenerating arms (II, red asterisk, scale bar 6 mm; III, red arrow). Regeneration can occur at any location of the arm depending only on the site of injury and will proceed towards the regeneration of a fully functional arm (II: early regenerating arm, III: late regenerating arm)

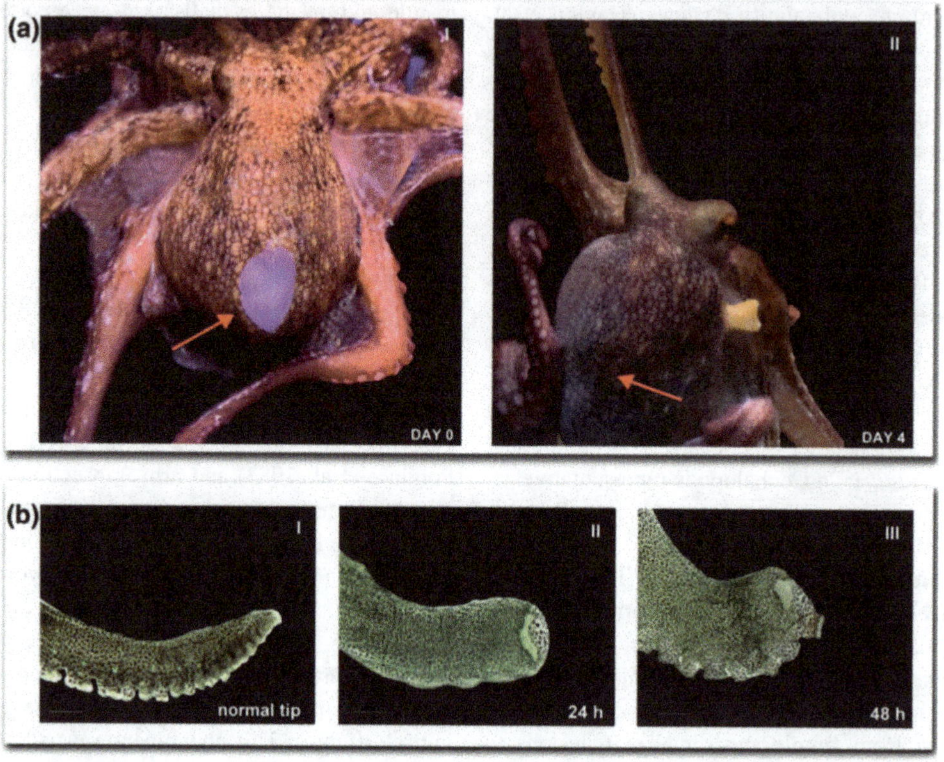

Fig. 14.2 Experimentally induced injury. **a** An animal showing a skin wound on the dorsal side of the mantle soon after experimental lesion (red arrow in I, Day 0). Four days later (II) the wound is almost completely closed, only a thin line (red arrow), due to intense muscular contraction and epidermis in-folding, is still visible around the site of injury. **b** Appearance of an arm tip uninjured (I), 24 h (II) and 48 h (III) after lesion. Scale bars: 2 mm. Soon after cut, the arm tip is interested by wound closure. 24 h' post injury, the majority of the exposed area is covered by skin (II). Two days post surgery (III) the wound is still visible but extremely reduced in size and suckers close to the lesion are brought toward the wound

At the tissue level, hemorrhagic areas and hemocytes invade the wound, producing swelling in the central part of the wound which is mainly observed 12 h post injury as a result of increased hemocytes diapedesis. Hemocytes aggregates on the injury site (between day 1 and 3) and temporary protect the wound, also containing abundant extracellular matrix and likely vesicles and/or mucous. Later, blood cells stratify in several layers and change their shape from round to fusiform, providing a first dermal plug covering the whole surface of the wound. In the arm, this represents the primary blastema that is supposed to supply material for the regenerating tip. Epidermal cells round up 2 weeks post lesion, while 3 weeks later the epidermis thickness increases (for a detailed description see (Shaw et al. 2016)). Time of healing can be greatly affected by bacterial infection that determines delays in muscle contraction and epidermal migration; this eventually results in an incomplete closure of the wound. In addition, an increase in hemocytes release and in their activity is observed compared to not infected wound. The majority of these cells become necrotic in proximity of the bacteria likely due to the effect of toxins released by the pathogens (Bullock et al. 1987).

Healing of the arm starts soon after the cut. In the example reported here, already 24 h' post injury, the majority of the exposed area is covered by skin and 2 days post surgery the wound is still visible but extremely reduced in size; suckers close to the lesion are brought toward the wound (compare Fig. 14.2b^{I}, b^{II}, b^{III}). The time required for the complete healing in the arm can go from less than 24 h up to 2 weeks on the base of several factors, mainly water temperature, animals' age and health status of the animals (Féral 1988; Lange 1920). In addition, healing appears also to depend on animal "self-abilities," as two different populations of healers have been identified for the common octopus, named slower and faster healers: in the latter case 80% of the wound is covered in 6 hours, 50–60% is observed instead for the slower group with modest increase in the following 18 h (Shaw et al. 2016).

14.3 Arm Regeneration

We will now describe more in details the histological modifications occurring at tissue level following arm injury and regeneration (Fig. 14.3).

Immediately after healing, the process of arm regeneration starts and already 3 days after injury a little knob at the cutting point is visible. This later elongates forming a small protrusion. The first well-identifiable structure has the shape of a hook and appears around 17 days after the injury (Fig. 14.3a^{I}). From histological analysis, a very thin layer of undifferentiated cells composes the first observed knob. A more defined and intensely proliferating "blastema" (bl) is then visible together with diffuse vascular components (v) at the arm tip (Fig. 14.3a^{II}). This structure then disappears, tissues enter in a differentiation state and the process of histogenesis starts. At later stages (between 50 and 60 days usually) a complete structure is visible with the restoration of a typical non-injured arm (Fig. 14.3b^{I}). At this stage both nervous (g) and muscle elements (m) become clearly visible and well-organized (Fig. 14.3b^{II}) (Fossati et al. 2011, 2013; Lange 1920; Zullo et al. 2017).

A special case of regeneration is represented by the aberrant arm regeneration where the injured arm forms bi- or trifurcation. It is not uncommon in literature to find examples of aberrant regeneration of cephalopods arms and tentacles (Alejo-Plata and Méndez 2014; González and Guerra 2008; Toll and Binger 1991). Here we report a case where the regenerating stump developed a tripartite arm composed by structurally normal arms (Fig. 14.4).

14.4 Pallial Nerve Degeneration and Regeneration

A pair of pallial nerves, connecting the subesophageal mass of the CNS to the mantle, is involved in the control of breathing and in the mantle skin pattering. If both nerves are damaged, the animal dies soon after as breathing is completely abolished (Fredericq 1878); however, if only one of

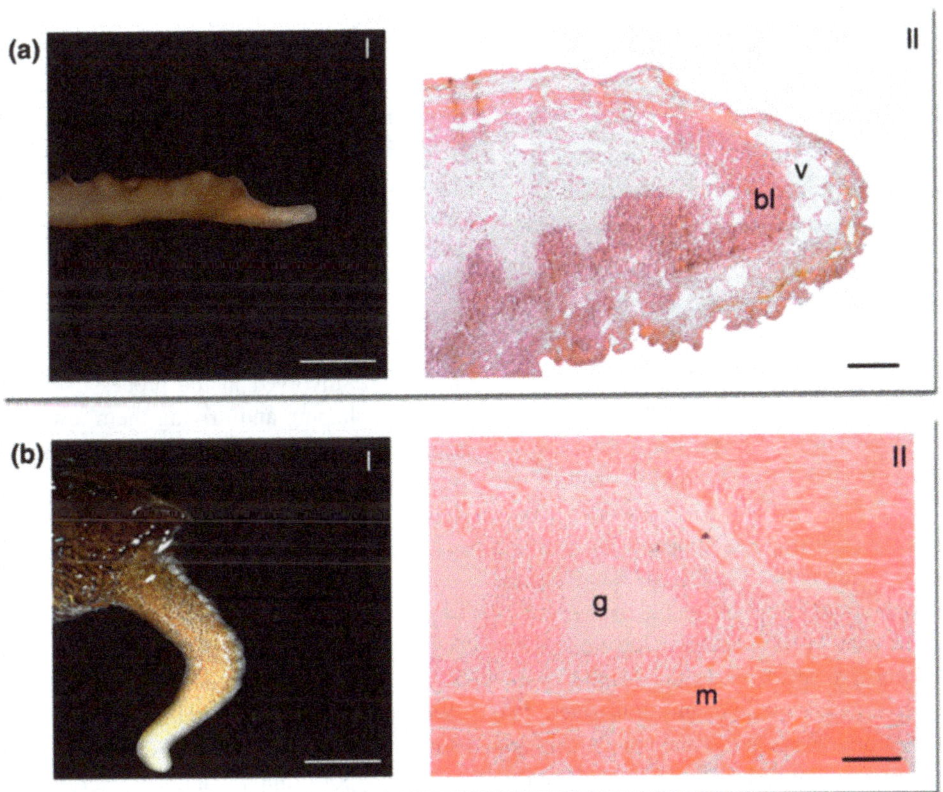

Fig. 14.3 Arm regeneration process. **a** Regenerating arm 17 days post injury. I: macroscopic image of the arm tip. *Scale bar* 5 mm. II: Hematoxylin and eosin stained longitudinal section showing the blastemal areas (bl) at the arm tip rich of vascular components (v). *Scale bar* 50 μm. At this stage of regeneration, a hook-like structure is visible and the tip is much unorganized. **b** Regenerating arm 55 days post injury. I, macroscopic image of the arm tip. Scale bar: 5 mm. II: Hematoxylin and eosin stained longitudinal section showing the well developed nervous (g: ganglia) and muscle (m) elements. *Scale bar* 100 μm. At this stage of regeneration, a normal arm structure is fully restored. Images A^{II}, B^{I} and B^{II} by courtesy of Dr. F. Carella

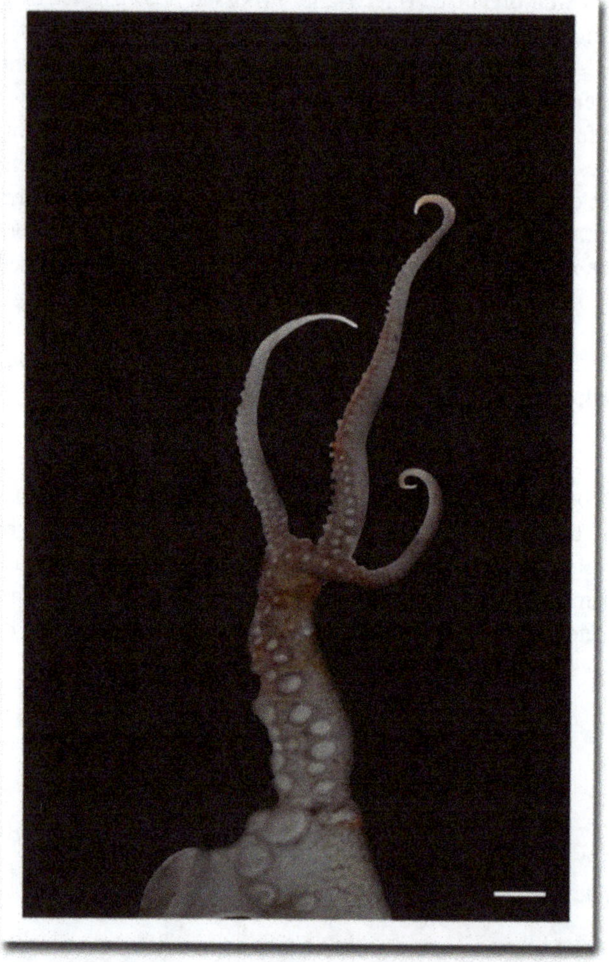

Fig. 14.4 Aberrant regeneration. Aberrant regeneration of an arm after lesion in the wild resulted in the formation of three morphologically normal tips. *Scale bar* 1 cm. *Source* Dr. Panagiotis Grigoriou (CretAquarium, Heraklion, Greece)

the two is subjected to injury, the animal is not only able to survive, but it also regenerates the nerve, recovering the lost functions (Imperadore et al. 2017, 2018; Sanders and Young 1974; Sereni and Young 1932). This lesion has never been described as a naturally occurring phenomenon, such as arm regeneration. The few accounts available depict it as the effect of surgical operations, through pallial nerve cut or crush. This might be due to the particular location of the nerves, which are well-protected inside the mantle cavity. When one of these nerves is experimentally transected, two immediate effects are obtained: paling of the mantle skin and paralysis of the respiratory muscles on the side ipsilateral to the lesion (Fig. 14.5a, b) (Fredericq 1878; Imperadore et al. 2017; Sanders and Young 1974; Sereni and Young 1932).

Despite this loss of functions, the animal appears healthy and active soon after recovery from anesthesia. An increase in self-grooming actions close to the injured area is the only alteration that might occur after lesion (Imperadore et al. 2017).

Complete functional recovery requires several months, but usually already after 3 to 4 days post surgery the denervated skin undergoes some peculiar changes (Sanders and Young 1974). First we can observe skin paling due to chromatophore muscles relaxation, as neural control between CNS and periphery is lost (Sereni and Young 1932). This is followed by dark color waves randomly and quickly crossing the skin of the affected side of the mantle. These have been named "wandering clouds" and are due to a state of chromatophores hyperexcitability (Imperadore et al. 2017; Packard 1992; Sanders and Young 1974). Three to five days after injury, the skin on the side of lesion appears, at rest, homogeneously colored and, seven to fourteen days later it is able to match the color pattern of the contralateral side. However, paling immediately returns on the injured side during rapid pattern changes, such as prey attack or escape. This effect cannot be the result of a lack in functional regeneration but it is more likely driven by local effects involving skin photoreceptors (Imperadore et al. 2017).

At the microscopical level, lesions of the nerves induce inflammation followed by the formation of a scar between the two nerve stumps, hemorrhagic areas, and additional cicatricial tissues in the muscles damaged. These scars are mainly formed by hemocytes, which rush to the site of lesion and invade the nerve stumps. The scar separating the stumps does not represent a barrier, as fibers of the central stump (still connected to the CNS) start immediately to regenerate, reaching the opposite stump, with a growth rate between 7 and 18 µm/h (Fig. 14.5c). Peripheral stump regeneration is observed after 10–14 days post lesion, it appears initially characterized only by degenerative phenomena, with axons swelling and fragmentation (Imperadore et al. 2017; Sereni and Young 1932). Connective tissue in the nerve appears also to be involved in the process, sealing the cut stumps initially, shaping and driving them toward each other a few days later. Both, hemocytes and connective tissue actively proliferate at the cut nerve and interestingly neural elements have also been suggested start differentiating as soon as two weeks after lesion (Imperadore et al. 2017).

14.5 Concluding Remarks

Arms and mantle skin wounds of various severity and even arm loss are common events experienced by cephalopods in nature. Upon injury, animals can manifest a series of responses going from mild aberration of the body coloration and patterning to severe behavioral modifications. Injury is often only the "first hit" while "second hits" are determined by a variety of processes such as inflammation and infection of the wound occurring hereinafter that can alter not only the aspect but also the functionality of the damaged tissues. Body skin appearance have been listed within the potential

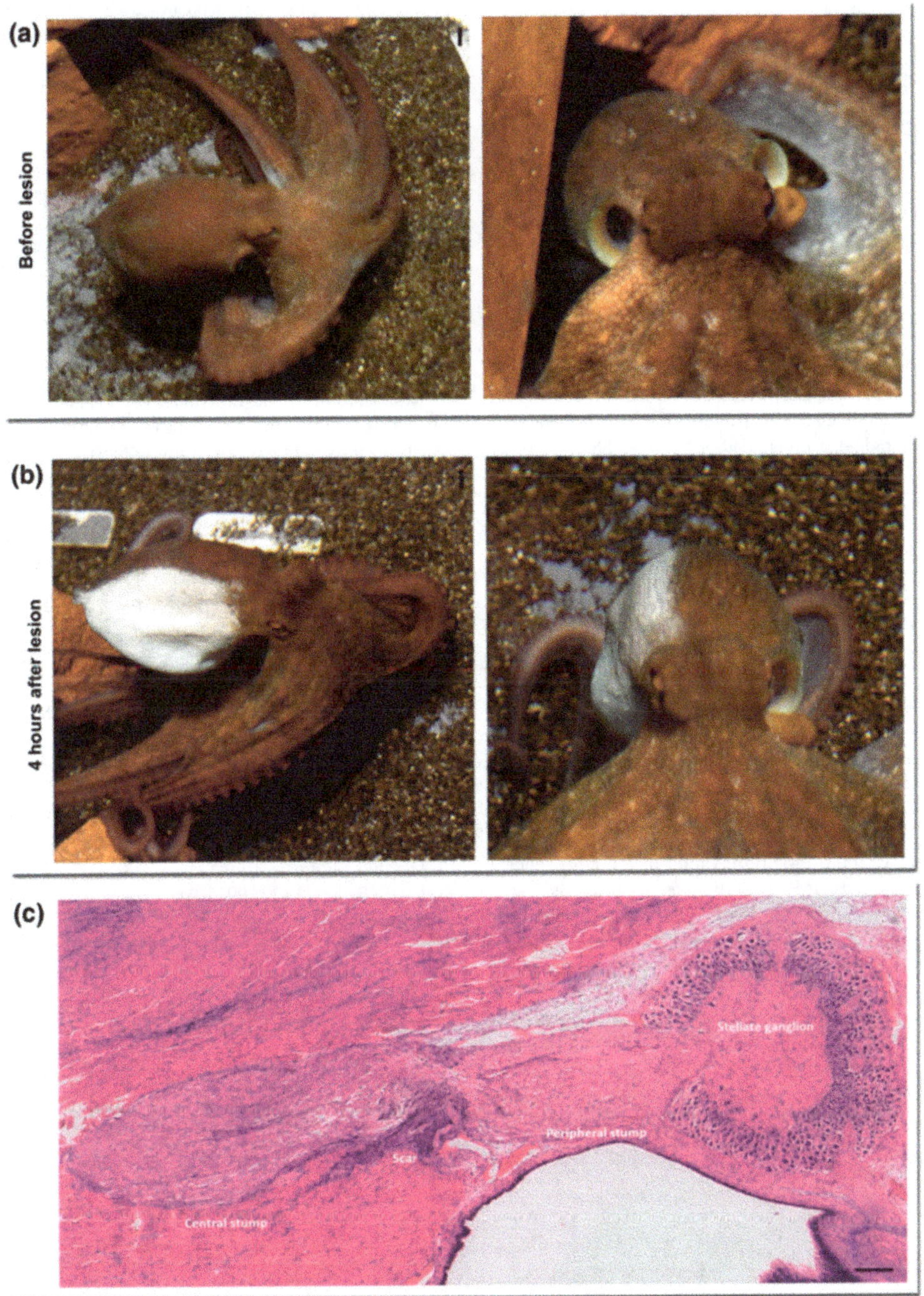

Fig. 14.5 Pallial nerve degeneration and regeneration. An animal before pallial nerve lesion (**a**) shows full ability in changing body pattern (I) and in controlling contraction of respiratory muscles on both sides of the mantle (II). Soon after lesion (**b**) the two functions are lost on the denervated side, which becomes completely pale (I) and flaccid (II). **c** Pallial nerve seven days post lesion presents a scar dividing the two nerve stumps (Central and Peripheral stumps), however the central stump is able to regenerate with fibers reaching the opposite side toward the stellate ganglion. *Scale bar* 0.2 mm

indicators of health and welfare in cephalopods (Fiorito et al. 2015) and thus represents a feature that have to be constantly monitored especially in captive animals. Moreover, it is fundamental to provide a constant assessment of experimental animals undergoing surgical procedures as the occurrence of secondary effects induced by tissue incisions might take place even days after experimentation. For most of these events, no special treatment has yet been established. It is therefore important, in the context of animal welfare, to early identify the occurrence and progress of regeneration/degeneration processes to avoid the possible occurrence of unhealthy conditions in captive animals.

References

Alejo-Plata MDC, Méndez OV (2014) Arm abnormality in *Octopus hubbsorum* (Mollusca: Cephalopoda: Octopodidae). Amer Malacolo Bull 32:217–219

Budelmann BU (1998) Autophagy in octopus. S Afri J Mar Sci 20:101–108

Bullock AM, Polglase JL, Phillips SE (1987) The wound healing and haemocyte response in the skin of the lesser octopus *Eledone cirrhosa* (Mollusca: Cephalopoda) in the presence of *Vibrio tubiashii*. J Zool 211:373–385

Bush SL (2006) Autotomy as a deep-sea squid defense. Integr Comp Biol 46:E19–E19

Bush SL (2012) Economy of arm autotomy in the mesopelagic squid Octopoteuthis deletron. Mar Ecol Progr Ser 458:133–140

Féral JP (1988) Wound healing after arm amputation in *Sepia officinalis* (Cephalopoda: Sepioidea). J Invert Pathol 52:380–388

Fiorito G, Affuso A, Basil J et al (2015) Guidelines for the Care and welfare of cephalopods in research—a consensus based on an initiative by CephRes, FELASA and the Boyd Group. Lab Anim 49:1–90

Fossati SM, Benfenati F, Zullo L (2011) Morphological characterization of the *Octopus vulgaris* arm. Vie Milieu 61:197–201

Fossati SM, Carella F, De Vico G, Et AL (2013) Octopus arm regeneration: role of Acetylcholine Esterase during morphological modification. J Exp Mar Biol Ecol 447:93–99

Fossati SM, Candiani S, Nodl MT et al (2015) Identification and expression of Acetylcholinesterase in *Octopus vulgaris* arm development and regeneration: a conserved role for ACHE? Mol Neurobiol 52:45–56

Fredericq L (1878) Recherches sur la Physiologie du poulpe commun. Arch Zool Exp Gen 7:535–583

González AF, Guerra A (2008) First observation of a double tentacle bifurcation in cephalopods. JMBA2—Biodiversity Records: 1–6

Hanlon RT, Hixon RF, Hulet WH (1983) Survival, growth, and behavior of the loliginid squids *Loligo plei*, *Loligo pealei*, and *Lolliguncula brevis* (Mollusca: Cephalopoda) in closed sea water systems. Biol Bull 165:637–685

Hanlon RT, Forsythe JW, Cooper KM, Dinuzzo AR, Folse DS, Kelly MT (1984) Fatal penetrating skin ulcers in laboratory-reared octopuses. J Invert Pathol 44:67–83

Imperadore P, Fiorito G (2018) Cephalopod tissue regeneration: consolidating over a century of knowledge. Front Physiol 9:593. https://doi.org/10.3389/fphys.2018.00593

Imperadore P, Shah SB, Makarenkova HP, Fiorito G (2017) Nerve degeneration and regeneration in the cephalopod mollusc *Octopus vulgaris*: the case of the pallial nerve. Sci Rep 7

Imperadore P, Uckermann O, Galli R, Steiner G, Kirsch M, Fiorito G (2018) Nerve regeneration in the cephalopod mollusc *Octopus vulgaris*: label-free multiphoton microscopy as a tool for investigation J R Soc Interface 15 https://doi.org/10.1098/rsif.2017.0889

Lange MM (1920) On the regeneration and finer structure of the arms of the cephalopods. J Exp Zool 31:1–57

Mather JA, Anderson RC (2007) Ethics and invertebrates: a cephalopod perspective. Diseas Aqua Org 75:119–129

Messenger JB (2001) Cephalopod chromatophores: neurobiology and natural history. Biol Rev 76:473–528

Packard A (1988) The skin of cephalopods (coleoids): general and special adaptations. In: Trueman ER, Clarke MR (eds) The Mollusca, form and functions, vol 11. Academic Pres, pp 37–67

Packard A (1992) A note on dark waves (wandering clouds) in the skin of *Octopus vulgaris*. J Physiol 446:40

Packard A, Hochberg FG (1977) Skin patterning in *Octopus* and other genera. Symp Zool Soc Lond 38:191–231

Polglase JL (1980) A Preliminary Report on the Thraustochytrid(s) and Labyrinthulid(s) Associated with a Pathological Condition in the Lesser Octopus *Eledone cirrosa*. Bot Mar XXIII: 699–706

Polglase JL, Bullock AM, Roberts RJ (1983) Wound healing and the haemocyte response in the skin of the Lesser octopus *Eledone cirrhosa* (Mollusca: Cephalopoda). J Zool 201:185–204

Sanders GD, Young JZ (1974) Reappearance of specific colour patterns after nerve regeneration in Octopus. Proc R Soc London B, Biol Sci, p 186

Sereni E, Young JZ (1932) Nervous degeneration and regeneration in Cephalopods. Pubbl Staz Zool Napoli 12:173–208

Shaw TJ, Osborne M, Ponte G, Fiorito G, Andrews PL (2016) Mechanisms of wound closure following acute arm injury in *Octopus vulgaris*. Zool Letters 2:8

Toll RB, Binger LC (1991) Arm anomalies: cases of supernumerary development and bilateral agenesis of arm pairs in Octopoda (Mollusca, Cephalopoda). Zoomorphol 110:313–316

Tressler J, Maddox F, Goodwin E, Zhang Z, Tublitz NJ (2014) Arm regeneration in two species of cuttlefish *Sepia officinalis* and *Sepia pharaonis*. Invert Neurosci 14:37–49

Zullo L, Fossati SM, Imperadore P, Nodl MT (2017) Molecular determinants of cephalopod muscles and their implication in muscle regeneration. Front Cell Dev Biol 5:53

Other Disorders

15

Camino Gestal, Santiago Pascual, and Sarah Culloty

Abstract

Neoplasia are growth disturbances characterized by excessive, abnormal proliferation of cells, independent of normal-regulating mechanisms of the animal and persisting after termination of the stimulus that initiated growth. Over lasts years there has been an increase in research into tumors of invertebrates. In cephalopods, reports on the incidence of the tumors or neoplasia are scarce. They have been described as hard compact and homogeneous nodules of connective tissue located in the mantle or at the base of suckers. The aetiological origin of tumors observed in cephalopods is unknown, but it could be related to aquarium maintenance. Other injurious agents, including infectious (virus, bacteria, or parasites) and xenobiotics, may also have produced the lesions. In occasions inflammatory processes have been associated with tumors with severe oedema associated. Inflammation is part of the biological response to body tissues to harmful stimuli such as pathogens, damaged cells or effect of xenobiotics. The inflammatory focus is characterized by exudation with interstitial fluid changes and hemocytic migration. Some inflammatory lesions include fibrosis and necrotic cells in the affected area, with loss of histological features and even organ architecture. All this changes have been observed in cephalopods in inflammatory reactions originated by infection with different pathogens. The chapter covers a selection of the reported cases of disorders related to neoplasia and inflammation.

Keywords

Neoplasia • Tumors • Inflammation • Haemocytic infiltration • Aedema

15.1 Introduction

Neoplasia are growth disturbances characterized by excessive, abnormal proliferation of cells, independent of normal-regulating mechanisms of the animal and persisting after termination of the stimulus that initiated growth (Sparks 1985). Similarly, tumors are ectopic masses of tissue formed by due to an abnormal cell proliferation. Over lasts years there has been an increase in research into tumors of invertebrates, since previously it was thought that tumors only occurred in vertebrates and invertebrates were not susceptible to developing neoplasia (Engel 1930). Nowadays the research in the area has increased and increasing number of tumors has been

C. Gestal (✉)
Aquatic Molecular Pathobiology Group, Institute of Marine Research, Spanish National Research Council (CSIC), 36208 Vigo, Pontevedra, Spain
e-mail: cgestal@iim.csic.es

S. Pascual
Ecology and Biodiversity Department, Institute of Marine Research, Spanish National Research Council (CSIC), 36208 Vigo, Pontevedra, Spain
e-mail: spascual@iim.csic.es

S. Culloty
Aquaculture & Fisheries Development Center, School of Biological, Earth and Environmental Sciences, University College Cork, The Cooperage, Distillery Fields, North Mall, Cork, Ireland
e-mail: s.culloty@ucc.ir

C. Gestal et al. (eds.), *Handbook of Pathogens and Diseases in Cephalopods*,
https://doi.org/10.1007/978-3-030-11330-8_15

detected in these organisms. Thus, histological and molecular research has provided a better understanding of the nature of these abnormal growths (Tascedda and Ottaviani 2014). In marine invertebrates, different types of tumors have been described, namely those emerged spontaneously, those due to hereditary phenomena, and those due to a wide range of environmental factors. Among those induced by environmental factors, different injurious agents including chemical toxins, physical stress, biological infections and potential carcinogenic substances, may produce that lesions (Hanlon and Forsythe 1990a). In molluscs, tumors, tumor-like growths or neoplasia have been described in gastropods, bivalves, and in some cases in cephalopods. In bivalves, sarcomas of hematopoietic origin such as disseminated neoplasia, or gonad neoplasia have been identified as causative of important mortalities (Carballal et al. 2015). Very few reports have been published in cephalopods.

Other disorder commonly observed in cephalopods is inflammation. It is part of the biological response to body tissues to harmful stimuli such as pathogens, damaged cells, or effect of xenobiotics. Inflammation is a protective response with a function of eliminates the initial cause of the cell injury, clear out necrotic cells and tissues damaged and initiate tissue repair. The description of the tissue modifications occurred in relation to infectious or non-infectious agents by histopathological analysis is essential for an accurate diagnosis of the disease.

15.2 Neoplasia and Tumors

In cephalopods, the incidence of the tumors or neoplasia is extremely low. In 1951 Jullien and Jullien (1951) reported cuttlefish with hard compact and homogeneous whitish nodules of connective tissue with loss of normal stratified appearance and highly vascularized at the periphery. In some cases, haemocytic infiltration is observed between the connective tissue and muscular fibers (Wauttier and Wautier 1955). Similar nodules were also observed in *Octopus vulgaris* (Figs. 15.1 and 15.2). Nigmatullin provided morphological data on tumors observed in *O. vulgaris* off the northwest coast of Africa with a prevalence of 1.6% of caught octopus. Pascual et al. (2006) described lesions characterized by consistent swelling of smooth surface nodules located at the sucker's base and mantle of *Octopus hubbsorum* (Figs. 15.3 and 15.4). At histological level, the lesions appear as mass proliferations of dense fibrous tissue between the dermis and muscle layers (Fig. 15.4a–c). Muscular tissue surrounding the lesions was degenerated and necrotic foci were observed (Figs. 15.2 and 15.4). The aetiological origin of tumors observed in cephalopods is

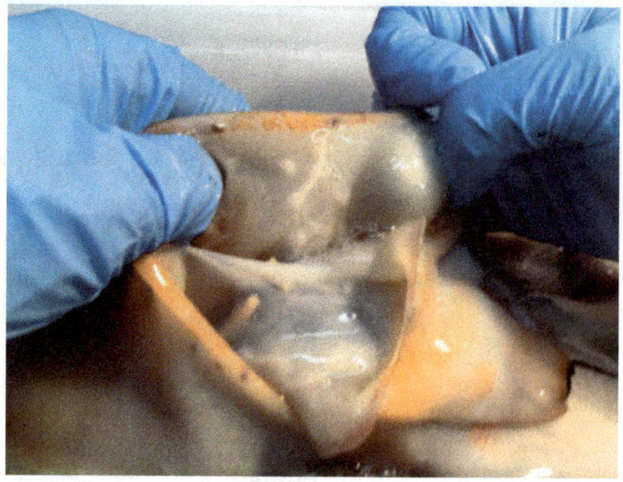

Fig. 15.1 Macroscopic aspect of nodules located at internal mantle side of *Octopus vulgaris*

unknown, especially in those observed in wild individual. However, different authors suggest that it could be the result of traumatic episodes related to aquarium maintenance (Hanlon and Forsythe 1990b). Other injurious agents, including infectious (virus, bacteria or parasites) and xenobiotics, may also have produced the lesions (Hanlon and Forsythe 1990a).

15.3 Inflammation

Histologically haemocytic infiltration with eosinophilic staining is observed in the intercellular space of a tissue with inflammation. The inflammatory focus is characterized by exudation with interstitial fluid changes and hemocytic migration. Some inflammatory lesions include fibrosis and necrotic cells in the affected area, with loss of histological features and even organ architecture. All this changes have been observed in cephalopods in inflammatory reactions originated by bacteria, parasites such as the coccidian *Aggregata* or metazoans such as *Anisakis* infections (Fig. 15.5). In occasions, inflammatory processes have been associated with tumors with severe oedema associated. Hanlon and Forsythe (1990a) described the presence of severe edema of the mantle and arms of *O. joubini* and *O. maya*, where epidermis and dermis are separated from the underlying muscle layers, or even the entire dermis of the mantle was separated from the muscle layers by a watery, almost gelatinous, layer of fluid. This condition was always fatal within 48 h. Similar lesions associated to inflammation process have been observed in *Octopus vulgaris* maintained for long period in aquarium installations also with fatal result within 48–72 h (pers. obs.) (Fig. 15.6).

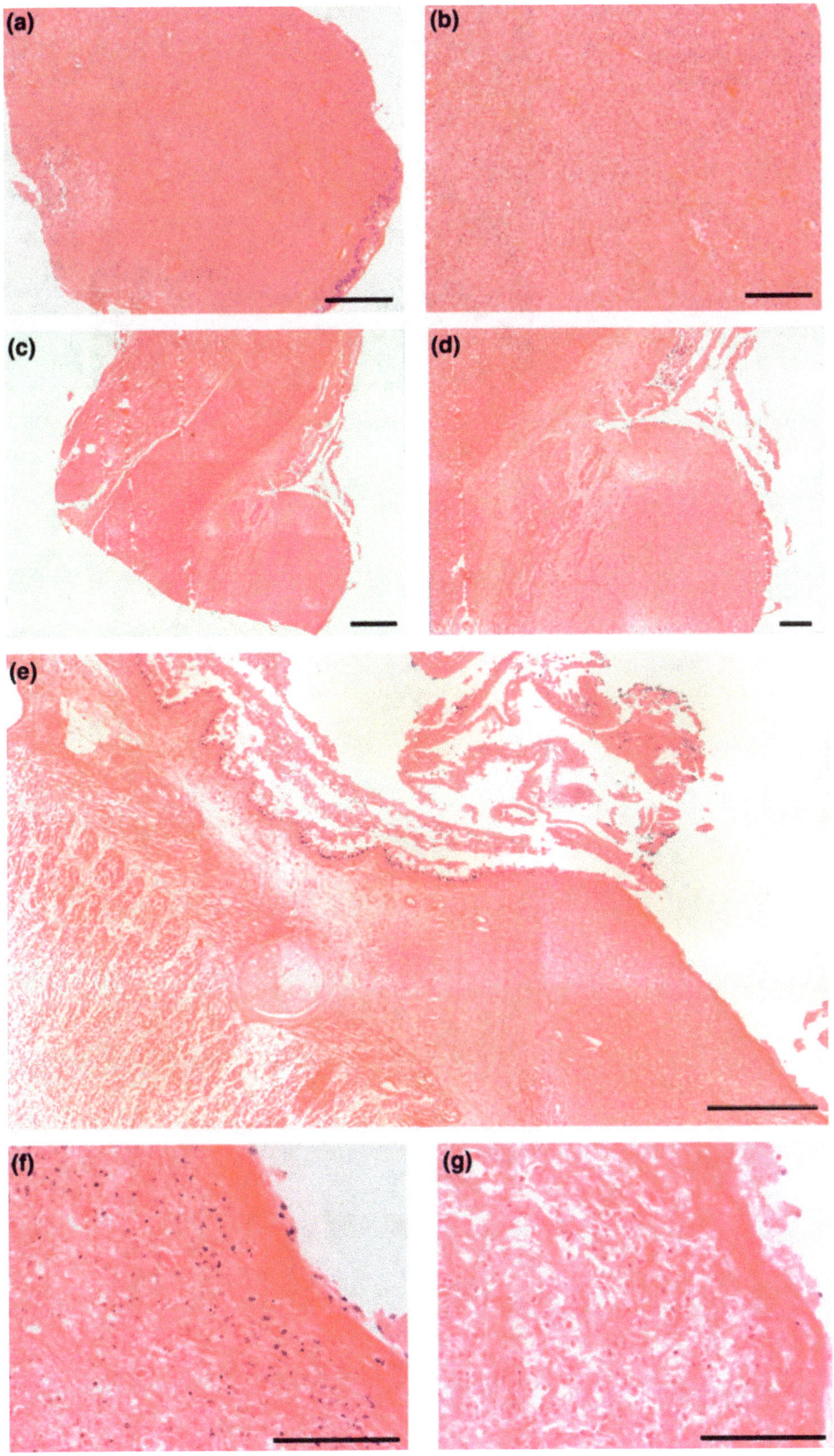

Fig. 15.2 Histological sections of nodules in *O. vulgaris* (**a–g**). **a–e** Detail of mass proliferations of dense fibrous tissue between the dermis and muscle layers. **f–g** Detail of necrotic foci also observed in **a** and **b**. *Scale bars* **a**, **d**, 200 μm; **b**, **f**, **g**, 100 μm; **c**, **e**, 500 μm

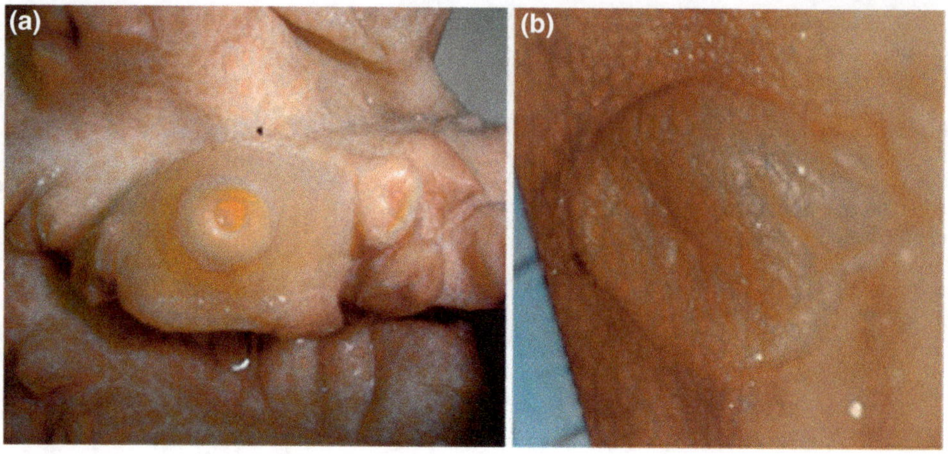

Fig. 15.3 Macroscopic aspect of nodules located at the sucker's base (**a**) and mantle (**b**) of *Octopus hubbsorum*

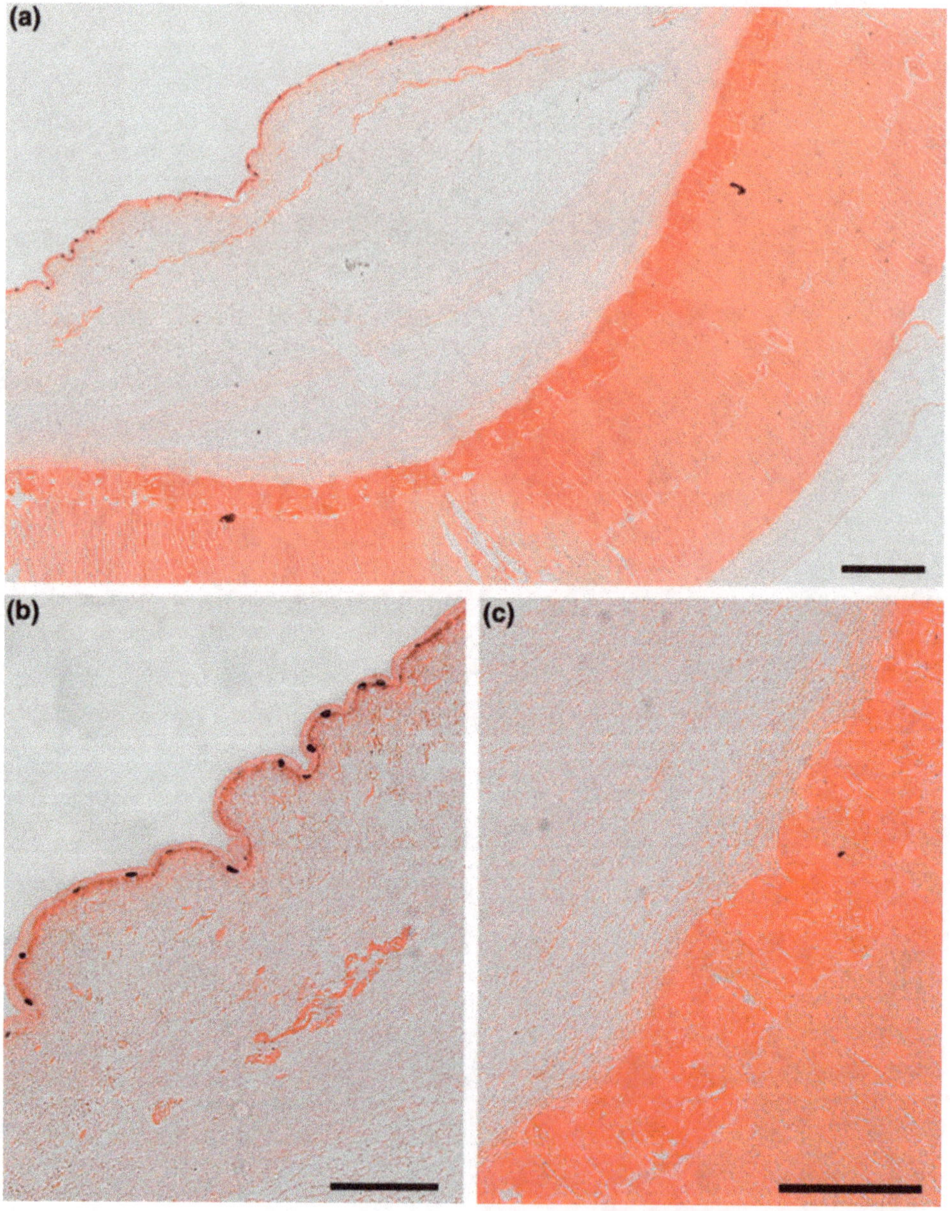

Fig. 15.4 Histological sections of nodules of *O. hubbsorum*. (**a–c**) Mass proliferations of dense fibrous tissue between the dermis and muscle layers. *Scale bars* **a**, 1 mm; **b**, **c**, 500 μm

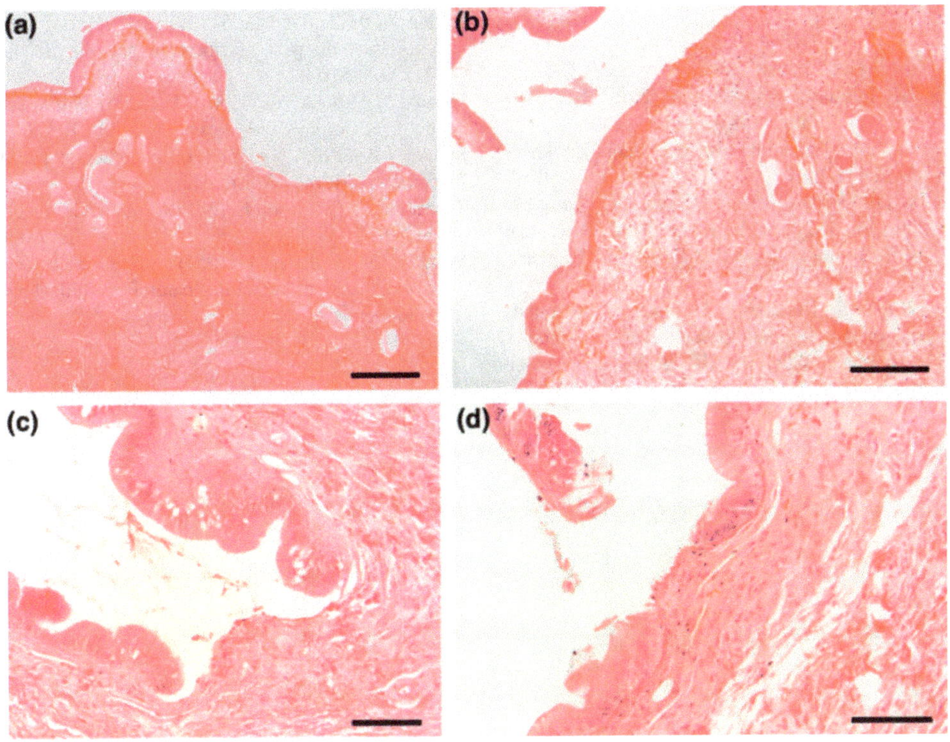

Fig. 15.5 Inflammatory focus in the mantle of *O. vulgaris* showing exudation with interstitial fluid and hemocytic migration (**a–b**). Fibrosis and necrotic cells is observed in the affected area (**b**), with loss of histological features (epithelium) (**c–d**) and even organ architecture (**a**). *Scale bars* **a**, 500 µm; **b**, 200 µm; **c**, **d**, 100 µm

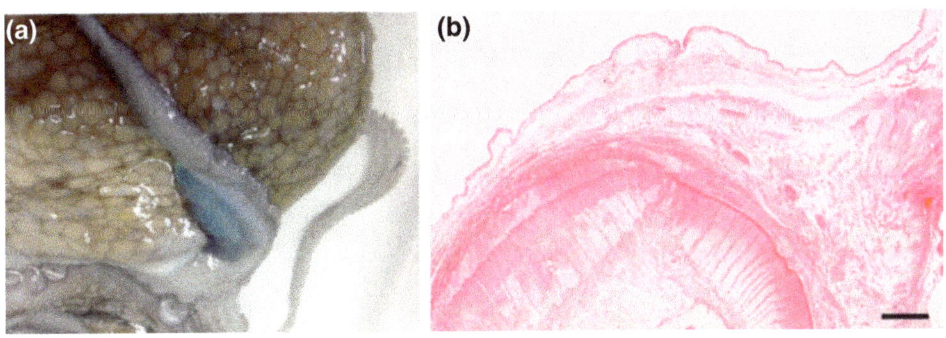

Fig. 15.6 Aedema in the arm of *O. vulgaris* maintained for long period in aquarium installations (**a–b**). **a** Macroscopic aspect of aedema focus at arm level characterized by exudation with interstitial fluid accumulation and hemocytic migration. **b** Histological detail showing the epidermis and dermis separated from the underlying muscle layers, by a watery, almost gelatinous, layer of fluid close to the sucker. *Scale bar* **b**, 1 mm

15.4 Concluding Remarks

While the study and identification of neoplasia has been increased in invertebrates and specifically in molluscs in the last years, the incidence of tumors in cephalopods is extremely low. Similarly occurs with histopathological descriptions of biological response or reactive processes of body tissues to harmful stimuli such as inflammatory reactions. The causes and effects of these disorders are not well studied. However, it is known that at least some of them could be the result of traumatic episodes, both in the wild or related to aquarium maintenance. Therefore, in the context of animal welfare, further research is needed in order to identify and to analyze the progress of those processes to avoid fatal results and to provide the best welfare conditions to the animals in captivity.

References

Carballal MJ, Barber BJ, Iglesias D, Villalba A (2015) Neoplastic diseases of marine bivalves. J Invert Pathol 131:83–106

Engel CS (1930) Warum erkraken wirbellose tiere nicht an krebs? Ztschr F Krebsforsch 32:531–543

Hanlon RT, Forsythe JW (1990a) Diseases of Mollusca: Cephalopoda. Structural abnormalities and neoplasia. In: Kinne O (ed) Diseases of marine annimals, vol III. Biologische Anstalt Helgoland, Hamburg, pp 47–227

Hanlon RT, Forsythe JW (1990b) Diseases of Mollusca: Cephalopoda. Diseases caused by protistans and metazoans. In: Kinne O (ed) Diseases of marine annimals, vol III. Biologische Anstalt Helgoland, Hamburg, pp 47–227

Jullien A, Jullien AP (1951) Sur un type de tumeur non provoquée expérimentalement et observée chez la Seiche. Acad Sci Paris 210:608–610

Pascual S, Rocha A, Guerra A (2006) Gross lesions in the Hubb octopus *Octopus hubbsorum*. Mar Biol Res 2:420–423

Sparks AK (1985) Synopsis of invertebrate pathology exclusive of insects. Elsevier, Amsterdam

Tascedda F, Ottaviani E (2014) Tumors in invertebrates. Int Sci J 11:197–203

Wauttier V, Wautier J (1955) Le cancer et les invertébrés, 1ére partie: réactions tumorales naturelles. Bull Mens Soc linnéde Lyon 3:76–96

16 Cephalopod Senescence and Parasitology

Katina Roumbedakis and Ángel Guerra

Abstract

In the majority of the shallow-water cephalopod species, senescence is a short stage of their lifespan, which takes place at the end of sexual maturity. Senescence is not a disease, although senescent cephalopods can be frequently mistaken with diseased animals. Senescence is accompanied by physiological, immunological and behavioural changes, which are briefly exposed in this chapter. A suppressed immune system may increase susceptibility to parasite infection in senescent cephalopods. High prevalence of infection by *Aggregata octopiana* was observed in *Octopus vulgaris* and *Aggregata* sp. in *Octopus maya*. In both cases, the infection was found in post-spawned females and was infecting different organs. Cestode larvae *Prochristianella* sp. were found in the buccal mass of post-spawned *O. maya* females.

Keywords

Senescence • Physiological changes • Immunological changes • Parasitology

16.1 Introduction

In the majority of the shallow-water cephalopod species, senescence is a short stage of their lifespan, which takes place at the end of sexual maturity (Tait 1986, 1987; Anderson et al. 2002). After mating, female octopuses adopt an 'extreme pattern of maternal care' (Wang and Ragsdale 2018). The mother abstains from food and exclusively takes care of the eggs, which will cost its own life; death usually occurs by the time of the offspring hatching (Wells 1978; Hanlon and Messenger 1996; Anderson et al. 2002). The senescence is reached still while the female breeds the eggs or soon after their hatching, while in males it usually begins after mating (Pascual et al. 2010).

K. Roumbedakis (✉)
Association for Cephalopod Research (CephRes), Naples, Italy
e-mail: katina.roumbedakis@gmail.com

Á. Guerra
Ecology and Biodiversity Department, Institute of Marine Research, Spanish National Research Council (CSIC), Eduardo Cabello 6, 36208 Vigo, Pontevedra, Spain
e-mail: angelguerra@iim.csic.es

Generally, males die approximately the same time as the females (Hanlon 1983; Mangold 1983; Van Heukelem 1983), but in some species, males may live longer than females, such as *Enteroctopus dofleini* (Hartwick 1983) or *Octopus vulgaris* (Mangold 1983).

The physiological process by which senescence occurs is not completely understood (Tait 1986, 1987; Anderson et al. 2002). Optic gland secretions, probably activated by environmental factors (e.g. light, temperature) and nutrition (Van Heukelem 1979), are involved in gonad maturation and in the inhibition of feeding (Tait 1986, 1987; Wodinsky 1977). Although a relatively small amount of information is available regarding the mechanisms that lead to senescence, it has been hypothesized that in species with terminal spawning (see Rocha et al. 2001 for a review of the reproductive strategies), the levels of hormonal secretions are high which would trigger the inhibition of feeding and lead to death. In species with intermittent spawning, the levels of hormonal secretions are lower, which would initiate spawning without inhibiting food intake and growth (Jackson and Mladenov 1994). Moreover, an attractive genetic mechanism of ageing, and therefore, senescence,

C. Gestal et al. (eds.), *Handbook of Pathogens and Diseases in Cephalopods*,
https://doi.org/10.1007/978-3-030-11330-8_16

was hypothesized by Guerra (1993) for all living cephalopods, except *Nautilus* species.

When sexual maturity occurs, the digestive gland ceases to function properly, leading to a gradual decrease in food intake until its cessation, consequently stopping growth (Mather 2006). A reduction of digestive enzymes in the posterior salivary glands and digestive gland observed in post-spawning octopuses is also assumed to contribute to starvation, body weight loss, and consequently, death (Sakaguchi 1968). Signs of degeneration in the nervous system and deterioration in the long-term memory process can also occur in senescent cephalopods (Chichery and Chichery 1992a).

16.2 Other Signs of Cephalopod Senescence

Senescence is accompanied by physiological, immunological and behavioural changes, which may include: (i) reduced or loss of appetite and feeding; (ii) retraction of the skin around the eyes; (iii) cloudy eyes; (iv) loss of coordination; and (iv) occurrence of skin lesions (Chichery and Chichery 1992a, b; Dumont et al. 1994; for reviews also see Anderson et al. 2002; Mather 2006).

Probably, one of the most remarkable consequences in senescent cephalopods is the loss of body weight as a consequence of starvation. A loss of body weight was observed in both male and female senescent octopuses: *Enteroctopus dofleini* (Cosgrove 1993; Anderson et al. 2002); *Octopus cyaneae* (Van Heukelem 1976); *Octopus maya* (Roumbedakis et al. 2018); *Octopus mimus* (Cortez et al. 1995); *Octopus vulgaris* (O'Dor and Wells 1987; Hernández-García et al. 2002) and *Octopus rubescens* (Anderson et al. 2002). According to these studies, in males the total loss of body weight varied between 4.3 and 32.1%, while in females larger percentages were observed, varying between 25 and 71%.

A decrease in both gonadosomatic and hepatosomatic indexes associated with the deterioration of general physiological condition occurs in post-spawned cephalopods (Tait 1986, 1987; Pollero and Iribarne 1988; Castro et al. 1992; Cortez et al. 1995; Zamora and Olivares 2004; Estefanell et al. 2010; Roumbedakis et al. 2018). Changes in gonads and the digestive gland appearance are also observed: ovaries and digestive glands became pale and opaque and oviductal glands darken (Fig. 16.1a–c), a reduction in size also occurs.

Mature and spent females of the deepwater squid *Moroteuthis ingens* showed advanced tissue breakdown with individuals having a tin mantle wall with inelastic, gelatinous appearance. Histological examination of the mantle wall revealed that tissue breakdown was due to a drastic histolysis of muscle tissue and to a lesser extent, collagen fibres (Jackson and Mladenov 1994). These features are considered by these authors in relation to the processes contributing to terminal maturation in *M. ingens*. Thus, because all the examined individuals had empty caecums, senescence and post-spawning death may be associated with starvation, as found in captive *Illex illecebrosus* (Rowe and Mangold 1975). Moreover, O'Dor and Wells (1978) noted that the tissue breakdown and death in *Octopus vulgaris* is not simply due to starvation and the energy demand of a developing ovary, because males also cease eating, show similar tissue degeneracy and die at approximately the same time as their mates. Therefore, they concluded that tissue degeneracy and death should be under the control of the optic hormone and that this hormone acted to inhibit protein synthesis. Nevertheless, it is probably that a developing ovary also produces a hormone that increases the release of muscle amino acids into the blood (O'Dor and Wells (1978).

The information on the effects of senescence in males is much scarcer than in females. Taitt experience (2013) with a senescent male Caribbean Reef Octopus (*O. briareus*) showed that its behaviour at the end of their life cycle is markedly different than that of females. Senescent males tend to be quite active, often at odd/uncharacteristic times of the day. Like females, males will generally refuse food offerings when they have approached the end of their life cycle. The male also exhibited a decline in his ability to control his chromatophores. The movement of both the male

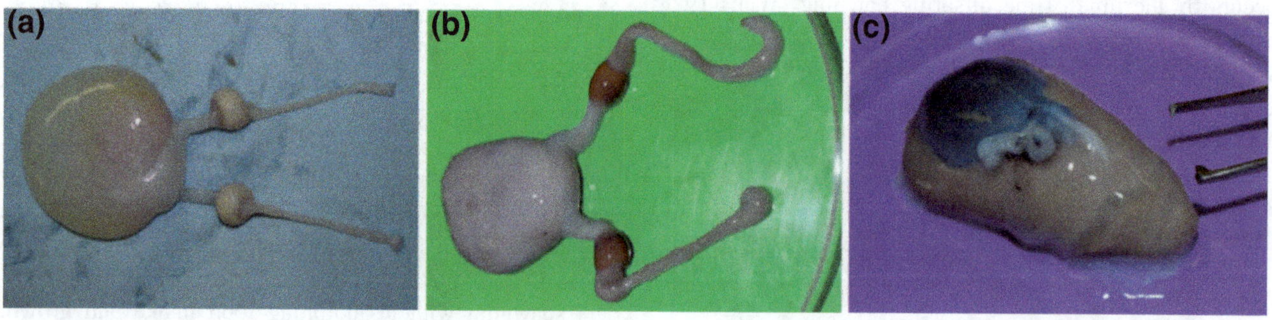

Fig. 16.1 Physiological changes in the gonad and in the digestive gland of post-spawning *Octopus maya*. **a** Gonad of a female octopus immediately after spawning; and **b** 40 days after spawning; **c** digestive gland of a female octopus 40 days after spawning

and the female are significantly less coordinated than in early stages of experimentation.

Parallel to body deterioration, a possible reduction in the immunological responses can occur during senescence (Pascual et al. 2010). However, studies evaluating the immunocompetence and health status of senescent cephalopods are rare (e.g. Roumbedakis et al. 2018). Although an immunological compensation through the cost of using energy reserves in female octopuses in the first period after spawning (i.e., until at least 40 days post-spawning) can occur (Roumbedakis et al. 2018), there is some evidence of an impairment of the immune system in senescent cephalopods. For instance, arm regeneration may not occur in injured senescent cuttlefish (Féral 1988) and host defence against parasite infection may be impaired in senescent octopuses (Pascual et al. 2010). The presence of 'unhealed wounds' in senescent female octopuses may be possibly related to an impairment of the immune responses (Wang and Ragsdale 2018).

Behavioural changes are also observed in senescent cephalopods. A recent study with sexually matured female *Octopus bimaculoides* described four stages of reproductive behavioural stages: (i) non-mated; (ii) feeding; (iii) fasting; and (iv) declining (Wang and Ragsdale 2018). The most remarkable characteristics commonly observed in senescent animals (e.g. skin lesions, retraction of skin around the eyes, missing arm tips or suckers) were seen in the fourth stage. The authors also identified that multiple signalling systems of the optic glands are involved in these behaviours.

16.3 Parasitology and Senescence

Senescence is not a disease, although senescent cephalopods can be frequently mistaken with diseased animals. For that reason, in order to be able to differentiate these conditions, it is important to recognize its signs (Anderson et al. 2002). Senescence-like symptoms due to poor animal welfare (e.g. changes in water quality parameters) can also occur (Budelmann 1998). Skin lesions caused by hits against the tank walls also are a common cause for bacterial infections (Hanlon and Forsythe 1990), which may eventually become a more likely occurrence due to the loss of coordination in senescent cephalopods.

Parasitological studies in senescent cephalopods are rare, however, they may provide important insights into host–parasite interactions. In senescent female cephalopods, the transmission of parasites through the food chain (e.g. trematodes digenea, cestodes, nematodes) might be reduced or inexistent, due to the reduction or lack of feeding in this period. Moreover, senescent cephalopods parasitized may eventually not properly activate immunological reactions, as observed in *Octopus vulgaris* infected with *Aggregata* (Pascual et al. 2010), in which low host reaction and no signs of inflammation were observed. A suppressed immune system may increase susceptibility to parasite infection in senescent cephalopods.

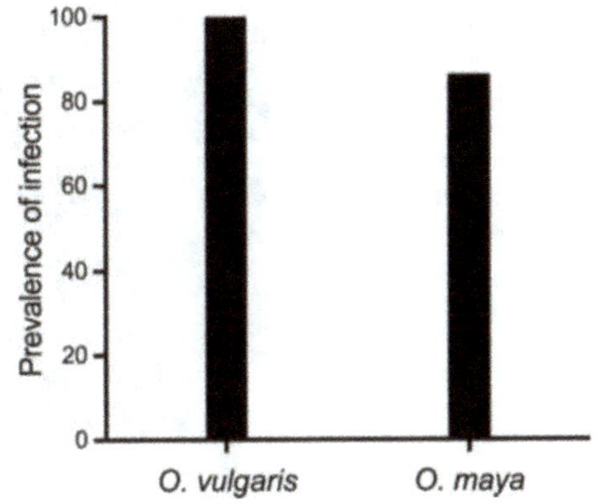

Fig. 16.2 Prevalence of infection of *Aggregata* spp. in post-spawned female octopuses: *Octopus vulgaris* (n = 4; compiled from Pascual et al. 2010) and *O. maya* (n = 22; original data)

As commonly observed in adult octopuses, post-spawned female octopuses also present high prevalence of infection by *Aggregata* spp. (Apicomplexa, Aggregatidae) (Fig. 16.2). In post-spawned female *O. vulgaris*, large numbers of sporogonial stages (infective forms) of *Aggregata octopiana* were highly spread in host tissues, probably to ensure the completion of parasite's life cycle (Pascual et al. 2010). In post-spawned female *O. maya* infections by *Aggregata* sp. were observed in the caecum (Fig. 16.3a), intestine, and gills of the hosts (Roumbedakis et al. 2017).

In addition, post-spawned female *O. maya* was also parasitized with cestode larvae *Prochristianella* sp. (Cestoda, Trypanorhyncha). This parasite was found in the buccal mass of the female octopuses (Fig. 16.3B), with 90.9% of prevalence and mean intensity of infection of 155.4 ± 107.73.

Both parasites, the coccidian *Aggregata* sp. and the thrypanorhynch cestode *Prochristianella* sp., are transmitted by the food chain. In this study, female octopuses were captured in the wild and acclimatized in the laboratory for approximately 1–2 months until sampling, which occurred immediately after or until 40 days after spawning. In the beginning of the acclimation period octopuses fed on frozen crabs or on an artificial diet and then feeding was gradually reduced until the spawning. This suggests that these animals were already infected with both parasites before capture.

16.4 Concluding Remarks

The degenerative process and death are so rapid in the majority of cephalopods that quantitative and qualitative changes are very important. For this and other reasons (e.g. excellent adaptation of some species to confinement

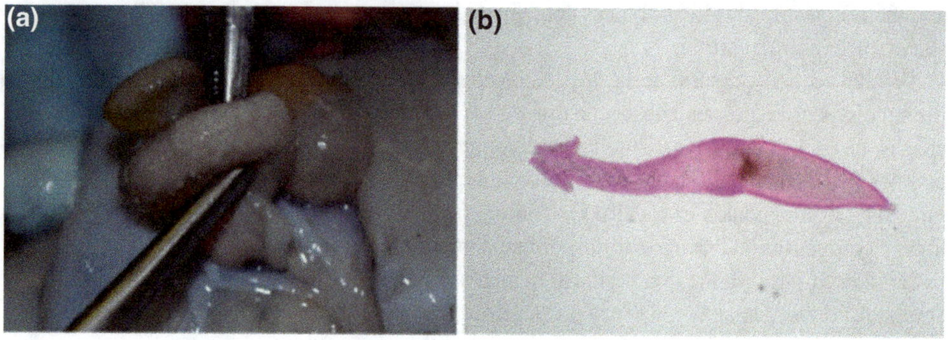

Fig. 16.3 Parasites of post-spawning female *O. maya*. **a** Caecum infected with the coccidian *Aggregata* sp. **b** Trypanorhynch cestode *Prochristianella* sp. collected from the buccal mass

conditions, and their capacity to tolerate well surgical operations) cephalopods are an excellent material for the study of mechanisms regulating ageing in laboratory models, and therefore in bio-gerontology. As pointed out by Nussey et al. (2012), the recent emergence of long-term field studies presents irrefutable evidence that senescence is commonly detected in nature. These authors found such evidence in 175 different animal species. The bulk of this evidence comes from birds and mammals, but senescence was also evidenced in other vertebrates and insects. It could surprise the absence of the cephalopods in this comprehensive review, but this may be due to the fact that senescence has hardly been observed in nature in these organisms. Parasitological studies in senescent cephalopods are rare, however, they may provide important insights into host–parasite interactions. For the above reasons, we consider that both the study of senescence in cephalopods and the relationship between this critical period of the life cycle and the pathological processes caused by infections is still in its infancy, and should be a field of research to be developed.

References

Anderson RC, Wood JB, Byrne RA (2002) Octopus senescence: the beginning of the end. J Appl Anim Welf Sci 5:275–283

Budelmann BU (1998) Autophagy in *Octopus*. In: Payne AIL, Lipinski MR, Clarke MR, Roeleveld MAC (eds) Cephalopod biodiversity, ecology and evolution. South Afri J Mar Sci 20:101–108

Castro BG, Garrido JL, Sotelo CG (1992) Changes in composition of digestive gland and mantle muscle of the cuttlefish *Sepia officinalis* during starvation. Mar Biol 114:11–20

Chichery MP, Chichery R (1992a) Behavioural and neurohistological changes in ageing *Sepia*. Brain Res 574:77–84

Chichery R, Chichery MP (1992b) Learning performances and aging in cuttlefish (*Sepia officinalis*). Exp Gerontol 27:233–239

Cortez T, Castro BG, Guerra A (1995) Reproduction and condition of female *Octopus mimus* (Mollusca: Cephalopoda). Mar Biol 123:505–510

Cosgrove JA (1993) In situ observations of nesting female *Octopus dofleini* (Wülker, 1910). J Cepha Biol 2:33–45

Dumont E, Chichery MP, Nouvelot A, Chichery R (1994) Variations of the lipid constituents in the central nervous system of the cuttlefish (*Sepia officinalis*) during aging. Comp Biochem Physiol Part A: Physiol 108(2–3):315–323

Estefanell J, Socorro J, Roo FJ, Fernández-Palacios H, Izquierdo M (2010) Gonad maturation in *Octopus vulgaris* during ongrowing, under different conditions of sex ratio. ICES J Mar Sci 67:1487–1493

Féral JP (1988) Wound healing after arm amputation in *Sepia officinalis* (Cephalopoda: Sepioidea). J Invert Pathol 52(3):380–388

Guerra A (1993) Ageing in cephalopods. In: Okutani T. et al (eds) The recent advances in cephalopod fisheries biology. Tokai University Press, pp 684–687

Hanlon RT (1983). *Octopus briareus*. In: Boyle PR (ed) Cephalopod life cycles: species accounts, vol 1. London Academic Press, pp 251–256

Hanlon RT, Forsythe JW (1990) Diseases caused by microorganisms. In: Kinne O (ed) Diseases of mollusca: cephalopoda. Biologische Anstalt Helgoland, Hamburg, pp 23–46

Hanlon RT, Messenger JB (1996) Cephalopod Behaviour. Cambridge University Press, Cambridge

Hartwick B (1983) *Octopus dofleini*. In: Boyle PR (ed) Cephalopod life cycles: species accounts, vol. 1. London Academic Press, pp 277–291

Hernández-García V, Hernández-López JL, Castro-Hernández JJ (2002) On the reproduction of *Octopus vulgaris* off the coast of the Canary Islands. Fish Res 57:197–203

Jackson GD, Mladenov PD (1994) Terminal spawning in the deepwater squid *Moroteuthis ingens* (Cephalopoda: Onychoteuthidae) J Zool Lond 234:189–201

Mangold KM (1983) *Octopus vulgaris*. In: Boyle PR (ed) Cephalopod life cycles: species accounts, vol. 1. London Academic Press, pp 335–364

Mather JA (2006) Behaviour development: a cephalopod perspective. Int J Comp Psychol 19(1):98–115

Nussey DH, Froy H, Lemaitre J-F, Gaillard J-M, Austad SN (2012) Senescence in natural populations of animals: widespread evidence and its implications for bio-gerontology. Ageing Res Rev 12(1):214–225

O'Dor RK, Wells MJ (1978) Reproduction *versus* somatic growth, hormonal control in *Octopus vulgaris*. J Exp Biol 77:15–31

O'Dor RK, Wells MJ (1987) Energy and nutrient flow. In: Boyle PR (ed) Cephalopod life cycles. London Academic Press, pp 109–133

Pascual S, González AF, Guerra A (2010) Coccidiosis during octopus senescence: preparing for parasite outbreak. Fish Res 106:160–162

Pollero RJ, Iribarne OO (1988) Biochemical changes during the reproductive cycle of the small Patagonian octopus, *Octopus tehuelchus*, d'Orb. Comp Bioch Physiol 90B(2):317–320

Rocha F, Guerra A, González AF (2001) A review of the reproductive strategies in cephalopods. Biol Rev 76:291–304

Roumbedakis K, Pascual C, Guillén-Hernández S, Rosas C. Martins ML (2017) Parasite fauna of post spawning female *Octopus maya* (Cephalopoda: Octopodidae) in the Yucatan Peninsula, Mexico. In: Cephs*In*Action & CIAC Meeting 'Cephalopod Science from Biology to Welfare', Heraklion, Greece, p 93

Roumbedakis K, Mascaró M, Martins ML, Gallardo P, Rosas C, Pascual C (2018) Health status of post-spawning *Octopus maya* (Cephalopoda: Octopodidae) females from Yucatan Peninsula, Mexico. Hydrobiologia 808:23–34

Rowe VL, Mangold K (1975) The effect of starvation on sexual maturation in *Illex illecebrosus* (Lesueur) (Cephalopoda: Teuthoidea). J Exp Mar Biol Physiol 17:157–163

Sakaguchi H (1968) Studies of digestive enzymes of devilfish. Bull Japan Soc Sci 34:716–721

Tait RW (1986) Aspects physiologiques de la sénescence post reproductive chez *Octopus vulgaris*. Ph D thesis. Universidad de Paris VI, France

Tait RW (1987) Why do octopus die? Cephalopod International Advisory Committee Newsletter 2:22–25

Taitt K (2013) End of *Octopus* life cycle https://kyletaitt.scienceblog.com/2013/11/26/end-of-female-octopus-life-cycle/with cephalopods (Visited on 25 Oct 2018)

Van Heukelem WF (1976) Growth, bioenergetics and lifespan in *Octopus cyanea* and *Octopus maya*. PhD thesis. University of Hawaii, Hawaii

Van Heukelem WF (1979) Environmental control of reproduction and life span in *Octopus*: an hypothesis. In: Stancyk SE (ed) Reproductive ecology of marine invertebrates. University of South Carolina Press, pp 123–133

Van Heukelem WF (1983) *Octopus maya*. In: Boyle PR (ed) Cephalopod life cycles: species accounts, vol. 1. London Academic Press, pp 311–323

Wang ZY, Ragsdale CW (2018) Multiple optic gland signalling pathways implicated in octopus maternal behaviors and death. J Exp Biol jeb-185751 pii: jeb185751; https://doi.org/10.1242/jeb.185751

Wells MJ (1978) Octopus: physiology and behaviour of an advanced invertebrate. Chapman and Hall, London, p 431

Wodinsky J (1977) Hormonal inhibition of feeding and death in *Octopus*: control by optic gland secretion. Science 198:948–951

Zamora MJ, Olivares A (2004) Variaciones bioquímicas e histológicas asociadas al evento reproductivo de la hembra de *Octopus mimus* (Mollusca: Cephalopoda). Int J Morphol 22(3):207–216

Pathogens and Related Diseases in Non-European Cephalopods: Central and South America

17

Yanis Cruz-Quintana, Jonathan Fabricio Lucas Demera, Leonela Griselda Muñoz-Chumo, Ana María Santana-Piñeros, Sheila Castellanos-Martínez, and Ma. Leopoldina Aguirre-Macedo

Abstract

Despite the economic and ecologic importance of Mexican four-eyed *Octopus maya* and the jumbo squid *Dosidicus gigas*, the pathogens and diseases in both species remain largely unknown. This chapter covers the pathogens and diseases, mainly protozoan and metazoan parasites, of these two non-European cephalopods.

Keywords

Mexico • Ecuador • Fisheries • Parasites • *Octopus maya* • *Dosidicus gigas*

17.1 Introduction

The Mexican four-eyed *Octopus maya* and the jumbo squid *Dosidicus gigas* are important fishery sources from Mexico and Ecuador, respectively. *Octopus maya* is an endemic species of the Yucatan peninsula, with a distribution range spanning from Ciudad del Carmen in Campeche State to Isla Mujeres in Quintana Roo State (Van Heukelem 1983). It is one of the most important commercially exploited species in Mexican fisheries, generating over 27 million dollars in revenue annually, with a high potential for aquaculture due to their good adaptability to captive conditions. On the other hand, *D. gigas* is an endemic species of the eastern Pacific, with a distribution range going from Alaska, USA, to Tierra del Fuego, Chile (Roper et al. 2010). It is commercially caught by the USA, México, Perú, and Chile. However, in early 2014, the Ecuador Government decided that *D. gigas* must be a new fishery target and the collection of biological data to improve the fisheries management began (Morales-Bojórquez and Pacheco-Bedoya 2016). In this chapter, an overview of the parasites and pathological conditions in two wild cephalopods, the Octopodidae *Octopus maya* from the Mexican Caribbean coast and the Ommastrephidae *Dosidicus gigas* from the Ecuadorian Pacific coast, is provided. Tissue slides collected from both species were stained with hematoxylin and eosin (H&E). The figures include the scale bar in micrometers, except in the majority of the macroscopic images which include the scale in millimeters. In this chapter, we will not go into detail on the anatomy and normal histology of *Octopus maya* or *Dosidicus gigas*, as these general aspects of cephalopods have been addressed previously in Chaps. 3 and 4. However, we will describe some anatomical and histological aspects of the affected organs or tissues, to facilitate the understanding of the tissue alterations.

Y. Cruz-Quintana (✉) · J. F. Lucas Demera · L. G. Muñoz-Chumo · A. M. Santana-Piñeros
Grupo de Investigación en Sanidad Acuícola, Inocuidad y Salud Ambiental. Escuela de Acuicultura y Pesquería, Facultad de Ciencias Veterinarias, Universidad Técnica de Manabí, Calle Gonzalo Loor Velasco, S/N., Ciudadela Universitaria, CP 130104 Bahía de Caráquez, Ecuador
e-mail: cqyanis@gmail.com

J. F. Lucas Demera
e-mail: jonathanlucas17@outlook.com

L. G. Muñoz-Chumo
e-mail: leitogris@gmail.com

A. M. Santana-Piñeros
e-mail: anasantana4@gmail.com

S. Castellanos-Martínez
Instituto de Investigaciones Oceanológicas UABC, Ensenada, Mexico
e-mail: mixtly2000@hotmail.com

Ma. L. Aguirre-Macedo
Laboratorio de Patología Acuática y Parasitología, CINVESTAV Unidad Mérida, Carretera Antigua a Progreso, Km 6, Cordemex, 97310 Mérida, Yucatán, Mexico
e-mail: leopoldina.aguirre@cinvestav.mx

C. Gestal et al. (eds.), *Handbook of Pathogens and Diseases in Cephalopods*,
https://doi.org/10.1007/978-3-030-11330-8_17

17.2 Pathogens and Related Diseases in the Mexican Four-Eyed Octopus *Octopus Maya*

The digestive tract of *O. maya*, like other octopuses, is rather short, consisting of a buccal mass, esophagus, crop, stomach, caecum, intestine, and digestive gland. The buccal mass, the first organ of the digestive system, is a roughly spherical structure that lies just in front of the brain, within a sinus formed by the base of the arms (Fig. 17.1a). It is loosely attached within the sinus by the esophagus and the enclosing buccal membrane, a pigmented web of folded skin that is attached to the arms. The buccal membrane surrounding the beaks is folded into inner and outer lips. Among other components like muscles, radula, and upper and lower beaks, the buccal mass involves the anterior salivary glands (Fig. 17.1b), a simple branched tubular gland surrounded by a thin capsule of lax connective tissue with scarce muscular fibers. The secretory epithelium of this gland is supported by a connective tissue membrane which forms trabecules within the tissue. Acinar spaces are formed and lined with secretory cells that vary in height, from cuboidal to columnar depending on the stage of secretion (Fig. 17.1c). The function of the mucus produced by the anterior salivary glands is not only limited to the provision of lubrication necessary for sliding and predigestion of the food but also provides support for eggs in spawning females.

Larval stages of the cestoda *Prochristianella hispida* infect the anterior salivary glands of *O. maya*, destroying the secretory tissue and producing fibrosis. In hosts with low infection (< 5 parasites), the cestodes cause focal necrosis of the tubules' epithelial tissue, with a slight proliferation of connective tissue (Fig. 17.1d). In moderate infections (6–20 parasites), damage is more noticeable, compromising larger areas (Fig. 17.2a), whereas in heavy infections (>20 parasites per host), the secretory epithelium is replaced by parasites and fibrous connective tissue (Fig. 17.2b), which reduces the functionality of the gland. The parasites also infect, although in less number, the scarce connective tissue between the internal and external epithelium and muscles of the buccal mass. The high prevalence of cestode larvae in the anterior salivary glands of *O. maya* and the severe damages associated with the infection level could cause reproductive and nutritional alterations, considering the functions of saliva in these two physiological processes.

Continuing through the digestive tract and posterior to the buccal mass, esophagus, crop, and stomach, the caecum is located; a tubular organ spirals around an axis or columella (Fig. 17.3a). The caecum shows longitudinal folds protruding into the lumen, increasing the surface area of the organ. In the external wall of the caecum, these folds are larger and more abundant than those in the internal wall near the columella. These primary folds that arise from the inner side of the external wall give way to secondary folds. They are all

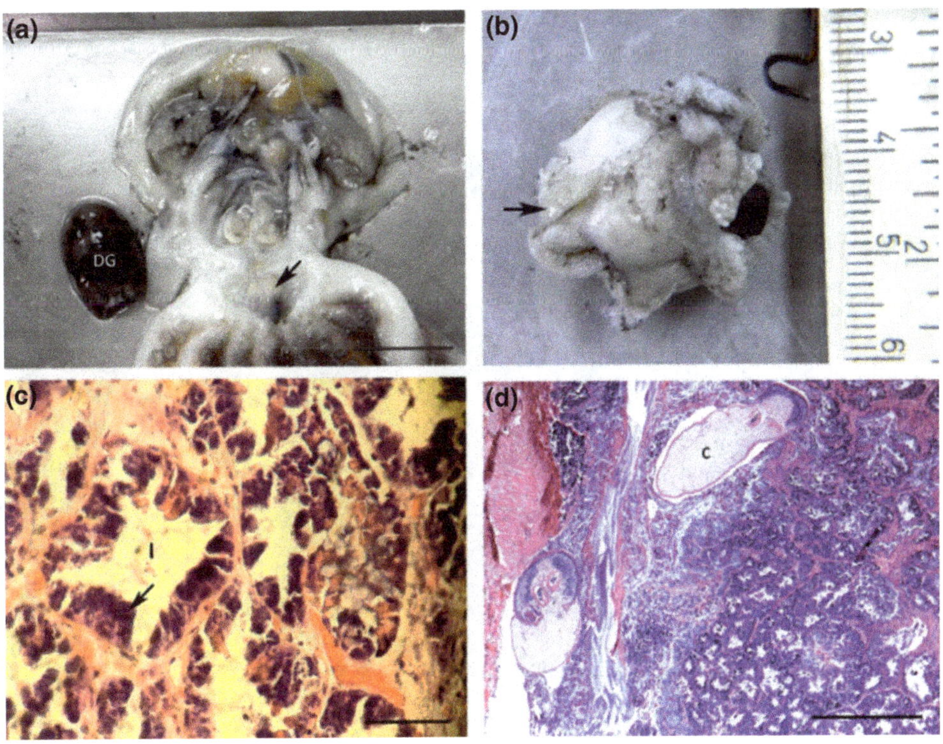

Fig. 17.1 **a** *Octopus maya* dissected, showing the digestive system: buccal mass (arrow), esophagus, posterior salivary glands, intestine, stomach, and caecum. The digestive gland (DG) was removed to facilitate the organs' visibility. Scale bar: 50 mm. **b** Buccal mass with anterior salivary glands (arrow). **c** Anterior salivary glands showing: cylindrical cells (arrows), lumen (l). Scale bar: 50 µm. **d** Anterior salivary glands with low cestode infection. Note the normal appearance of the secretory tissue (lower right) despite the presence of two cestodes (c). Scale bar: 500 µm

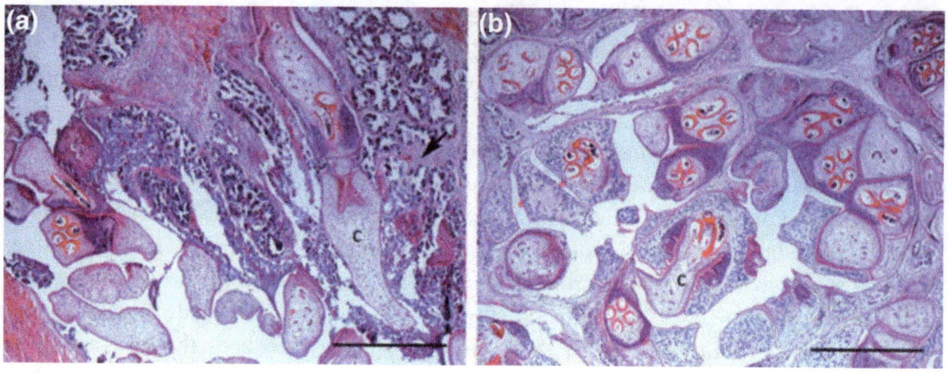

Fig. 17.2 Anterior salivary glands with cestode (c) infection. **a** Moderate infection, observing the proliferation of connective tissue (arrow) and loss of secretory tissue (lower left). Scale bar: 500 µm. **b** Heavy infection where secretory tissue has been replaced by cestodes and fibrous connective tissue. Scale bar: 500 µm

lined by a simple, cylindrical, and ciliated epithelium, and have a central axis of loose connective tissue (or corion) with high vascularization (Fig. 17.3b). The mucosa is underlined by scarce connective tissue and thin fascicles of longitudinal muscle fibers. A similar architecture is shown in the intestine, which has longitudinal folds protruding into the lumen mainly in the proximal and medial zones. The mucosa is lined by a pseudostratified and ciliated epithelium that lies on a loose, highly vascularized connective tissue with some muscle fibers. Behind the connective tissue, a thin muscular wall comprised by an external circular layer and an internal longitudinal one provides the support and elasticity to the intestine.

As found in *Octopus vulgaris* (Estévez et al. 1996; Gestal et al. 1999, 2002), coccidian of the genus *Aggregata* infects the wall and primary folds in the caecum and intestine of *Octopus maya*. Small and whitish cysts containing *Aggregata* sporocysts are easily distinguished in the external wall of both organs by gross observation (Fig. 17.3a). Histologically, gamogony and sporogony of *Aggregata* sp. are observed in the loose connective tissue and epithelium of the primary folds. The presence of macro- and microgametes cause enlargement, not only in the infected cells but also in the primary folds (Fig. 17.4a). Frequently, these marked enlargements cause rupture of the basal membrane with the detachment of the epithelium.

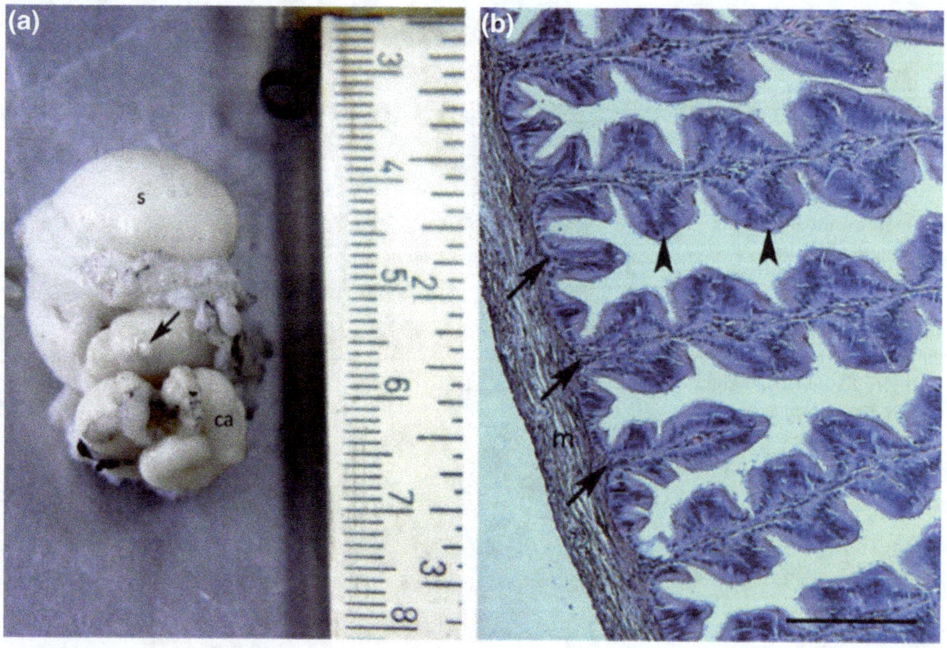

Fig. 17.3 **a** Dorsal view of the stomach(s) and caecum coiled (ca) of *O. maya*. Oocyst of *Aggregata* sp. (arrow) in the external wall of the caecum coiled. **b** Normal histology of the caecum coiled showing the external wall with primary longitudinal folds, with different heights (arrows), and secondary folds (arrowhead). (m) Muscle of external wall. Scale bar: 200 µm

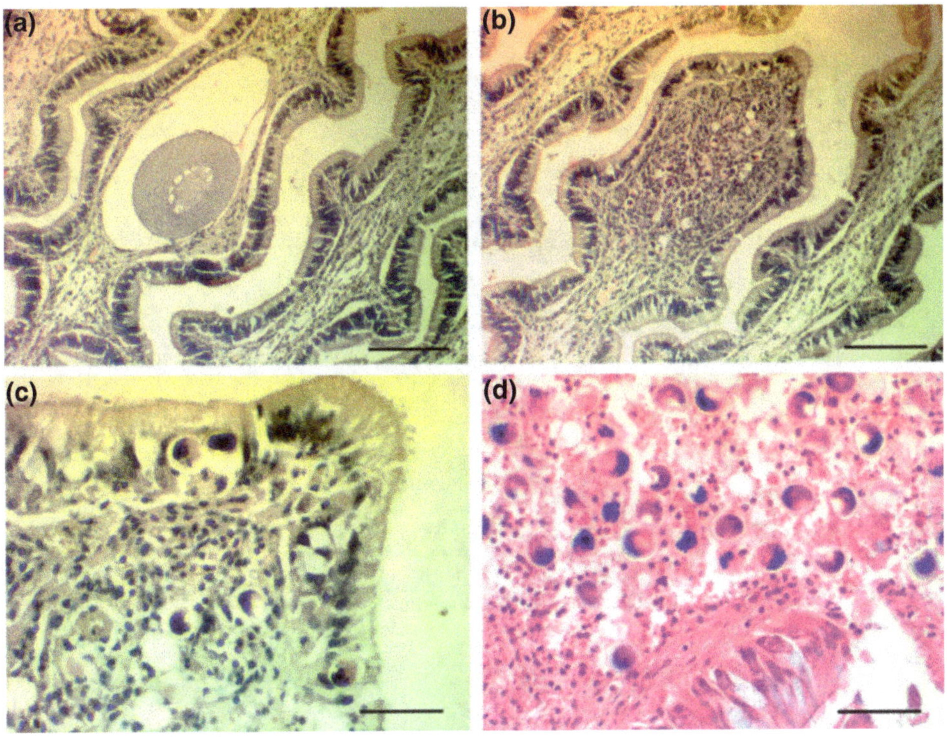

Fig. 17.4 **a** Histological section of macrogametes on an infected caecum of *O. maya*. Scale bar: 200 µm. **b** Histological section of sporocyst located on the loose connective tissue of an infected caecum of *O. maya*. The presence of sporocysts causes hemocytic infiltration and distension of the primary folder. Scale bar: 200 µm. **c** The histological section at a higher magnification of the infected caecum as shown in Fig. 17.4b. Note the sporocysts in the loose connective tissue of the primary folder and throughout the epithelium. Scale bar: 50 µm. **d** Histological section of sporocysts located on the loose connective tissue of an infected intestine of *O. maya*. Note the destruction of the tissue organ architecture and loss of intestinal epithelium. Scale bar: 50 µm

Individual sporocysts not enclosed in cysts are located within epithelial cells of the mucous membrane and in the submucosal connective tissue of the caecum and intestine of *O. maya* (Fig. 17.4b–d). Pericyst reactions of connective tissue and hemocytic infiltration produce marked distension in the affected area (Fig. 17.4b). In the mucous membrane of the digestive tract, the sporocysts containing the infective stages (sporozoites) migrate through the epithelium causing degenerating and the death of the invaded cell (Fig. 17.4c). Periodically, necrotic portions of the caecum and infected intestinal epithelium are sloughed off and eliminated. In heavily infected hosts, most of the tissue is replaced by parasites, and loss of caecum, intestinal epithelium, and destruction of the organ tissue architecture can be observed (Fig. 17.4d). The damage may have detrimental effects on gastrointestinal function and a malabsorption syndrome is probably the result in a heavily infected host, which agrees with the observations by Gestal et al. (2002).

The digestive gland, the most prominent organ of *O. maya*, is brown in color and is located in the anterior half of the body (Fig. 17.5a). This is a branched tubular organ enclosed in a capsule of loose connective tissue with scarce smooth muscular fibers. Each tubule represents a functional unit and is composed of highly vacuolated polyhedral cells, which are seated in a thin basal lamina and defined apically the lumen of the tubule (Fig. 17.5b). The organ's function is related to the digestive process, supplying most of the digestive enzymes (Domíngues et al. 2007; Aguila et al. 2007).

The presence of *Aggregata* sp. in the digestive gland of *O. maya* is less frequent than in the caecum and intestine. However, sporogony stages can be seen in the epithelial cells of the hepatopancreatic tubes. Focal necrosis of the tubular epithelium and hemocytic infiltrations in the intertubular spaces are caused by the presence of sporogony stages. The severity of the damage is related to the infection level, which can cause degeneration of epithelial cells and atrophy of the organ (Fig. 17.5c, d).

As in other coleoids, a single pair of well-vascularized gills suspended in the mantle cavity permits the respiratory exchange of *O. maya* with the environment (Fig. 17.6a). The gill has primary lamellae that extend perpendicularly to the gill axis, forming inner and outer demibranches supported by cartilaginous rods. Each primary lamella is folded to form

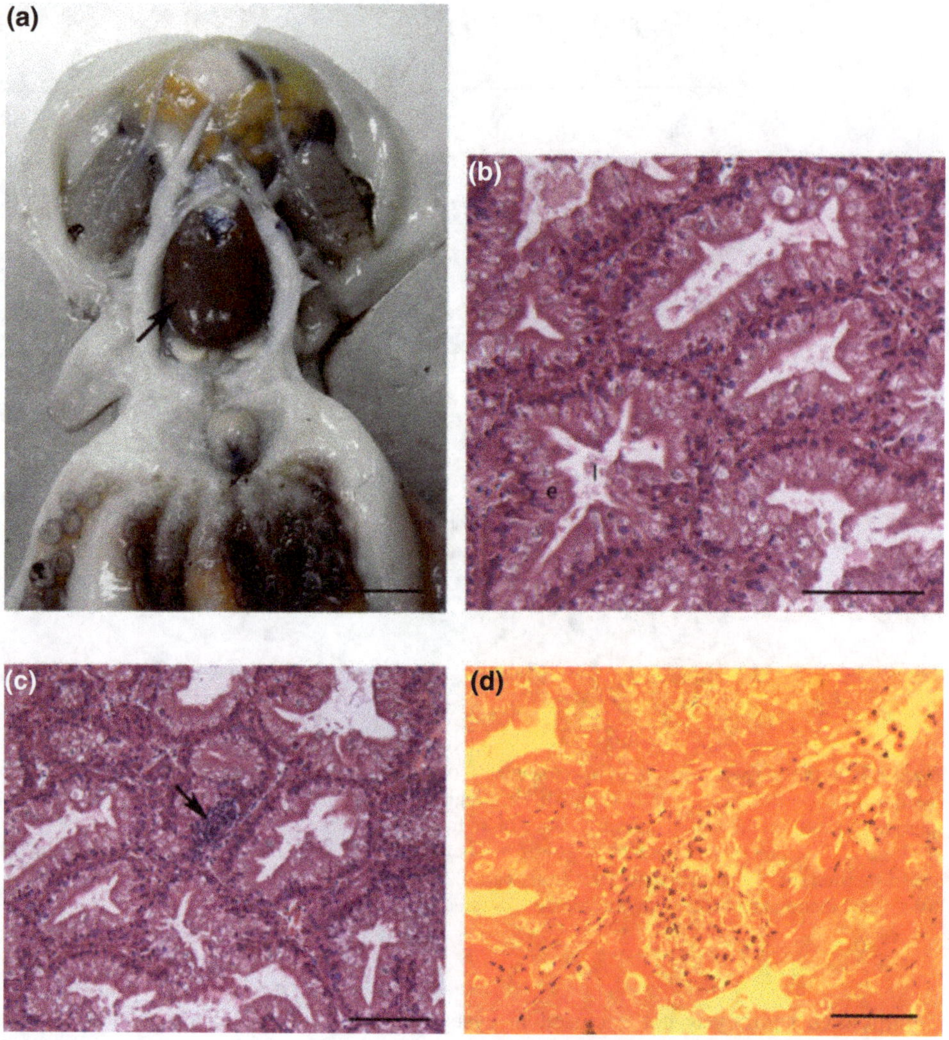

Fig. 17.5 **a** Digestive gland (arrow) in *O. maya*. Scale bar: 50 mm. **b** Histological section of the digestive gland on a healthy *O. maya*. The lumen (l) of the tubules is lined by the epithelium (e) that it is supported by the basal lamina. Scale bar: 100 µm. **c** Histological section of the digestive gland showing a focal necrosis (arrow) in the tubular epithelium. Scale bar: 100 µm. **d** Histological section of the digestive gland on an infected *O. maya* with *Aggregata* sp. Note the focal necrosis and uninucleate sporoblasts on the epithelium. Scale bar: 50 µm

secondary lamellae that are partially partitioned by a septum. A branched arrangement of the secondary lamellae originates the tertiary lamellae (Fig. 17.6b). The secondary and tertiary lamellae are lined by a thin epithelium in a concave inner and convex outer side. Between inner and outer parts, the hemolymph runs in lacunae facilitating the gas exchange (Fig. 17.6c).

The gills are the target organs of most parasite species in *O. maya*. Copepods of the genus *Octopicola* are frequent parasites of the gill tissue. The number of parasites varies according to locality and climatic season, but generally, the abundance is high. Infections by these copepods cause hemocytic infiltration between the inner and outer layers of the secondary and tertiary lamellae, with connective tissue proliferation and lamella fusion (Figs. 17.7a, b). The damage is greater when the abundance of parasites increases, compromising large areas of gill tissue. The second more frequent parasite that infects the gills of *O. maya* is an unidentified larval cestode. The presence of plerocercoids in the gill tissue is more frequent in primary lamellae and less frequent in secondary lamellae, where the cestodes induce connective tissue proliferation with hemocytic infiltration (Fig. 17.7c, d). The compromised area depends on the number of cestodes and the magnitude of host tissue reaction, but in heavily infected hosts the hemolymph flow may be reduced considerably, affecting physiological processes.

A *Cryptogonimidae* trematode has been identified in gills from *O. maya*. This parasite is less frequent than copepods and cestodes, and the histological damage associated with it is more focal. The metacercariae show a preference for the primary lamellae, producing distention and hemocytic infiltration (Fig. 17.8a, b).

Extraintestinal sporogonia of *Aggregata* sp. have been observed in the gills of *O. maya*. The infected hosts show

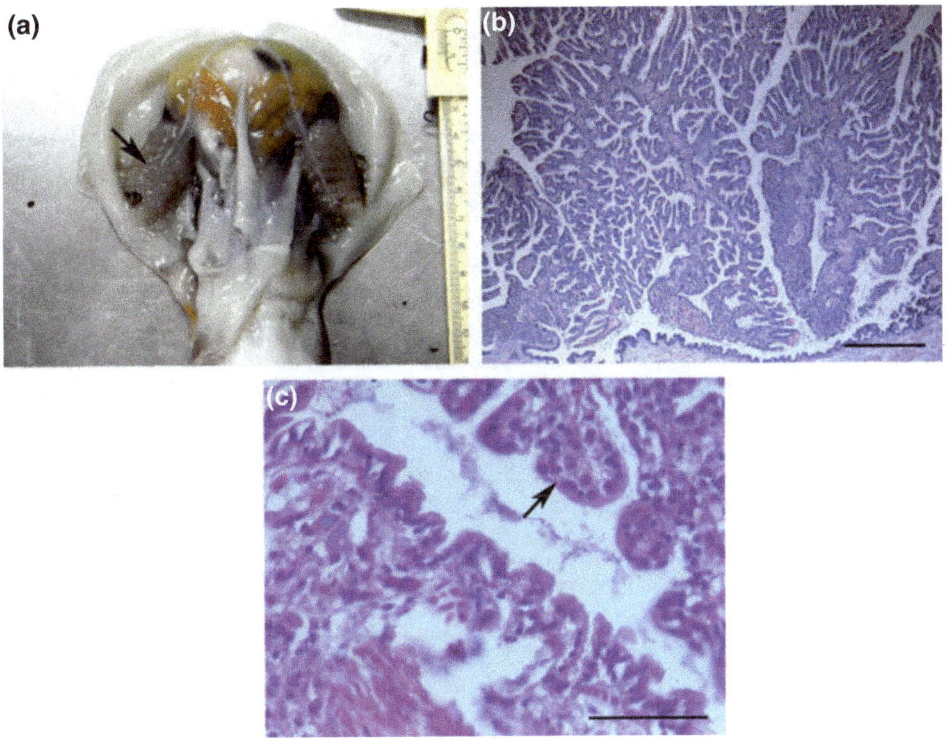

Fig. 17.6 **a** Gills in *O. maya* (arrow). **b** Histological section of gill on a healthy *O. maya*. Note the branching arrangement of the lamellae. Scale bar: 500 µm. **c** Histological section of a gill of a healthy *O. maya* showing the epithelium (arrow). Scale bar: 100 µm

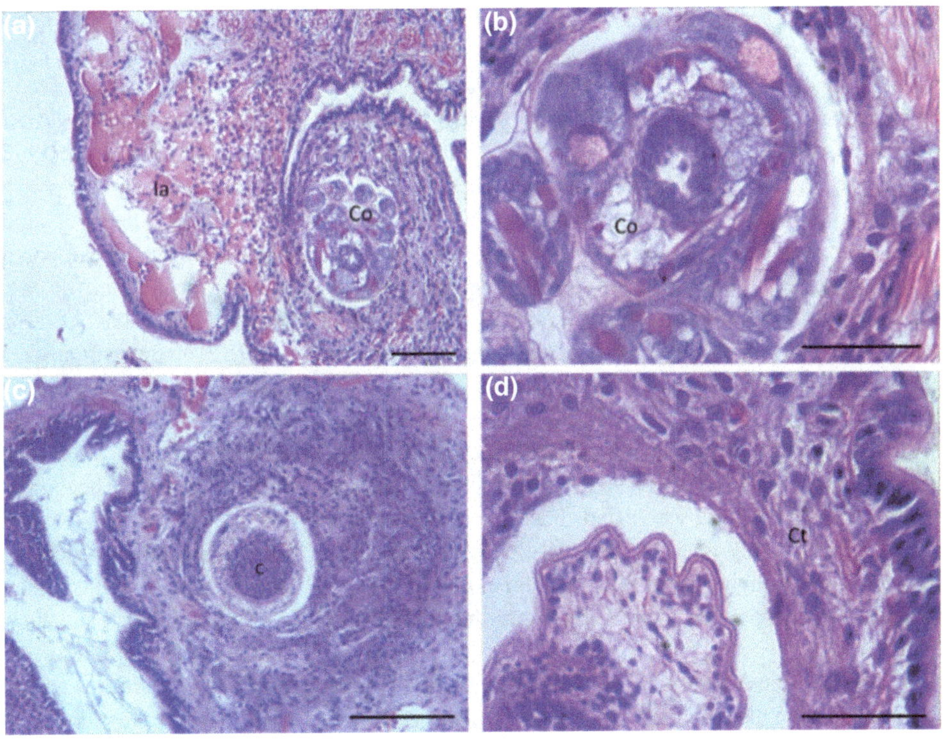

Fig. 17.7 **a** Gill section of *O. maya* with an *Octopicola* copepod (Co) producing distention of lacunae (la) and hemocytic infiltration. Scale bar: 100 µm. **b** Higher magnification of Fig. 17.7a. Note the arrangement of the host tissue to encapsulate the copepod (Co). Scale bar: 50 µm. **c** Gill section of *Octopus maya* with a strong hemocytic reaction around an unidentified larval cestode (c). Scale bar: 200 µm. **d** Higher magnification of the gill tissue, showing proliferation of connective tissue (Ct) around unidentified larval cestode. Scale bar: 50 µm

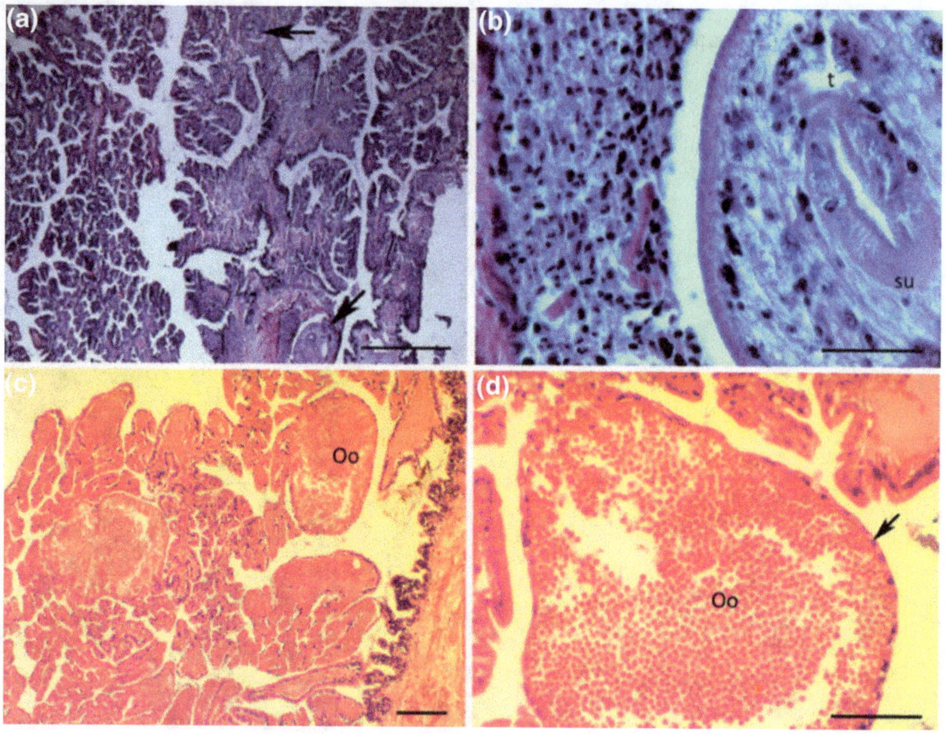

Fig. 17.8 **a** Gill section of *O. maya* with a *Cryptogonimidae* gen. sp. (arrows) producing distention of primary lamellae and hemocytic infiltration. Scale bar: 500 μm. **b** Higher magnification of Fig. 17.8a showing the sucker (su) of *Cryptogonimidae* trematode (t). The tissue shows autolysis by poor fixation. Scale bar: 50 μm. **c** Gill section of *Octopus maya* with oocysts (Oo) of *Aggregata* sp. Scale bar: 200 μm. **d** Higher magnification of Fig. 17.8c showing distention of the lamellar epithelium (arrow) caused by the presence of numerous uninucleate sporoblasts inside the oocyst (Oo). Scale bar: 500 μm

numerous oocysts in the gills' secondary and tertiary lamellae (Fig. 17.8c). Each oocyst containing high numbers of uninucleate and less binucleate sporoblasts is surrounded by a thin wall and grows among inner and outer epithelium of secondary and tertiary lamellae (Fig. 17.8d). The larger oocysts disrupt the normal branched pattern of the gill and can cause mechanical compression in adjacent lamellae, likely affecting hemolymph flow. The impact of *Aggregata* sp. infections in *O. maya* has not been yet studied. However, the histological damages observed in the intestine and gills suggest a high pathogenic capability of *Aggregata* sp. that may affect the physiology and body condition on the infected hosts.

Like other cephalopods (Hochberg 1990), the excretory organs of *O. maya* exhibit dicyemids attached principally to the renal appendages (Fig. 17.9a, b). The presence of these vermiform stages is not associated to excretory tissue damages (Fig. 17.9c), and it is generally accepted that the dicyemids are symbionts that may facilitate host excretion of nitrogenized compounds by contributing to the acidification of the urine.

Idiopathic focal necrosis in the epithelium of renal tubules has been observed in *O. maya* at very low prevalence (Fig. 17.9d). However, no pathogen has been observed in the histological sections of affected organs, and there are no precedent studies pointing to a pathogen responsible for the latter. Therefore, further investigations to clarify the etiology of idiopathic necrosis in the renal appendages of *O. maya* are still needed.

17.3 Pathogens and Related Diseases in the Jumbo Squid *Dosidicus Gigas*

The jumbo flying squid *Dosidicus gigas*, the other non-European cephalopod treated in this chapter, also harbors some parasites and diseases that affect tissues and organs (Pardo-Gandarillas et al. 2009; Iannacone and Alvariño 2009). The buccal mass, the first organ of the digestive system, is heavily infected by an unidentified larval cestode. Plerocercoids can be observed among the acini of anterior salivary glands and under the mucosal epithelium (Fig. 17.10a, d). The damages on affected tissue are related to the infection level. At low parasite numbers, the damages are local, consisting of focal modifications of tissue architecture and proliferation of connective tissue (Fig. 17.10b, c). Higher parasite numbers can cause degeneration and necrosis in the secretory epithelium of anterior salivary glands, which is replaced by parasites and fibro-connective tissue (Fig. 17.10 d). In severe infections (>20 parasites per host), the secretory tissue of the salivary gland may be severely affected, greatly reducing saliva production. This could have a negative effect on nutrition and therefore on the body weight and general physiological condition of the host.

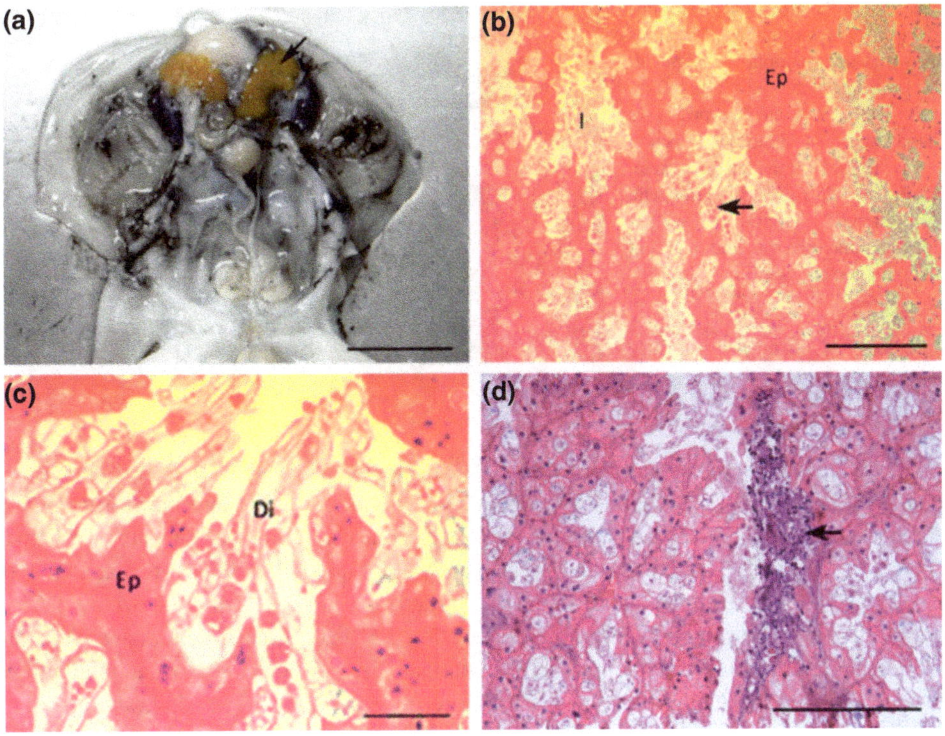

Fig. 17.9 **a** Renal organs in *O. maya* (arrow). Scale bar: 50 mm. **b** Section of renal tissue of healthy *O. maya* showing dicyemids symbionts (arrow) in the lumen of the tubules. (Ep) Epithelium of the renal tubules. Scale bar: 250 µm. **c** Higher magnification of Fig. 17.9b showing the nucleus of epithelial cells (Ep) of the renal tubules and the presence of dicyemids (Di) in the lumen. Scale bar: 50 µm. **d** Section of renal tissue with idiopathic focal necrosis (arrow) in the excretory epithelium. Scale bar: 200 µm

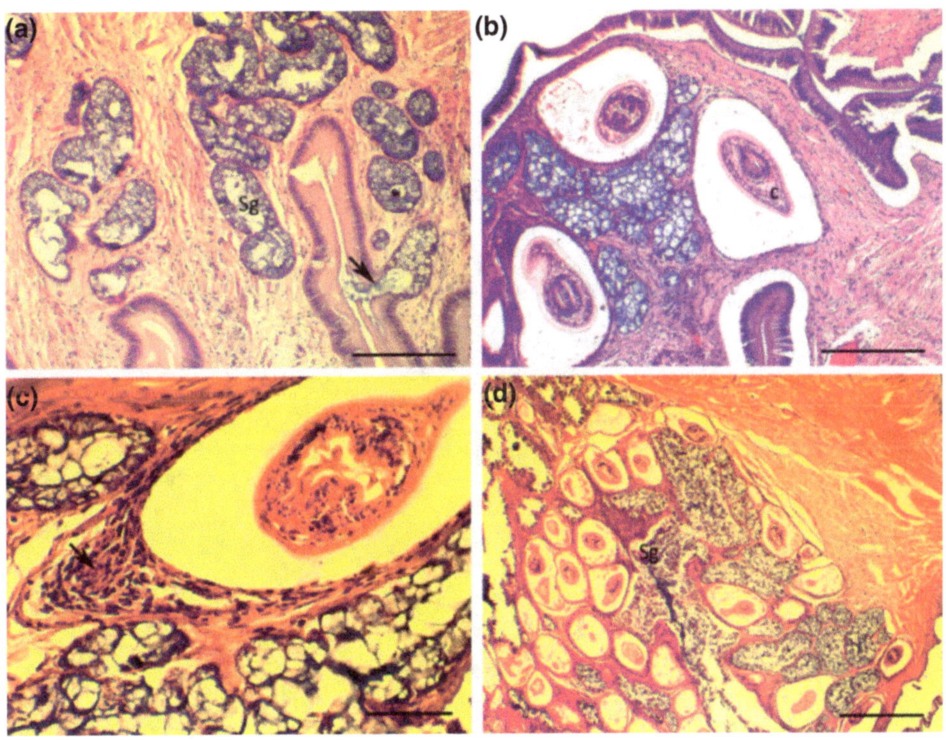

Fig. 17.10 Histological section of buccal mass from *Dosidicus gigas*. **a** Acini of the anterior salivary gland (Sg); one of them is discharging the mucous secretion through the epithelium (arrow). Scale bar: 250 µm. **b** Anterior salivary gland with moderate infection by larval cestode (c). Scale bar: 250 µm. **c** Anterior salivary gland showing proliferation of connective tissue (arrow) around a larval cestode. Scale bar: 100 µm. **d** Anterior salivary gland (Sg) heavily infected with larval cestodes. Secretory tissue is strongly reduced and has been replaced by parasites and fibro-connective tissue (left). Scale bar: 500 µm

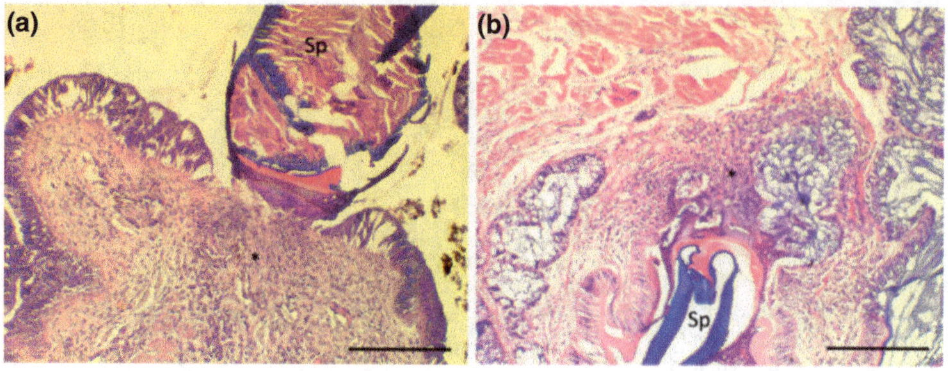

Fig. 17.11 Histological sections of buccal mass from male *D. gigas* showing spermatophores (Sp) attached to the mucosa. **a** The epithelium and lamina propria are damaged and a hemocytic reaction (*) is visible in the affected area. Scale bar: 250 µm. **b** Hemocytic infiltration (*) around the epithelium, lamina propria and adjacent acinus, affected. Scale bar: 250 µm

In males of *D. gigas*, some spermatophores can be found attached to the mucosa of the buccal mass (also in the gills, see below) causing ulcers that penetrate into the submucosa (Fig. 17.11a, b). The epithelium and basal lamina are damaged at the site of attachment, and hemocytic infiltration can be seen around the injury. A plausible explanation for this interesting and unusual condition is that the spermatophores probably belong to another male and act as foreign bodies when coming into contact with the tissues of the receptor host.

The general morphology of the caecum in *D. gigas* is similar to that of *O. maya*. Primary folds arise from the inner margin of the caecum wall and are protruded into the lumen. The secondary folds stem from both sides of the primary folds and perpendicularly to their axes (Fig. 17.12a). Two kinds of parasites, nematode and cestode, infect the caecum. *Anisakidae* nematodes have been found encysted in the caecum wall, where a hemocytic infiltration causes distention of the connective tissue (Fig. 17.12b). In contrast, plerocercoids of an unidentified cestode are very frequent in the basal, medial, and apical zones of the primary folds of the caecum causing degeneration and focal necrosis (Fig. 17.12c, d).

In the intestine, two morphotypes of an unidentified cestode were found (Fig. 17.13a, b). One large morphotype

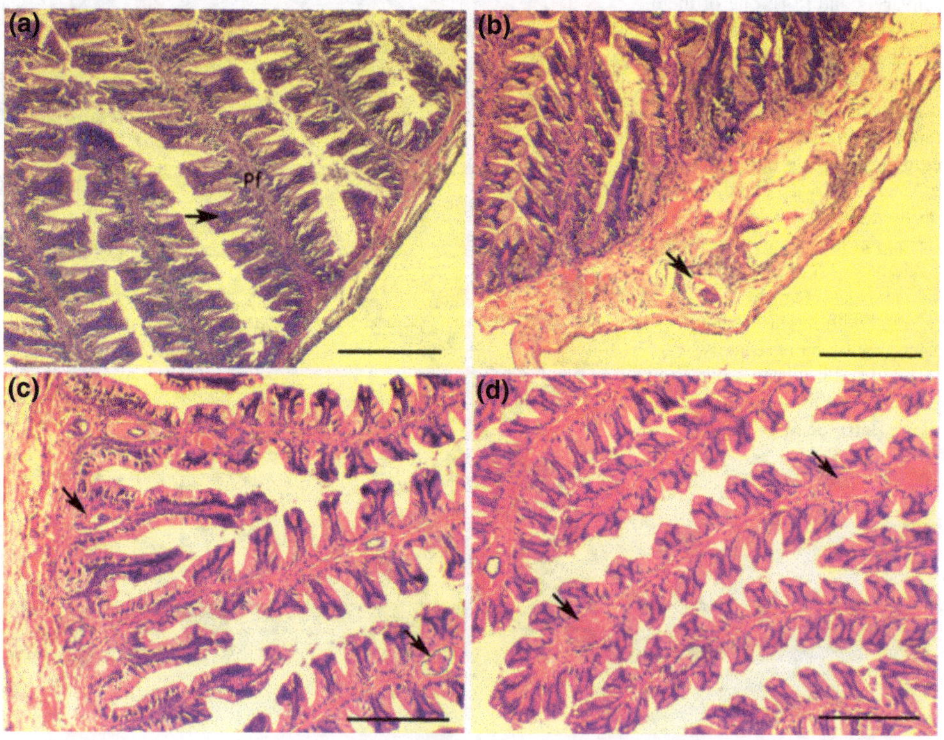

Fig. 17.12 Histological section of the coiled caecum of *D. gigas*. **a** Healthy tissue showing the external wall with primary longitudinal folds (Pf) and secondary folds (arrow). Scale bar: 250 µm. **b** A larvae of *Anisakidae* nematode (arrow) encysted in the wall of the coiled caecum. Scale bar: 250 µm. **c** Coiled caecum showing unidentified larval cestodes (arrow) infecting the loose connective tissue of primary fold. Scale bar: 250 µm. **d** Primary fold showing degenerated tissue and focal necrosis (arrow) in the loose connective tissue. Scale bar: 250 µm

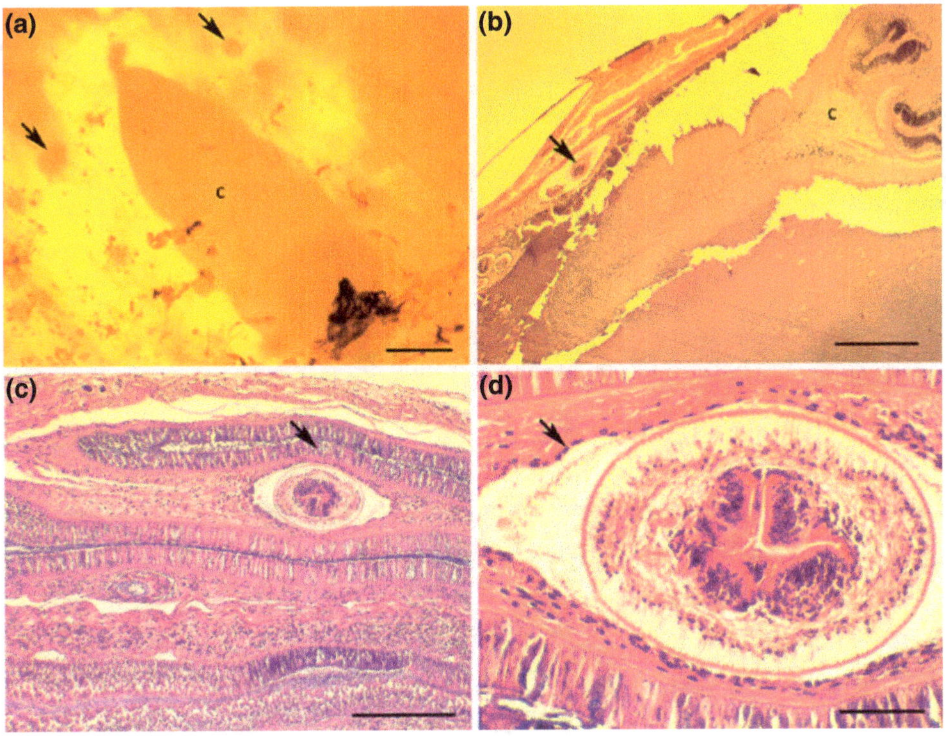

Fig. 17.13 Wet mount and histological sections of intestine from *D. gigas*. **a** Fresh intestine infected with two morphotypes of unidentified larval cestodes. One larger morphotype (c) inside the intestine, and second smaller morphotype (arrows) encysted in the intestine wall. Scale bar: 500 µm. **b** Histological section of the intestine from Fig. 17.13a showing the two morphotypes of unidentified larval cestodes. Scale bar: 500 µm. **c** Larval cestode of the smaller morphotype infecting the intestinal submucosa. Note the protruded intestinal epithelium (arrow) by expansion of subjacent connective tissue. Scale bar: 250 µm. **d** Higher magnification of Fig. 17.13c showing the flattened nuclei of fibroblastic cells organized around the larval cestode. Scale bar: 100 µm

can be found in the lumen of the intestine, while a smaller and more abundant morphotype infects not only the intestinal wall and folds but also the caecum primary folds and digestive gland. No damage has been associated with the presence of the larger morphotype cestode in the intestinal lumen. The smaller morphotype produces a protrusion of the intestinal epithelium by an expansion of a subjacent connective tissue (Fig. 17.13c). The presence of plerocercoids in the corion of the intestinal fold triggers the host's cellular response, and the fibroblastic cells come to organize themselves around the parasite to encapsulate it, causing distention (Fig. 17.13d). Like in the caecum, focal necrosis and degenerated tissue can be seen near the plerocercoid, probably caused by the secretions of the parasite. The presence of this smaller morphotype of plerocercoid in digestive gland was infrequent, and no damage or alteration of the normal tissue architecture was related to the presence of parasite (Fig. 17.14a, b).

Despite the macroscopic differences in gill morphology between *D. gigas* and *O. maya*, microscopically they share a similar basic morphology. The primary lamellae form the secondary ones, and these form the tertiary ones on a continuous fold pattern. The main morphological difference is the fanlike fold pattern in *D. gigas* in comparison to the branched arrangement pattern in *O. maya* (Fig. 17.15a, b). As mentioned above, spermatophores were found attached to the gills of male specimens (Fig. 17.15c). The number of spermatophores in the gills varies greatly but is generally high, causing compression and modification of the fanlike folded pattern of lamellae (Fig. 17.15d).

Nodular lesions in the epithelium of secondary and tertiary lamellae were observed and associated with the presence of coccidian (Fig. 17.16a). *Aggregata* sp. sporocysts are phagocytized by hemocytes and surrounded by strong hemocytic infiltration (Fig. 17.16b). The space between inner and outer epithelium in the infection sites is distended and filled with proliferative connective tissue, reducing its gas exchange capability. In addition, oocysts containing numerous uninucleate sporoblasts are present and produce distention of the lamellae (Fig. 17.16c). Multiple oocysts of

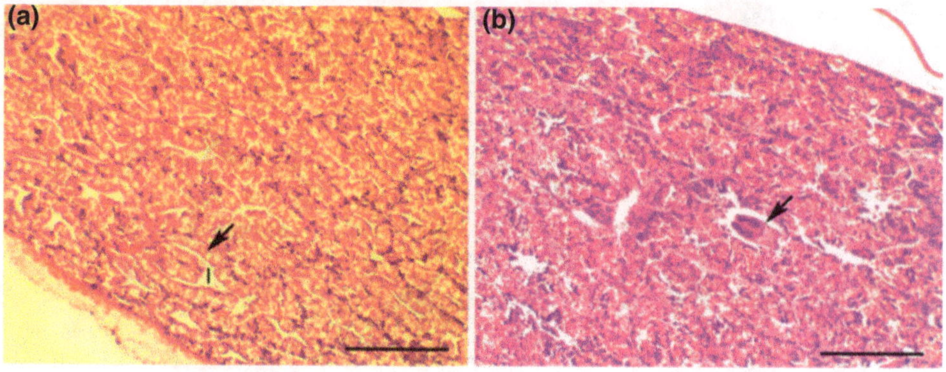

Fig. 17.14 Histological sections of digestive gland from *D. gigas*. **a** Healthy tissue showing the tubular epithelium (arrow) and the lumen of the tubules (l). Scale bar: 250 μm. **b** Unidentified larval cestode (arrow) among tubules of the digestive gland. Scale bar: 250 μm

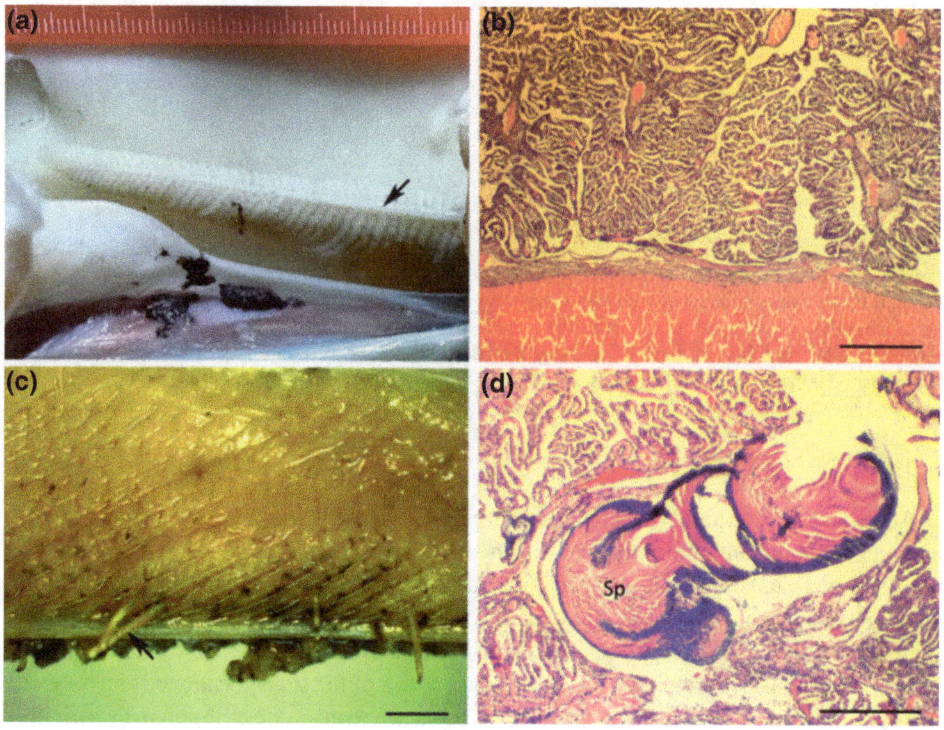

Fig. 17.15 Macroscopic view and histological section of gill from *D. gigas*. **a** Macroscopic view of fold pattern and primary efferent vessel (arrow) in gill. **b** Histological section showing the fold pattern and primary efferent vessel (lower view). Scale bar: 500 μm. **c** Spermatophores (arrow) attached to the gill in mature male of *D. gigas*. Scale bar: 5 mm. **d** Histological section showing the modified architecture of the gill caused by the attached spermatophore (Sp). Scale bar: 250 μm

different sizes are present in the same lamella, separated by a thin wall (Fig. 17.16d).

The mantle of *D. gigas*, as in other cephalopods, is mainly a muscular layer lined with a delicate yet sophisticated skin, which functions as the primary barrier against pathogens and environmental stressors. For this reason, some pathogens settle in this organ as the first site of infection, facilitating the entry of opportunistic pathogens. This is the case of *Anisakidae* nematodes, whose larvae penetrate through the skin and encyst in the mantle musculature until the final host devours the squid and the life cycle is completed. Whitish and slightly protuberant nodules containing *Anisakidae* nematodes are visible by gross observation in the mantle of *D. gigas* (Fig. 17.17a). A connective tissue reaction and hemocytic infiltration surround the nematodes (Fig. 17.17b), but the organization of the host's tissue response may be associated to the time of permanence of the larva. A less organized inflammatory response could be associated with newly migrating larvae (Fig. 17.17c).

In the musculature of the mantle, and to some extent in that of the tentacles, there are also nodules of variable size, well delimited, and brown in color (Fig. 17.18a). These nodules contain a homogeneous hyaline material, with very

Fig. 17.16 Histological section of gill from *D. gigas*. **a** Nodular lesion (arrow) and oocysts of *Aggregata* sp. (arrowhead) in gill. Scale bar: 500 μm. **b** Proliferative reaction around the free sporocysts of *Aggregata* sp. (arrow). Scale bar: 30 μm. **c** Oocysts (Oo) of *Aggregata* sp. among inner and outer epithelium (arrow). Scale bar: 100 μm. **d** Higher magnification of Oocysts (Oo) in gill. Each oocyst, containing many uninucleate and some binucleate sporoblasts, are delimited by a thin wall (arrow). Scale bar: 30 μm

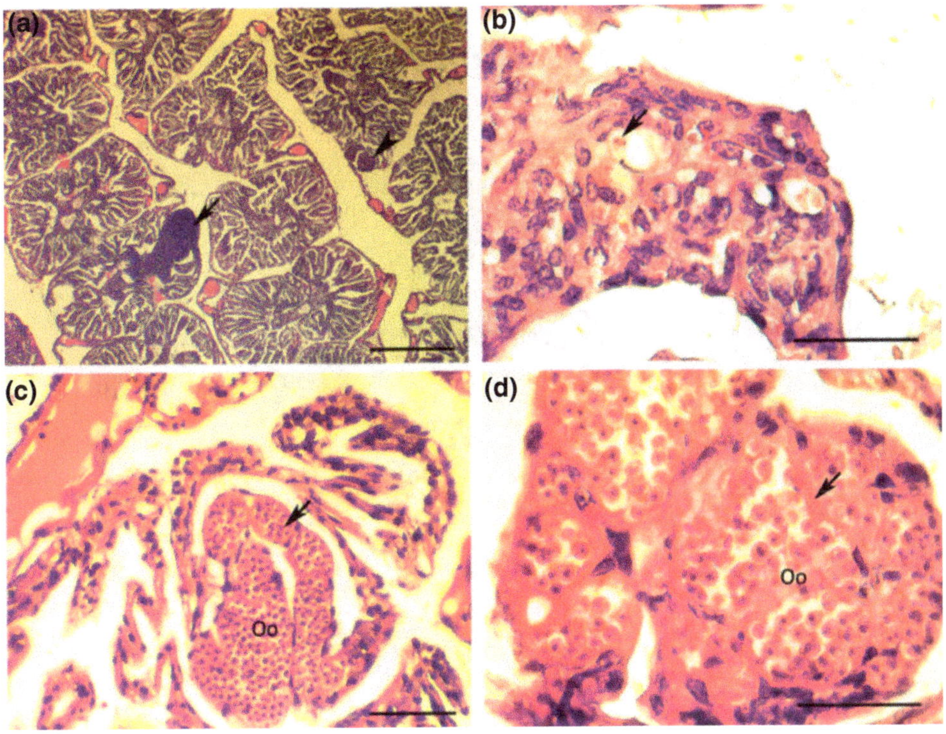

Fig. 17.17 Macroscopic view and histological sections of mantle from *D. gigas*. **a** A larva of *Anisakidae* nematode (arrow) encysted in the mantle musculature. Note the host's tissue response forming a white ring around the nematode. Scale bar: 100 μm. **b** Histological section of the tissue that was showed in Fig. 17.17a. The nematode (central view), sectioned transversally, is rounded by an organized connective tissue and hemocytic infiltration. Scale bar: 500 μm. **c** Degeneration of muscular fibers and focal necrosis with hemocytic infiltrate in the mantle muscle (M) caused by the presence of *Anisakidae* nematodes (arrow). Scale bar: 250 μm

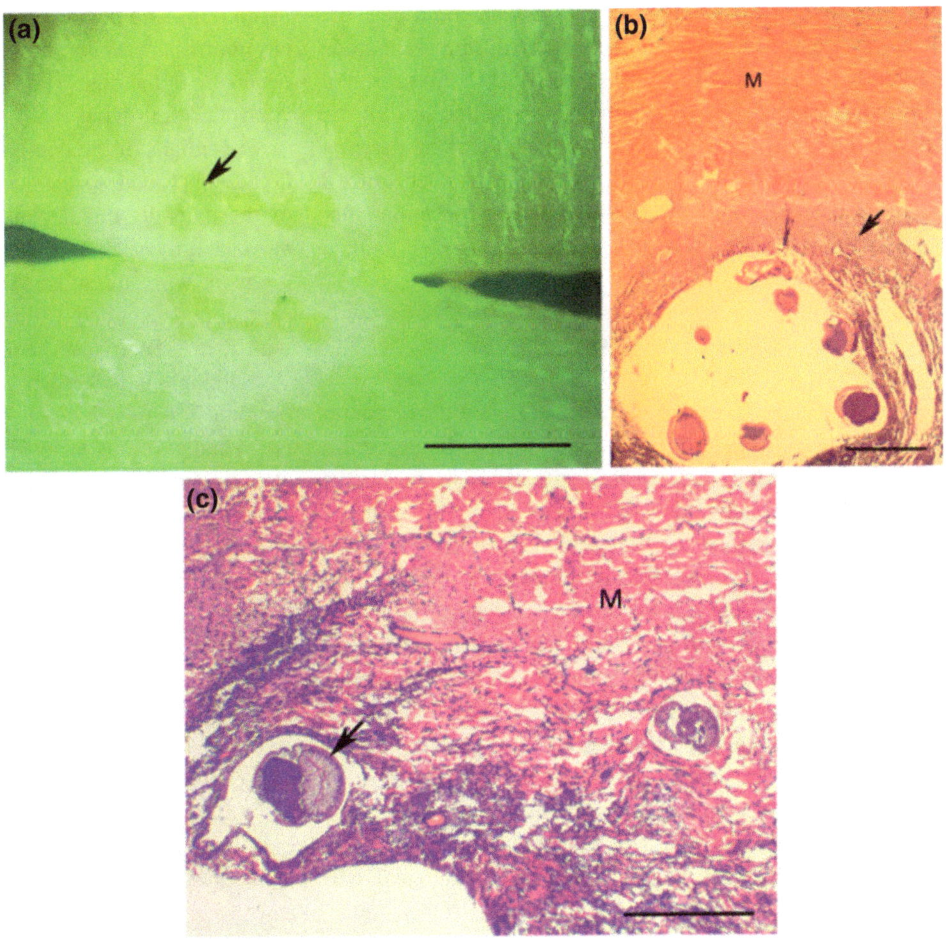

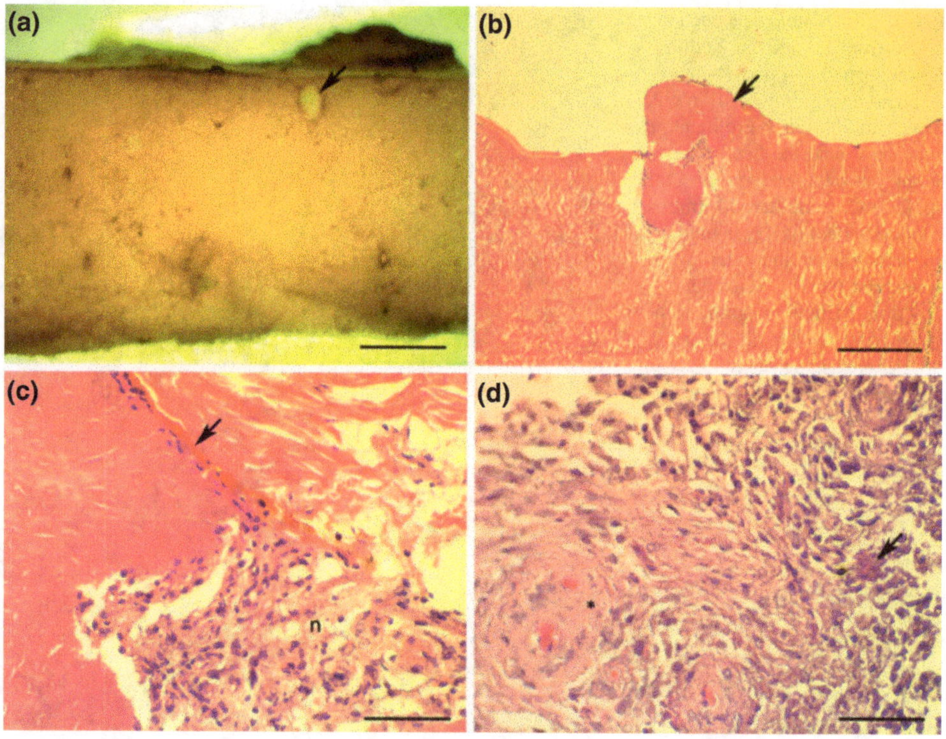

Fig. 17.18 Macroscopic view and histological sections of mantle from *D. gigas*. **a** Macroscopic view of a nodule in the mantle (arrow), just below the epithelium. The tissue has been cut transversally to facilitate the view. Scale bar: 500 μm. **b** Histological section of the mantle showing a hyaline nodule (arrow). Scale bar: 500 μm. **c** Higher magnification of Fig. 17.18b showing the hyaline material (left) and focal necrosis (n) surrounded by fibroblasts and pigmented cells (arrow). Scale bar: 100 μm. **d** Giant cells with phagocytized bacteria (*) and colonies of bacteria (arrow) free among connective tissue fibers. Note the organization of the tissue around the bacterial colonies. Scale bar: 100 μm

few cells inside of them (Fig. 17.18b), which could be some type of degraded residue generated during nematode migration. The nodules are covered by a layer of fibro-connective tissue and pigmented cells that give it the brown color (Fig. 17.18c). In some areas, foci of necrosis and connective tissue proliferation can be observed around bacterial colonies, suggesting a subsequent infection after nematode larvae migration (Fig. 17.18d).

17.4 Concluding Remarks

It is evident that there are severe pathological affections in wild cephalopods, with the most serious being those occurring in the digestive system, particularly in the buccal mass. In both cephalopods studied here, heavy infection of cestodes was identified as the etiological origin. Although the severity of infection depends directly on the infection degree, higher parasite numbers can cause degeneration and necrosis in the secretory epithelium and salivary glands, so that nutrients absorption can be affected and in consequence the entire host condition. This affection, nonetheless, can be easily avoided in captive cephalopods. The cephalopods in these infections are playing as second intermediate host of the cestodes; being copepods or small crustaceans the first intermediate hosts and sharks or rays the definitive host, so that water quality control and captivity food control will avoid reinfections that are undoubtedly happening in natural environments. With cestodes, most metazoan parasites occurring in the digestive system any other host tissue can be controlled following the same practices.

Coccidians of the genus *Aggregata* were also common to both cephalopod species, similarly to cestodes, the severity of the damage will depend on the infection degree. In *O. maya,* the most affected organ was the intestine while in *D. gigas* it was the gills. *Aggregata* are common to most cephalopods studied till now and the diseases associated with its presence have been addressed in several hosts.

Although it is known that in captivity an ectoparasitic protozoan *Ichthyobodo necator* can infect the skin of *O. maya* and several species of bacteria including Vibrionaceae also represent a major threat, we did not find histopathological evidence of their presence in wild octopus *O. maya* or the jumbo squid *Dosidicus gigas*.

References

Aguila J, Cuzon G, Pascual C, Domingues PM, Gaxiola G, Sánchez A, Maldonado T, Rosas C (2007) The effects of fish hydrolysate (CPSP) level on *Octopus maya* (Voss and Solis) diet: digestive enzyme activity, blood metabolites, and energy balance. Aquaculture 273:641–655

Boyle P, Rodhouse P (2005). Cephalopods: ecology and fisheries. Blackwell Science, p 467

Domingues PM, López N, Muñoz JA, Maldonado T, Gaxiola G, Rosas C (2007) Effects of a dry pelleted diet on growth and survival of the Yucatan octopus, *Octopus maya*. Aquacul Nutr 13:273–280

Estévez J, Pascual S, Gestal C, Soto M, Rodríguez H, Arias C (1996) *Aggregata octopiana* (Apicomplexa: Aggregatidae) from *Octopus vulgaris* off NW Spain. Dis Aquat Org 27:227–231

Gestal C, Abollo E, Pascual S (2002) Observations on associated histopathology with *Aggregata octopiana* infection (Protista: Apicomplexa) in *Octopus vulgaris*. Dis Aquat Org 50:45–49

Gestal C, Pascual S, Corral L, Azevedo C (1999) Ultrastructural aspects of the sporogony of *Aggregata octopiana* (Apicomplexa, Aggregatidae), a coccidian parasite of *Octopus vulgaris* (Mollusca, Cephalopoda) from NE Atlantic Coast. Eur J Protistol 35:417–425

Hochberg FG (1990) Diseases of Mollusca: Cephalopoda. Diseases caused by protistans and metazoans. In: Kinne O (ed) Diseases of marine annimals, vol III. Biologische Anstalt Helgoland, Hamburg, pp 47–227

Iannacone J, Alvariño L (2009) Catastre of endoparasite fauna of jumbo flying squid *Dosidicus gigas* (Cephalopoda) in the north of Peru. Neotropl Helminthol 3:89–100

Morales-Bojórquez E, Pacheco-Bedoya J (2016) Jumbo squid *Dosidicus gigas*: a new fishery in Ecuador. Rev Fish Sci Aquacul 24:98–110

Pardo-Gandarillas M, Lohrmann K, Valdivia A, Ibañez C (2009) First record of parasites of *Dosidicus gigas* (d'Orbigny, 1835) (Cephalopoda: Ommastrephidae) from the Humboldt Current system off Chile. Rev Biol Mar Oceanogr 44:397–408

Roper C, Nigmatullin C, Jereb P (2010) Family Ommastrephidae. In: Jereb P, Roper CFE (eds) Cephalopods of the World. An annotated and illustrated catalogue of species known to date. FAO Species catalogue for Fisheries Purposes. No 4, vol 2, FAO Rome, pp 269–347

Van Heukelem WF (1983) *Octopus maya*. In: Boyle PR (ed) Cephalopod Life Cycles, vol I. Academic Press, London, pp 311–323

18 Pathogens and Related Diseases in Non-European Cephalopods: Asia. A Preliminary Review

Jing Ren, Xiaodong Zheng, Yaosen Qian, and Qingqi Zhang

Abstract

Parasitic diseases and other abnormalities play critical roles in causing morbidity in the majority of Cephalopoda. However, to date, reports of cephalopod diseases from Asia are scarce and lack detailed information on the description of specific characters. This paper presents a brief overview of various pathogens and produced diseases in Asian cephalopods, including coccidiosis by *Aggregata,* Anisakiasis, infection by the copepods *Octopicola,* and other abnormalities such as edema and broken skin. The coccidian *Aggregata* sp. that infects the definitive host *Amphioctopus fangsiao* is a heteroxenous parasite transmitted through the food web. Anisakids play an important role in Asia as parasitic disease for cephalopods and it is even transmitted to humans. Concerning the infection by copepods, *Octopicola* sp. is the only species of the family Octopicolidae reported from North Pacific waters. Other abnormalities like edema or broken skin may have been the result of bacterial infections, so that abnormalities could cause the degeneration and death observed in *A. fangsiao*.

Keywords

Cephalopoda • Pathology • Diseases • *Amphioctopus fangsiao* • *Aggregata* • Anisakis • Octopicola • Asian waters

J. Ren · X. Zheng (✉)
Institute of Evolution & Marine Biodiversity, Ocean University of China, Qingdao 266003, China
e-mail: xdzheng@ouc.edu.cn

J. Ren
e-mail: renjing@stu.ouc.edu.cn

J. Ren · X. Zheng
Key Laboratory of Mariculture, Ministry of Education, Ocean University of China, Qingdao 266003, China

Y. Qian
Ganyu Institute of Fishery Science, Lianyungang 222100, China
e-mail: gysks6089@163.com

Q. Zhang
Ganyu Jiaxin Fishery Technical Development Co., Ltd., Lianyungang 222100, China
e-mail: lygjx158@163.com

C. Gestal et al. (eds.), *Handbook of Pathogens and Diseases in Cephalopods*,
https://doi.org/10.1007/978-3-030-11330-8_18

18.1 Introduction

Cephalopoda is the most complex in the invertebrate phyla. Cephalopods include exclusively marine animals that live in all oceans of the world except the Black Sea. In Asia, many cephalopods are important economic species for human beings. Octopods were reported the highest production for 2010, at 217,506 tones, while European production of octopuses was only 42,945 tones (Norman et al. 2014), which are also one of the most important commercial cephalopod groups in China (Zheng et al. 2014; Xu and Zheng 2018). Cuttlefish, such as *Sepia pharaonis* and *Sepiella japonica,* were also an important fishery in the northern part of the Indian Ocean and southeastern Asia

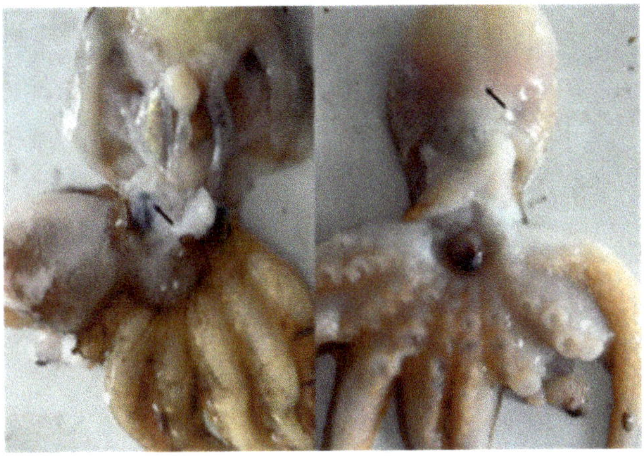

Fig. 18.1 Distribution of parasites on *Amphioctopus fangsiao*. Arrows showing disseminated cysts in the epidermis

(Nesis, Yin et al. 2018). However, to date, reports of cephalopod diseases from Asia are scarce and lack of detailed information on the description of specific characters.

18.2 *Aggregata* Sp.

Cephalopods are specifically infected by coccidians of the genus *Aggregata*, which were heteroxenous parasites transmitted through the food web. Sexual stages (including gamogony and sporogony) occur inside the digestive tract of the definitive cephalopod host (Dobell 1925; Gestal et al. 2002). Coccidian infection at pathological level has not been previously reported in Asia and data of its prevalence and distribution are currently scarce. Protozoan parasites of the genus *Aggregata* affecting *Amphioctopus fangsiao* in natural environment have been associated with large-scale concentrated deaths occurred in the process of artificial temporarily culture facility in China. White cysts were found in the body surface representing the 43% of the total number of *A. fangsiao* inspected (95/220) (unpublished data) (Fig. 18.1).

Histological sections of intestinal tissue revealed destruction of the organ architecture and substitution of the tissue by parasite cysts (Fig. 18.2a). Through histological sections observation, the oocysts were spherical, in the range of 249.75–501.75 μm (mean 360.76 ± 70.39 μm) and 116.84–350.87 μm (mean 231.67 ± 74.89 μm) ($n = 20$) with plenty of sporocysts in each oocyst. The size of sporocysts was measured as follows: 17.69–20.72 μm (mean 19.20 ± 0.93 μm) by 15.97–20.00 μm (mean 18.31 ± 1.19 μm) ($n = 20$). The surface of sporocysts was smooth. The histological results are shown in Fig. 18.2b (unpublished data).

18.3 Anisakidae

The life cycle of Anisakidae is rather complex involving small crustaceans as the first intermediate host; fishes and cephalopods as the second host; and marine mammals which act as the definitive host (Nesis et al. 1987; dos Santos and Howgate 2011; Sangaran and Sundar 2016). Thus, anisakiasis is a parasitic disease of cephalopods in Asia. In Japan, where raw squids are consumed as an integral part of the Japanese diet, Anisakid transmission to humans has been reported, producing a strong pathology (Oshima 1972; Tomoo and Kliks 1987; Sakanari and Mckerrow 1989). In China, natural infection of Anisakidae larvae was investigated in squids (2 species, 29 specimens) caught in the yellow sea and the East China Sea (Koyama 1969).

18.4 Octopicola

To date, the genus *Octopicola* contains five species parasitizing octopuses (Humes 1957, 1963, 1974; Du et al. 2018). *Octopicola huanghaiensis* (Fig. 18.3) is the first species reported in *A. fangsiao* and *Octopus minor*, and the only species of the family Octopicolidae known in Asia (Du et al. 2018).

Fig. 18.2 Histological sections of *A. fangsiao* intestines infected by *Aggregata* sp. **a** Oocysts infecting the intestinal tissue. **b** Sporocysts inside the oocyst. Scale bars: A, 50 μm B, 20 μm

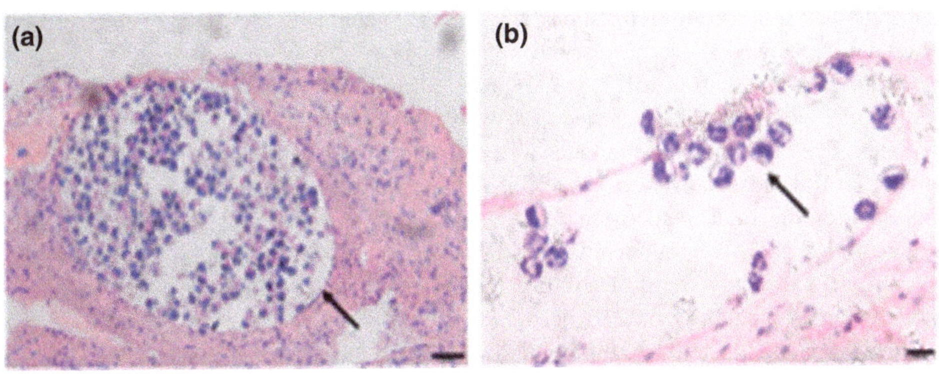

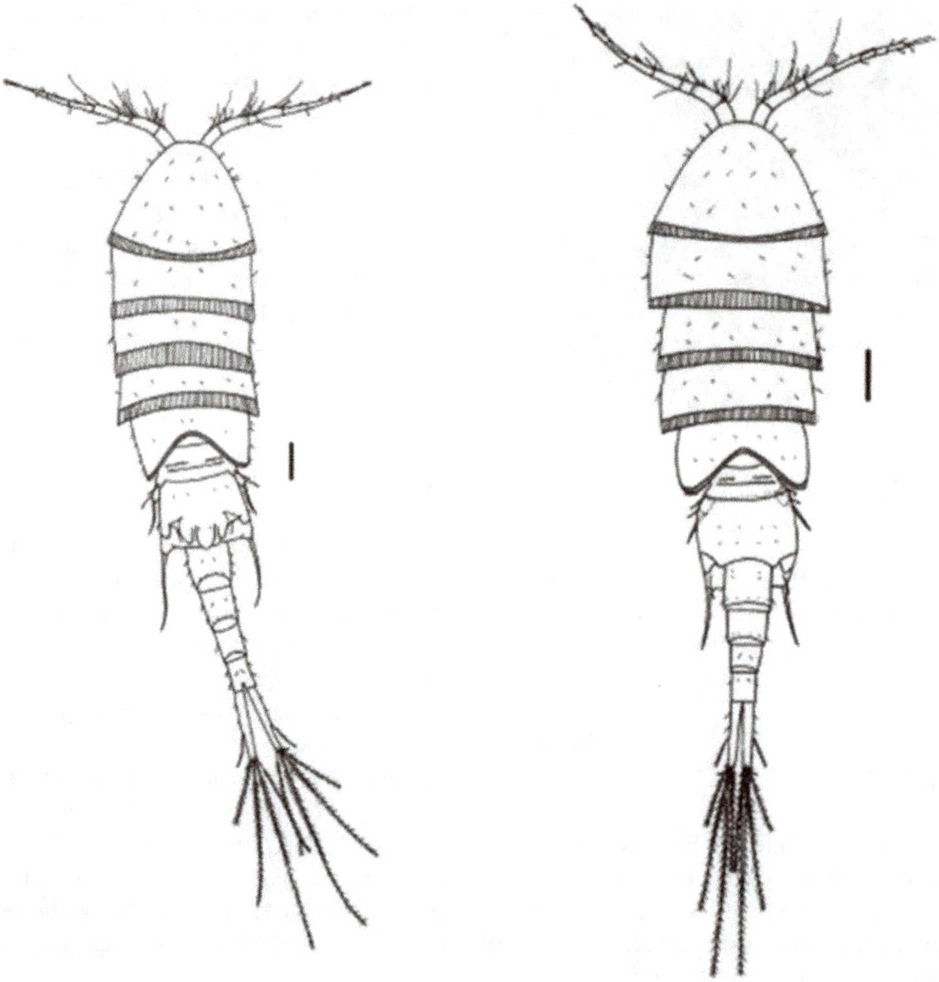

Fig. 18.3 *Octopicola huanghaiensis* (Scale-bar: 100 μm) (Du et al. 2018)

18.5 Other Abnormalities

There are some other abnormalities recorded in Asian octopuses (Fig. 18.4). During our study, wild specimens of *A. fangsiao* were caught in March 2017 in the Yellow Sea (off Lianyungang, Jiangsu Prov.). The specimens were temporarily reared indoors of the Ganyu Jiaxin Fishery Technical Development Co., Ltd. Individuals were placed in concrete tanks, under the conditions of 11.8 °C, natural photoperiod, as well as plastic suspensors for shelter.

From March 16 to April 2, 1303 dead *A. fangsiao* individuals were sampled in order to separate males and females. The total number of females was 836, accounting for 64% of all deaths. There were 467 males, accounting for 36% of the total deaths; the female death rate was much higher than that of the male in breeding season, which was extremely weird. Therefore, further examination by gross pathology of 220 dead individuals (body surface) was conducted from March 24 to April 2 to analyze the death situation. Eventually, it was found that skin surface of dead individuals includes mainly edema and edema with coccidian (individuals of edema only amount to 16% of the total number of inspection), broken skin (37% of the total number of inspection), and broken arms (4% of the total number of inspection). Those

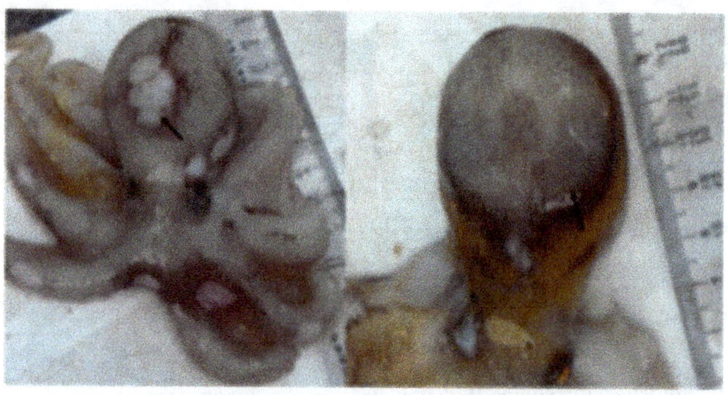

Fig. 18.4 Abnormalities of *A. fangsiao*. Arrows showing exfoliation of the mantle and edema

abnormalities may have been the results of bacterial infection so that abnormalities could cause degeneration and death of the species.

18.6 Concluding Remarks

As summarized above, only handful studies have been documented for cephalopod diseases from Asia currently, including coccidiosis by *Aggregata* sp., Anisakiasis, *Octopicola*, edema, and broken skin. However, further characterization and functional studies are needed to confirm the effect of diseases on the cephalopods health. Finally, the results obtained in the chapter provide a brief overview of parasitic diseases in Asian waters.

Acknowledgements This work was supported by research grants from National Natural Science Foundation of China (No. 31672257) and the Fundamental Research Funds for the Central Universities (No. 201822022).

References

Dobell C (1925) The life-history and chromosome cycle of *Aggregata eberthi* (Protozoa: Sporozoa: Coccidia). Parasitology 17(1):1–136

dos Santos CAL, Howgate P (2011) Fishborne zoonotic parasites and aquaculture: a review. Aquaculture 318(3–4):253–261

Du X, Dong C, Sun SC (2018) *Octopicola huanghaiensis* n. sp. (Copepoda: Cyclopoida: Octopicolidae), a new parasitic copepod of the octopuses *Amphioctopus fangsiao* (d'Orbigny) and *Octopus minor* (Sasaki) (Octopoda: Octopodidae) in the Yellow Sea. Syst Parasitol 95(8–9):905–912

Gestal C, Guerra A, Pascual S, Azevedo C (2002) On the life cycle of *Aggregata eberthi* and observations on *Aggregata octopiana* (Apicomplexa, Aggregatidae) from Galicia (NE Atlantic). Eur J Protistol 37(4):427–435

Humes AG (1957) *Octopicola superba* ng, n. sp., Copepode Cyclopoide parasite d'un Octopus de la Mediterranee. Vie et Milieu Env 8:1–8

Humes AG (1963) *Octopicola stocki* n. sp. (Copepoda, Cyclopoida), associated with an octopus in Madagascar. Crustaceana 5(4):271–280

Humes AG (1974) *Octopicola regalis*, n. sp. (Copepoda, Cyclopoida, Lichomolgidae) associated with *Octopus cyaneus* from New Caledonia and Eniwetok Atoll. Bull Mar Sci 24(1):76–85

Koyama T (1969) Morphological and taxonomical studies on Anisakidae larvae found in marine fishes and squids. Jap J Parasitol 18 (5):466–487

Nesis KN, Burgess LA, Levitov BS (1987) Cephalopods of the world: squids, cuttlefishes, octopuses, and allies. TFH, p 351

Norman MD, Finn JK, Hochberg FG, Jereb P, Roper CFE (2014) Cephalopods of the world. An annotated and illustrated catalogue of cephalopod species known to date. FAO Species Catalogue for Fishery Purposes, vol 3(4), pp 1–22

Oshima T (1972) Anisakis and anisakiasis in Japan and adjacent area. Prog Med Parasit, Japan, pp 301–393

Sakanari J, Mckerrow JH (1989) Anisakiasis. Clin Microbiol Rev 2 (3):278–284

Sangaran A, Sundar S (2016) Fish and shell fish borne parasitic infections-a review. Int J Sci Environ Technol 5(5):2954–2958

Tomoo O, Kliks M (1987) Effects of marine mammal parasites on human health. Int J Parasitol 17(2):415–421

Xu R, Zheng XD (2018) Selection of reference genes for quantitative real-time PCR in *Octopus minor* (Cephalopoda: Octopoda) under acute ammonia stress. Environ Toxicol Phar 60:76–81

Yin SJ, Zhang LM, Zhang LL, Wan JX, Song W, Jiang XM, Park YD, Si YX (2018) Metabolic responses and arginine kinase expression of juvenile cuttlefish (*Sepia pharaonis*) under salinity stress. Int J Biol Macromol 113:881–888

Zheng XD, Qian YS, Liu C, Li Q (2014) *Octopus minor*. In: Iglesias J, Fuentes L, Villanueva R (eds) Cephalopod Culture. Springer, Dordrecht, pp 415–426

www.ingramcontent.com/pod-product-compliance
Lightning Source LLC
LaVergne TN
LVHW082219200926
848484LV00008B/2277